ychiatry

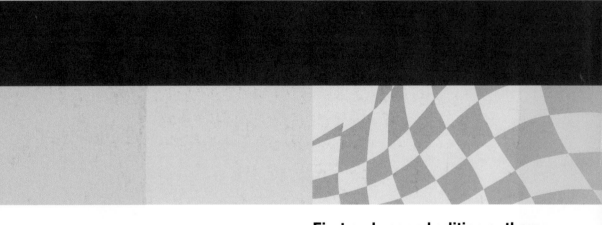

First and second edition authors:

Darran Bloye

Simon Davies

Alisdair D Cameron

Third edition authors:

Julius Bourke

Matthew Castle

Fourth edition authors:

Katie Marwick

Steven Birrell

5th Edition
CRASH COURSE

SERIES EDITORS

Philip Xiu
MA, MB BChir, MRCP
GP Registrar
Yorkshire Deanery
Leeds, UK

Shreelata Datta
MD, MRCOG, LLM, BSc (Hons), MBBS
Honorary Senior Lecturer
Imperial College London,
Consultant Obstetrician and Gynaecologist
King's College Hospital
London, UK

FACULTY ADVISOR

Steven Birrell
MBChB, MRCPsych, PGCertClinEd, AFHEA
Consultant Psychiatrist
Queen Margaret Hospital, Dunfermline, Fife, UK

Psychiatry

Katie Marwick

MA (Hons), MB ChB (Hons), MRCPsych, PhD
Honorary Specialty Registrar in General Adult Psychiatry,
NHS Lothian
Clinical Lecturer in Psychiatry, University of Edinburgh
Edinburgh, UK

For additional online content visit StudentConsult.com

ELSEVIER

ELSEVIER

Content Strategist: Jeremy Bowes
Content Development Specialist: Alexandra Mortimer
Project Manager: Andrew Riley
Design: Christian Bilbow
Illustration Manager: Karen Giacomucci
Illustrator: MPS North America LLC
Marketing Manager: Deborah Watkins

First edition 1999
Second edition 2004
Third edition 2008
Reprinted 2010
Fourth edition 2013
Updated Fourth edition 2015
Fifth edition 2019

Notices

Practitioners and researchers must always rely on their own experience and knowledge in evaluating and using any information, methods, compounds or experiments described herein. Because of rapid advances in the medical sciences, in particular, independent verification of diagnoses and drug dosages should be made. To the fullest extent of the law, no responsibility is assumed by Elsevier, authors, editors or contributors for any injury and/or damage to persons or property as a matter of products liability, negligence or otherwise, or from any use or operation of any methods, products, instructions, or ideas contained in the material herein.

ISBN: 978-0-7020-7383-0
eISBN: 978-0-7020-7350-2

 your source for books,
journals and multimedia
in the health sciences

www.elsevierhealth.com

  Working together
to grow libraries in
developing countries

www.elsevier.com • www.bookaid.org

The
publisher's
policy is to use
**paper manufactured
from sustainable forests**

Printed in Poland
Last digit is the print number: 9 8 7 6 5 4 3 2 1

Series Editors' foreword

The *Crash Course* series was conceived by Dr Dan Horton-Szar who as series editor presided over it for more than 15 years – from publication of the first edition in 1997, until publication of the fourth edition in 2011. His inspiration, knowledge and wisdom lives on in the pages of this book. As the new series editors, we are delighted to be able to continue developing each book for the twenty-first century undergraduate curriculum.

The flame of medicine never stands still, and keeping this all-new fifth series relevant for today's students is an ongoing process. Each title within this new fifth edition has been re-written to integrate basic medical science and clinical practice, after extensive deliberation and debate. We aim to build on the success of the previous titles by keeping the series up-to-date with current guidelines for best practice, and recent developments in medical research and pharmacology.

We always listen to feedback from our readers, through focus groups and student reviews of the *Crash Course* titles. For the fifth editions we have reviewed and re-written our self-assessment material to reflect today's 'single-best answer' and 'extended matching question' formats. The artwork and layout of the titles has also been largely re-worked and are now in colour, to make it easier on the eye during long sessions of revision. The new on-line materials supplement the learning process.

Despite fully revising the books with each edition, we hold fast to the principles on which we first developed the series. *Crash Course* will always bring you all the information you need to revise in compact, manageable volumes that still maintain the balance between clarity and conciseness, and provide sufficient depth for those aiming at distinction. The authors are junior doctors who have recent experience of the exams you are now facing, and the accuracy of the material is checked by a team of faculty editors from across the UK.

We wish you all the best for your future careers!

Shreelata Datta and Philip Xiu

Author

The ability to diagnose and manage mental health problems is an increasingly valued skill. Greater scientific understanding of mental illness is reducing the stigma associated with it, in turn allowing its impact to be greater recognised: mental illness is the single largest cause of disability in the UK (28%), the leading cause of sickness absence, costs the UK economy 4.5% of GDP, and the life expectancy of people with severe mental illness is reduced by 15–20 years. Despite its importance, mental illness is typically under-recognised and undertreated: around three quarters of people with a mental illness in England receive no treatment (compared with around a quarter of people with a physical illness). Mental and physical health problems are frequently comorbid and exacerbate each other, meaning you will have the opportunity to improve the lives of people with mental illness in almost any branch of medicine you choose.

This book is designed to equip you with the core knowledge and skills you need to help people with mental health problems, both to pass your exams and to be a holistic and skilled future doctor. The already popular 4th edition has been updated to be in line with contemporary guidelines, classification systems and self-assessment formats. This edition also includes two brand new chapters on neurodevelopmental disorders, an increasingly common clinical presentation in children and adults.

Psychiatry can be a challenging speciality but it is also one where you can make a real difference to people's lives – old or young, rich or poor, in hospital or at home. Psychiatry is also a rapidly changing speciality, however, I have done my best to ensure this book will provide a solid foundation to help you effectively diagnose and treat mental illness in the patients and people you care for in the future. I wish you the best of luck!

Katie Marwick

Faculty Advisor

As a proud co-author of the fourth edition of the book, it has been a privilege to work in an advisory role on this title. The fifth edition of *Crash Course: Psychiatry* builds upon the success of previous incarnations of the book, being fully up to date with regards contemporary psychiatric practice, the current classification systems, evidence base and guidelines, and medico-legal information. It also includes an expanded and improved self-assessment section. As with all titles within the *Crash Course* series, the perfect balance of attention to detail and concise accessibility means this book will be perfect for you whether you are a medical student on placement or studying for exams, a junior doctors hoping to refresh their knowledge, or indeed anyone interested in a career in psychiatry. Enjoy!

Steven Birrell

Acknowledgements

I would firstly like to thank my faculty advisor, Dr Steve Birrell, who has provided consistently sound and sensible advice on all topics as well as being a supportive and kind colleague.

This textbook has drawn strength from expert feedback on specialist chapters on a goodwill basis; I have done my best to accurately convey the reviewers' expertise and judgement. I am very grateful to: Dr Lucy Stirland (Clinical Research Fellow in Older Adult Psychiatry, University of Edinburgh), Dr Rebecca Lawrence (Consultant Psychiatrist in Addictions, NHS Lothian), Dr Rachel Petrie (Consultant Psychiatrist in Addictions, NHS Lothian), Dr Premal Shah (Consultant Psychiatrist, Adult ADHD and ASD team, NHS Lothian), Dr Rob Stewart (Consultant Perinatal Psychiatrist, NHS Lothian), Dr Leah Jones (ST5 in Forensic Psychiatry, NHS Lothian) and Dr Senem Sahin (ST4 General Adult Psychiatry, Camden & Islington NHS Foundation Trust). I am particularly grateful to Dr Jennifer Cumming (ST6 in Child and Adolescent Psychiatry, NHS Lothian) who also co-authored the Child and Adolescent Mental Health chapter. Representatives of the Royal College of Psychiatrists (RCPsych) were very helpful in providing detailed advice on some specific aspects of UK Mental Health Acts (Dr Gerry Lynch, Consultant Psychiatrist, Chair of RCPsych in Northern Ireland and Vice President of RCPsych, and Helen Phillips, Senior Policy Administrator, RCPsych). I am also grateful to Dr Liana Romaniuk (CT1 Psychiatry, NHS Lothian) who provided early input into the book's reorganisation.

This is the first edition of this textbook to contain Objective Structured Clinical Exams (see accompanying resources on studentconsult.com). I have been greatly helped in crafting their structure and content by the other members of the Edinburgh University Psychiatry Undergraduate OSCE writing team (2015-2017), in particular my co-chair Dr Chris O'Shea (Clinical Teaching Fellow, NHS Lothian) and Dr Jennie Higgs (Clinical Teaching Fellow, NHS Lothian).

I am also grateful to those who have taught me, those whom I have taught, and patients I have met. I hope I have distilled some of their wisdom and outlook into the clinical cases and tips throughout the book.

I am deeply thankful to my husband, Jonathan Shutt, and to my family, for their support and understanding during the epic process of writing a textbook - again.

Katie Marwick

Dedication

Author

To my mother, Dr Helen Marwick (Developmental Psychologist and Senior Lecturer, University of Strathclyde), who helped to shape my early interest in understanding people and neuroscience and who has been much in my thoughts during the preparation of this book.

Katie Marwick

Faculty Advisor

To my wife, children, family, friends, colleagues, and patients who all continue to inspire, challenge, and support me.

Steven Birrell

Series Editors' acknowledgements

We would like to thank the support of our colleagues who have helped in the preparation of this edition, namely the junior doctor contributors who helped write the manuscript as well as the faculty editors who check the veracity of the information.

We are extremely grateful for the support of our publisher, Elsevier, whose staffs' insight and persistence has maintained the quality that Dr Horton-Szar has set-out since the first edition. Jeremy Bowes, our commissioning editor, has been a constant support. Alex Mortimer and Barbara Simmons our development editors has managed the day-to-day work on this edition with extreme patience and unflaggable determination to meet the ever looming deadlines, and we are ever grateful for Kim Benson's contribution to the online editions and additional online supplementary materials.

Shreelata Datta and Philip Xiu

Contributor:

Jennifer Cumming
Dr Jennifer Cumming BSc (Hons) MBChB MRCPsych AFHEA
ST6 Child and Adolescent Psychiatry & NHS Lothian Clinical Educator
Royal Edinburgh Hospital
Edinburgh, UK
Chapter 30. Child and Adolescent Psychiatry

Contents

Contents

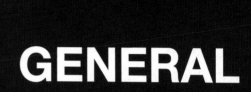

GENERAL

GENERAL

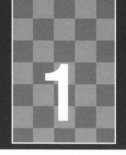

Psychiatric assessment and diagnosis

The psychiatric assessment is different from a medical or surgical assessment in that: (1) the history taking is often longer and requires understanding each patient's unique background and environment; (2) a mental state examination (MSE) is performed; and (3) the assessment can in itself be therapeutic. Fig. 1.1 provides an outline of the psychiatric assessment, which includes a psychiatric history, MSE, risk assessment, physical examination and formulation.

INTERVIEW TECHNIQUE

- Whenever possible, patients should be interviewed in settings where privacy can be ensured – a patient who is distressed will be more at ease in a quiet office than in an accident and emergency cubicle.

- Chairs should be at the same level and arranged at an angle, so that you are not sitting directly opposite the patient.
- Establishing rapport is an immediate priority and requires the display of empathy and sensitivity by the interviewer.
- Notes may be taken during the interview; however, explain to patients that you will be doing so. Make sure that you still maintain good eye contact.
- Ensure that both you and the patient have an unobstructed exit should it be required.
- Carry a personal alarm and/or know where the alarm in the consulting room is, and check you know how to work the alarms.
- Introduce yourself to the patient and ask them how they would like to be addressed. Explain how long the interview will last. In examination situations, it may

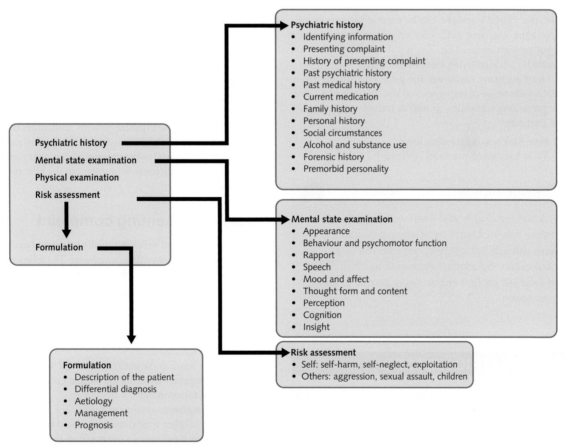

Fig. 1.1 Outline of the psychiatric assessment procedure.

prove helpful to explain to patients that you may need to interrupt them due to time constraints.
- Keep track of and ration your time appropriately.
- Flexibility is essential (e.g. it may be helpful to put a very anxious patient at ease by talking about their background before focusing in on the presenting complaint).

HINTS AND TIPS

Arrange the seating comfortably, and in a way that allows everyone a clear exit, before inviting the patient into the room.

Make use of both open and closed questions when appropriate:

Closed questions limit the scope of the response to one- or two-word answers. They are used to gain specific information and can be used to control the length of the interview when patients are being over-inclusive. For example:

- Do you feel low in mood? (Yes or no answer)
- What time do you wake up in the morning? (Specific answer)

Note that closed questions can be used at the very beginning of the interview, as they are easier to answer and help to put patients at ease (e.g. 'Do you live locally?'; 'Are you married?'; see Identifying information later).

Open questions encourage the patient to answer freely with a wide range of responses and should be used to elicit the presenting complaint, as well as feelings and attitudes. For example:

- How have you been feeling lately?
- What has caused you to feel this way?

COMMUNICATION

Rapport building is vital when working in mental health. Always think why a patient may have difficulty establishing one with you (e.g. persecutory delusions, withdrawal, apathy). Failure to establish rapport should never be due to the interviewer.

PSYCHIATRIC HISTORY

The order in which you take the history is not as important as being systematic, making sure you cover all the essential subsections. A typical format for taking a psychiatric history is outlined in Fig. 1.1 and is described in detail below.

Identifying information

- Name
- Age
- Marital status and children
- Occupation
- Reason for the patient's presence in a psychiatric setting (e.g. referral to out-patient clinic by family doctor, admitted to ward informally having presented at casualty)
- Legal status (i.e. if detained under mental health legislation)

For example:

Mrs LM is a 32-year-old married housewife with two children aged 4 and 6 years. She was referred by her family doctor to a psychiatric out-patient clinic.

Presenting complaint

Open questions are used to elicit the presenting complaint. Whenever possible, record the main problems in the patient's own words, in one or two sentences, instead of using technical psychiatric terms. For example:

Mrs LM complains of 'feeling as though I don't know who I am, like I'm living in an empty shell'.

Patients frequently have more than one complaint, some of which may be related. It is helpful to organize multiple presenting complaints into groups of symptoms that are related; for instance, 'low mood', 'poor concentration' and 'lack of energy' are common features of depression. For example:

Mrs LM complains firstly of 'low mood', 'difficulty sleeping' and 'poor self-esteem', and secondly of 'taking to the bottle' associated with withdrawal symptoms of 'shaking, sweating and jitteriness' in the morning.

It is not always easy to organize patients' difficulties into a simple presenting complaint in psychiatry. In this case, give the chief complaint(s) as the presenting complaint, and cover the rest of the symptoms or problems in the history of the presenting complaint.

History of presenting complaint

This section is concerned with eliciting the nature and development of each of the presenting complaints. The following headings may be helpful in structuring your questioning:

- *Duration*: when did the problems start?
- *Development*: how did the problems develop?
- *Mode of onset*: suddenly, or over a period of time?
- *Course*: are symptoms constant, progressively worsening or intermittent?
- *Severity*: how much is the patient suffering? To what extent are symptoms affecting the patient's social and occupational functioning?
- *Associated symptoms*: certain complaints are associated with clusters of other symptoms that should be enquired about if patients do not mention them spontaneously. This is the same approach as in other

Table 1.1 Typical questions used to elicit specific psychiatric symptoms

Questions used to elicit...	Chapter
Suicidal ideas	6
Depressive symptoms	11
Mania/hypomania	10
Delusions	9
Hallucinations	9
Symptoms of anxiety	12
Dissociative symptoms	14
Obsessions and compulsions	13
Somatoform disorders	15
Memory and cognition	7
Problem drinking	8
Symptoms of anorexia and bulimia	16
Symptoms of insomnia	25

specialties; for example, enquiring about nausea, diarrhoea and distension when someone reports abdominal pain. When 'feeling low' is a presenting complaint, biological, cognitive and psychotic features of depression, as well as suicidal ideation, should be asked about. You can also ask about symptom clusters for psychosis, anxiety, eating problems, substance use and cognitive problems, among others. Also, certain symptoms are common to many psychiatric conditions, and these should be screened for (e.g. a primary complaint of insomnia may be a sign of depression, mania, psychosis or a primary sleep disorder).

- *Precipitating factors:* psychosocial stress frequently precipitates episodes of mental illness (e.g. bereavement, moving house and relationship difficulties).

Table 1.1 directs you to the relevant chapters with example questions for different components of the history and MSE.

HINTS AND TIPS

It is useful to learn how to screen patients for common symptoms. This is especially so with patients who are less forthcoming with their complaints. Remember to ask about:

- Low mood (depression)
- Elevated mood and increased energy (hypomania and mania)
- Delusions and hallucinations (psychosis)
- Free-floating anxiety, panic attacks or phobias (anxiety disorders)
- Obsessions or compulsions (obsessive-compulsive disorder)
- Alcohol or substance abuse

HINTS AND TIPS

Depression and obsessive-compulsive symptoms often coexist (>20%), with onset of obsessive-compulsive symptoms occurring before, simultaneously with or after the onset of depression. You may find it useful to have a set of screening questions ready to use.

Past psychiatric history

This is an extremely important section, as it may provide clues to the patient's current diagnosis. It should include:

- Previous or ongoing psychiatric diagnoses
- Dates and duration of previous mental illness episodes
- Previous treatments, including medication, psychotherapy and electroconvulsive therapy
- Previous contact with psychiatric services (e.g. referrals, admissions)
- Previous assessment or treatment under mental health legislation
- History of self-harm, suicidal ideas or acts

Past medical history

Enquire about medical illnesses or surgical procedures. Past head injury or surgery, neurological conditions (e.g. epilepsy) and endocrine abnormalities (e.g. thyroid problems) are especially relevant to psychiatry.

Current medication

Note all the medication patients are using, including psychiatric, nonpsychiatric and over-the-counter drugs. Also enquire how long patients have been on specific medication and whether it has been effective. Nonconcordance, as well as reactions and allergies, should be recorded.

Family history

- Enquire about the presence of psychiatric illness (including suicide and substance abuse) in family members, remembering that genetic factors are *when talking about her lack of self-esteem. After this her posture relaxed, her eye contact improved and there were moments when she smiled. There were no abnormal movements.*

The term 'psychomotor' is used to describe a patient's motor activity as a consequence of their concurrent mental processes. Psychomotor abnormalities include *retardation* (slow, monotonous speech; slow or absent body movements) and *agitation* (inability to sit still; fidgeting, pacing or hand-wringing; rubbing or scratching skin or clothes).

Note whether you can establish a good rapport with patients. What is their attitude towards you? Do they make good eye contact, or do they look around the room or at the floor? Patients may be described as cooperative, cordial, uninterested, aggressive, defensive, guarded, suspicious, fearful, perplexed, preoccupied or disinhibited (that is, a lowering of normal social inhibitions; e.g. being overfamiliar or making sexually inappropriate comments), amongst many other adjectives.

HINTS AND TIPS

Observations of appearance and behaviour may also reveal other useful information (e.g. extrapyramidal side-effects from antipsychotic medication). It is useful to remember to look for:

- *Parkinsonism:* drug-induced signs are most commonly a reduced arm swing and unusually upright posture while walking. Tremor and rigidity are late signs, in contrast to idiopathic parkinsonism.
- *Acute dystonia:* involuntary sustained muscular contractions or spasms.
- *Akathisia*: subjective feeling of inner restlessness and muscular discomfort, often manifesting with an inability to sit still, 'jiggling' of the legs (irregularly, as opposed to a tremor, which would be regular) or apparent psychomotor agitation.
- *Tardive dyskinesia:* rhythmic, involuntary movements of head, limbs and trunk, especially chewing, grimacing of mouth and making protruding, darting movements with the tongue.

Speech

Speech should be described in terms of:

- *Rate of production:* pressure of speech in mania; long pauses and poverty of speech in depression
- *Quality and flow of speech:* volume, dysarthria (articulation difficulties), dysprosody (unusual speech rhythm, melody, intonation or pitch), stuttering
- *Word play:* punning, rhyming, alliteration (generally seen in mania)

COMMON PITFALLS

Note that disorganized, incoherent or bizarre speech (e.g. flight of ideas) is usually regarded as a thought disorder and is described later in the thought form section.

Mood and affect

Mood refers to a patient's sustained, subjectively experienced emotional state over a period of time. *Affect* refers to the transient ebb and flow of emotion in response to stimuli (e.g. smiling at a joke or crying at a sad memory).

Mood is assessed by asking patients how they are feeling and might be described as depressed, elated, anxious, guilty, frightened, angry, etc. It is described subjectively (what the patient says they are feeling) and objectively (what your impression of their prevailing mood is during the interview) For example, *her mood was subjectively 'rock bottom' and objectively low.* Affect is assessed by observing patients' posture, facial expression, emotional reactivity and speech. There are two components to consider when assessing affect:

1. The appropriateness or congruity of the observed affect to the patient's subjectively reported mood (e.g. a woman with schizophrenia who reports feeling suicidal but has a happy facial expression would be described as having an *incongruous* affect).
2. The range of affect or range of emotional expressivity. In this sense, affect may be:
   - Within the normal range
   - Blunted/flat: a noticeable reduction in the normal intensity of emotional expression, as evidenced by a monotonous voice and minimal facial expression

Note that a *labile* mood refers to a fluctuating mood state that alternates between extremes (e.g. a young man with a mixed affective episode alternates between feeling overjoyed, with pressure of speech, and miserable, with suicidal ideation).

Thoughts

Problems with thinking are considered under two headings: thought form (abnormal patterns of thinking) and thought content (abnormal beliefs).

Thought form

Disordered thinking includes circumstantial and tangential thinking, loosening of association (derailment/knight's move thinking), flight of ideas and thought blocking (see Chapter 9 for the definitions of these terms). Whenever possible, record patients' disorganized speech word for word, as it can be very difficult to label disorganized thinking with a single technical term, and written language may be easier to evaluate than spoken language.

Thought content: delusions, obsessions and overvalued ideas

It is diagnostically significant to classify delusions as:

- Primary or secondary
- Mood congruent or mood incongruent
- Bizarre or nonbizarre
- According to the content of the delusion (summarized in Table 9.1)

See Chapter 9 for a detailed description of these terms.

An obsession is an involuntary thought, image or impulse that is recurrent, intrusive and unpleasant and enters the mind against conscious resistance. Patients recognize that the thoughts are a product of their own mind. See Chapter 13 for more information.

COMMUNICATION

Some psychiatrists include thoughts of self-harm, suicide or harm to others under thought content, while others mention it only under risk assessment. As long as you mention it, it doesn't matter where.

Perception

Hallucinations are often mentioned during the history. However, this is not always the case, so it is important that you specifically enquire about abnormal perceptual experiences (perceptual abnormalities are defined and classified in Chapter 9). If patients admit to problems with perception, it is important to ascertain:

- Whether the abnormal perceptions are hallucinations, pseudohallucinations, illusions or intrusive thoughts
- From which sensory modality the hallucinations appear to arise (i.e. are they auditory, visual, olfactory, gustatory or somatic hallucinations – see Chapter 9)
- Whether auditory hallucinations are elementary (a very simple abnormal perception; e.g. a flash or a bang) or complex. If complex, are they experienced in the first person (audible thoughts, thought echo), second person (critical, persecutory, complimentary or command hallucinations) or third person (voices arguing or discussing the patient, or giving a running commentary)?

It is also important to note whether patients seem to be responding to hallucinations during the interview, as evidenced by them laughing inappropriately as though they are sharing a private joke, suddenly tilting their head as though listening or quizzically looking at hallucinatory objects around the room.

RED FLAG

Elementary hallucinations are more common in delirium, migraine and epilepsy than in primary psychiatric disorders.

Cognition

The cognition of all patients should be screened by checking orientation to place and time. Depending on the circumstances, a more thorough cognitive assessment may be required. Cognitive tests, including tests of generalized cognitive abilities (e.g. consciousness, attention, orientation) and specific abilities (e.g. memory, language, executive function, praxis, perception), are discussed fully in Chapter 7. Figure 7.1 and Tables 7.1, 7.2 and 7.6 describe methods of testing cognition.

Insight

Insight is not an 'all or nothing' attribute. It is often described as good, partial or poor, although patients really lie somewhere on a spectrum and vary over time. The key questions to answer are:

- Does the patient believe they are unwell in any way?
- Do they believe they are mentally unwell?
- Do they think they need treatment (pharmacological, psychological or both)?
- Do they think they need to be admitted to hospital (if relevant)?

RISK ASSESSMENT

Although it is extremely difficult to make an accurate assessment of risk based on a single assessment, clinicians are expected, as far as is possible, to establish some idea of a patient's risk to:

- *Self*: through self-harm, suicide, self-neglect or exploitation by others. Chapter 6 explains the assessment of suicide risk in detail.
- *Others*: includes violent or sexual crime, stalking and harassment. Chapter 32 discusses key principles in assessing dangerousness.
- *Children*: includes physical, sexual or emotional abuse, as well as neglect or deprivation. Child abuse is discussed in more detail in Chapter 30.
- *Property*: includes arson and physical destruction of property.

PHYSICAL EXAMINATION

The psychiatric examination includes a general physical examination, with special focus on the neurological and endocrine systems. Always remember to look for signs relevant to the psychiatric history (e.g. signs of liver disease in patients who misuse alcohol, ophthalmoplegia or ataxia in someone withdrawing from alcohol (indicating Wernicke encephalopathy), signs of self-harm in patients with a personality disorder and signs of intravenous drug use (track marks) in patients who use drugs). Also, examine for side-effects of psychiatric medication (e.g. parkinsonism, tardive dyskinesia, dystonia, hypotension, obesity and other cardiometabolic sequelae, signs of lithium toxicity). It may not be possible to complete a detailed physical examination in an exam situation, but you should always recommend that it should be done. Always make a point of mentioning your positive physical findings when summarizing the case.

THE FORMULATION: PRESENTING THE CASE

'Formulation' is the term psychiatrists use to describe the integrated summary and understanding of a particular patient's problems. The formulation usually includes:

- Description of the patient
- Differential diagnosis
- Aetiology
- Management
- Prognosis

Description of the patient

The patient may be described: (1) in detail by recounting all the information obtained under the various headings in the psychiatric history and MSE; or (2) in the form of a case summary. The case summary consists of one or two paragraphs and contains only the salient features of a case, specifically:

- Identifying information
- Main features of the presenting complaint

- Relevant background details (e.g. past psychiatric history, positive family history)
- Positive findings in the MSE and physical examination

Table 1.2 shows a case summary as a formulation.

Differential diagnosis

The differential diagnosis is mentioned in order of decreasing probability. Only mention conditions that you have obtained evidence about in your assessment, as you should be able to provide reasons for and against all the alternatives on your list. Table 1.2 provides an example of a typical differential diagnosis.

Aetiology

The exact cause of most psychiatric disorders is often unknown, and most cases seem to involve a complex interplay of biological, social and psychological factors. In clinical practice, psychiatrists are especially concerned with the question: 'What factors led to this patient presenting with this specific problem at this specific point in time?' That is, what factors predisposed to the problem, what factors precipitated the problem, and what factors are perpetuating the problem? Table 1.2 illustrates an aetiology grid that is very helpful in structuring your answers to these questions in terms of biological, social and psychological factors – the emphasis should be on *considering* all the blocks in the grid, not necessarily on filling them.

Management

Investigations

Investigations are considered part of the management plan and are performed based on findings from the psychiatric assessment. Appropriate investigations relevant to specific conditions are given in the relevant chapters. Familiarize yourself with these, as you should be able to give reasons for any investigation you propose.

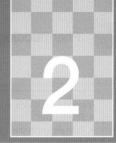
Psychotropic (mind-altering) medications can be divided into the following groups:

- Antidepressants
- Mood stabilizers
- Antipsychotics
- Anxiolytics and hypnotics
- Other

Despite its simplicity, this method of grouping drugs by the disorder they were first used to treat is flawed, because many drugs from one class are now used to treat disorders in another class (e.g. antidepressants are first-line therapies for many anxiety disorders, and some antipsychotics also have mood stabilizing and antidepressant effects).

ANTIDEPRESSANTS

History

Antidepressants were first used in the late 1950s, with the appearance of the tricyclic antidepressant (TCA) imipramine and the monoamine oxidase inhibitor (MAOI) phenelzine. Research into TCAs throughout the 1960s and 1970s resulted in the development of many more tricyclic agents and related compounds. A major development in the late 1980s was the arrival of the first selective serotonin reuptake inhibitor (SSRI) fluoxetine (Prozac). There has since been considerable expansion of the SSRI class, as well as the development of antidepressants such as mirtazapine and agomelatine that have other mechanisms of action.

Classification and mechanism of action

At present, antidepressants are classified according to their pharmacological actions, as there is not yet an adequate explanation as to what exactly makes antidepressants work. Although there are many different classes of antidepressants, their common action is to elevate the levels of one or more monoamine neurotransmitters in the synaptic cleft. Some predominantly influence serotonin, some noradrenaline and some dopamine, with many influencing the transporters or receptors for multiple neurotransmitters. It is likely that the combination of effects on multiple neurotransmitter pathways acts synergistically in causing the antidepressant effect. For example, agomelatine is both a melatonin receptor agonist and a 5-HT$_{2C}$ (serotonin 2C) receptor antagonist, but neither of these actions alone have an antidepressant effect. Fig. 2.1 illustrates the mechanism of action of antidepressants at synapses, and Table 2.1 summarizes their classification and pharmacodynamics.

The latest research has focused on monoamine neurotransmitter activation of 'second messenger' signal transduction mechanisms. This results in the production of transcription factors that lead to the activation of genes controlling the expression of downstream targets such as brain-derived neurotrophic factor (BDNF). BDNF is neuroprotective, and might be a key target of antidepressant action.

HINTS AND TIPS

When recommending antidepressants to trial in a patient with treatment-resistant depression, it makes sense to try those with different pharmacodynamic properties to antidepressants that have been trialled before. See Table 2.1.

Indications

SSRIs are used in the treatment of:

- Depression
- Anxiety disorders
- Obsessive-compulsive disorder

Mirtazapine is used in the treatment of:

- Depression (particularly where sedation or increased oral intake is desirable)

TCAs are used in the treatment of:

- Depression
- Anxiety disorders
- Obsessive-compulsive disorder (clomipramine)
- Other: chronic pain, nocturnal enuresis, narcolepsy

MAOIs are used in the treatment of:

- Depression (especially atypical depression, which is characterized by hypersomnia, overeating and anxiety)
- Anxiety disorders
- Other: Parkinson disease, migraine prophylaxis, tuberculosis

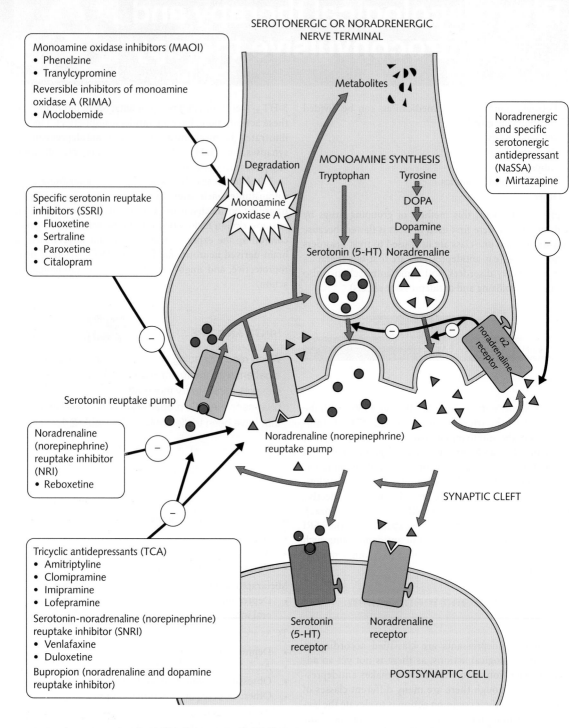

Note: the serotonin and noradrenaline (norepinephrine) pathways are presented together for convenience; they do not occur in the same nerve terminal

Fig. 2.1 Mechanism of action of antidepressants at the synaptic cleft.

Table 2.1 Classification and pharmacodynamics of the antidepressants

Class of antidepressant	Examples	Mechanism of action
Commonly used		
Selective serotonin reuptake inhibitor (SSRI)	Fluoxetine, sertraline, paroxetine, citalopram, fluvoxamine	Selective presynaptic blockade of serotonin reuptake pumps.
Serotonin and noradrenaline reuptake inhibitor (SNRI)	Venlafaxine, duloxetine	Presynaptic blockade of both noradrenaline (norepinephrine) and serotonin reuptake pumps (also dopamine in high doses), but with negligible effects on muscarinic, histaminergic or α-adrenergic receptors (in contrast to tricyclic antidepressants).
Noradrenergic and specific serotonergic antidepressant (NaSSA)	Mirtazapine	Presynaptic alpha 2 receptor blockade (results in increased release of noradrenaline (norepinephrine) and serotonin from presynaptic neurons). Also 5-HT$_{2A/C}$ and 3 receptor antagonist and histamine 1 receptor antagonist.
5-HT$_{2A/C}$ antagonist/serotonin reuptake inhibitor (SARI)	Trazodone	Also antagonist at alpha 1 adrenergic receptors, histamine type 1 receptors and T-type calcium channels. Which of its actions is important in inducing its sedative and anxiolytic effects is unclear.
Tricyclic antidepressant	Amitriptyline, lofepramine, clomipramine, imipramine	Presynaptic blockade of both noradrenaline (norepinephrine) and serotonin reuptake pumps (to a lesser extent - dopamine). Also, blockade of muscarinic, histaminergic and α-adrenergic receptors.
Less commonly used		
Monoamine oxidase inhibitor (MAOI)	Phenelzine, tranylcypromine, isocarboxazid	Nonselective and irreversible inhibition of monoamine oxidase A and B.
Reversible inhibitor of monoamine oxidase A (RIMA)	Moclobemide	Selective and reversible inhibition of monoamine oxidase A.
Noradrenaline and dopamine reuptake inhibitor	Bupropion	Dopamine and noradrenaline reuptake pump inhibitor.
Dopamine agonist	Pramipexole, ropinirole	Dopamine receptor agonist (D_2, D_3, D_4).
Selective noradrenaline reuptake inhibitor (NRI)	Reboxetine	Selective presynaptic blockade of noradrenaline (norepinephrine) reuptake pumps.
Melatonin agonist and serotonin antagonist	Agomelatine	Melatonin receptor 1 and 2 agonist and 5-HT$_{2C}$ receptor antagonist.
Serotonin modulator and stimulator	Vortioxetine	Selective serotonin reuptake inhibitor, plus varied effects on different 5-HT receptor subtypes (1A agonist, 1B partial agonist, 1D, 3 and 7 antagonist).

Side-effects and contraindications

SSRIs and SNRIs

SSRIs have fewer anticholinergic effects than the TCAs and are not sedating. The majority of patients find them alerting, so they are prescribed to be taken in the morning. Soon after initiation, or when taken at high doses, some patients can feel alerted to the point of agitation/anxiety. This may be associated with an increased risk for suicide, particularly in adolescents (see Chapter 30 for recommendations on use in young people). Due to their low cardiotoxicity, SSRIs are the antidepressant of choice in patients with cardiac disease and in those who are at risk for taking an overdose. However, they do have their own side-effects that may be unacceptable to some patients. These are summarized in Box 2.1. Selective serotonin and noradrenaline reuptake inhibitors (SNRIs) such as venlafaxine have similar side-effects to SSRIs, but they tend to be more severe.

Contraindications: mania, poorly controlled epilepsy and prolonged QTc interval (for citalopram and escitalopram).

BOX 2.1 COMMON SIDE-EFFECTS OF SSRIs

Gastrointestinal disturbance (nausea, vomiting, diarrhoea, pain) – early[a]

Anxiety and agitation – early[a]

Loss of appetite and weight loss (sometimes weight gain)

Insomnia

Sweating

Sexual dysfunction (anorgasmia, delayed ejaculation)

[a] Gastrointestinal and anxiety symptoms occur on initiation of treatment and resolve with time.

Mirtazapine

Mirtazapine is very commonly associated with increased appetite, weight gain and sedation (via histamine antagonism). These side-effects can be used to advantage in many patients. It is also associated with headache, dry mouth and, less commonly, dizziness, postural hypotension, tremor and peripheral oedema. It has negligible anticholinergic effects.

Contraindications: mania.

Tricyclic antidepressants

Table 2.2 summarizes the common side-effects of TCAs, most of which are related to the multireceptor blocking effects of these drugs. The sedative side-effect can be useful if patients have insomnia. TCAs with prominent sedative effects include amitriptyline and clomipramine. Those with less sedative effects include lofepramine and imipramine. Due to their cardiotoxic effects, TCAs are dangerous in overdose, although lofepramine (a newer TCA) has fewer antimuscarinic effects, and so is relatively safe compared with other TCAs.

Contraindications: recent myocardial infarction, arrhythmias, acute porphyria, mania and high risk for overdose.

Table 2.2 Common side-effects of tricyclic antidepressants

Mechanism	Side-effects
Anticholinergic: muscarinic receptor blockade	Dry mouth Constipation Urinary retention Blurred vision
α-Adrenergic receptor blockade	Postural hypotension (dizziness, syncope)
Histaminergic receptor blockade	Weight gain Sedation
Cardiotoxic effects	QT interval prolongation ST segment elevation Heart block Arrhythmias

Trazodone

Trazodone is a relatively weak antidepressant but a good sedative. It is relatively safe in overdose and has negligible anticholinergic side-effects. It is often used as an adjunctive antidepressant in those receiving a nonsedative primary antidepressant (e.g. an SSRI).

Contraindications: as TCAs (closely related structurally).

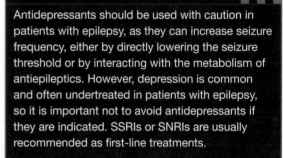

RED FLAG

Antidepressants should be used with caution in patients with epilepsy, as they can increase seizure frequency, either by directly lowering the seizure threshold or by interacting with the metabolism of antiepileptics. However, depression is common and often undertreated in patients with epilepsy, so it is important not to avoid antidepressants if they are indicated. SSRIs or SNRIs are usually recommended as first-line treatments.

MAOIs/RIMAs

Due to the risk for serious interactions with certain foods and other drugs, the MAOIs have become second-line antidepressants. Their inhibition of monoamine oxidase A results in the accumulation of amine neurotransmitters and impairs the metabolism of some amines found in certain drugs (e.g. decongestants) and foodstuffs (e.g. tyramine). Because MAOIs bind irreversibly to monoamine oxidase A and B, amines may accumulate to dangerously high levels, which may precipitate a life-threatening hypertensive crisis. An example of this occurs when the ingestion of dietary tyramine results in a massive release of noradrenaline (norepinephrine) from endogenous stores. This is termed the 'cheese reaction,' because some mature cheeses contain high levels of tyramine. Box 2.2 lists the drugs and foodstuffs that should be avoided in patients taking MAOIs.

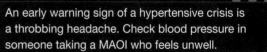

RED FLAG

An early warning sign of a hypertensive crisis is a throbbing headache. Check blood pressure in someone taking a MAOI who feels unwell.

The reversible inhibitor of monoamine oxidase A (RIMA) moclobemide reversibly inhibits monoamine oxidase A. Therefore the drug will be displaced from the enzyme as amine levels start to increase. So, although there is a small risk for developing a hypertensive crisis if high levels of tyramine are ingested, dietary restrictions are much less onerous.

BOX 2.2 DRUGS AND FOODS THAT MAY PRECIPITATE A HYPERTENSIVE CRISIS IN COMBINATION WITH MAOIS

Tyramine-rich foods

Cheese – especially mature varieties (e.g. Stilton)

Degraded protein: pickled herring, smoked fish, chicken liver, hung game

Yeast and protein extract: Bovril, Oxo, Marmite

Chianti wine, beer

Broad bean pods

Soya bean extract

Overripe or unfresh food

Medication or Substances

Adrenaline (epinephrine), noradrenaline (norepinephrine)

Amphetamines

Cocaine

Ephedrine, pseudoephedrine, phenylpropanolamine (cough mixtures, decongestants)

L-dopa, dopamine

Local anaesthetics containing adrenaline (epinephrine)

Note: the combination of MAOIs and antidepressants or opiates (especially pethidine or tramadol) may result in serotonin syndrome. Opiates have some serotonin reuptake inhibitory activity.

RED FLAG

When other antidepressants that have a strong serotonergic effect (e.g. SSRIs, clomipramine, imipramine) are administered simultaneously with an MAOI, the risk for developing the potentially lethal 'serotonin syndrome' is increased (see Table 2.8). Therefore antidepressant wash-out periods are required if starting or stopping an MAOI – check guidance for the specific switch you are considering.

MAOIs may have further side-effects similar to those induced by TCAs, including postural hypotension and anticholinergic effects.

Contraindications (MAOIs): phaeochromocytoma, cerebrovascular disease and mania.

HINTS AND TIPS

The abrupt withdrawal of any antidepressant may result in a discontinuation syndrome with symptoms such as gastrointestinal disturbance, agitation, dizziness, headache, tremor and insomnia. SSRIs with short half-lives (e.g. paroxetine, sertraline) and venlafaxine are particular culprits. Therefore all antidepressants (with the exception of fluoxetine, which has a long half-life and many active metabolites) should be gradually tapered down before being withdrawn completely.

COMMUNICATION

Although certain antidepressants may cause a discontinuation syndrome, they do not cause a dependence syndrome or 'addiction,' in that patients do not become tolerant to them or crave them.

MOOD STABILIZERS

These include lithium and the anticonvulsants valproate, carbamazepine and lamotrigine. Antipsychotics such as quetiapine and olanzapine are also increasingly used in treating episodes of mania and in prophylactic mood stabilization (these are covered in the next section; see also Chapter 22).

History

In 1949, John Cade discovered that lithium salts caused lethargy when injected into animals, and later reported lithium's antimanic properties in humans. Trials in the 1950s and 1960s led to the drug entering mainstream practice in 1970.

Valproate was first recognized as an effective anticonvulsant in 1962. Along with carbamazepine and lamotrigine, it was later shown to be effective in treating patients with bipolar affective disorder.

Mechanism of action

It is not known how any of the mood stabilizers work. Lithium appears to modulate the neurotransmitter-induced activation of second messenger systems. Valproate, carbamazepine and lamotrigine all inhibit the activity voltage-gated sodium channels, and also enhance GABA-ergic neurotransmission.

Indications

Lithium is used in the treatment of:

- Acute mania
- Prophylaxis of bipolar affective disorder (prevention of relapse)
- Treatment-resistant depression (lithium augmentation)

Valproate is used in the treatment of:

- Epilepsy
- Acute mania
- Prophylaxis of bipolar affective disorder (second-line)

Carbamazepine is used in the treatment of:

- Epilepsy
- Prophylaxis of bipolar affective disorder (third-line)

Lamotrigine is used in the treatment of:

- Epilepsy
- Prophylaxis of depressive episodes in bipolar affective disorder (third-line)

HINTS AND TIPS

Valproate is available in formulations as sodium valproate, valproic acid and semisodium valproate (Depakote), which comprises equimolar amounts of sodium valproate and valproic acid. Different formulations have different equivalent doses, so prescribe by brand.

Side-effects and contraindications

Lithium

Lithium has a narrow therapeutic window between non-therapeutic and toxic blood levels. Lower levels can be toxic in older patients.

- Therapeutic levels: 0.4–0.8 mmol/L when used adjunctively for depression; 0.6–1.0 mmol/L for treatment of acute mania and for bipolar disorder prophylaxis
- Toxic levels: >1.5 mmol/L
- Dangerously toxic levels: >2 mmol/L

Lithium is only taken orally and is excreted almost entirely by the kidneys. Clearance of lithium is decreased with renal impairment (e.g. in older adults, dehydration) and sodium depletion. Certain drugs such as diuretics (especially thiazides), nonsteroidal antiinflammatory drugs (NSAIDs) and angiotensin-converting enzyme (ACE) inhibitors can also increase lithium levels and should ideally be avoided or prescribed with caution and frequent checks of lithium levels during initiation. Furthermore, antipsychotics may

Table 2.3 Side-effects and signs of toxicity of lithium[a]

Side-effects	Signs of toxicity
Thirst, polydipsia, polyuria, weight gain, oedema	**1.5–2 mmol/L:** nausea and vomiting, apathy, coarse tremor, ataxia, muscle weakness
Fine tremor	
Precipitates or worsens skin problems	
Concentration and memory problems	**>2 mmol/L:** nystagmus, dysarthria, impaired consciousness, hyperactive tendon reflexes, oliguria, hypotension, convulsions, coma
Hypothyroidism	
Hyperparathyroidism	
Impaired renal function	
Cardiac: T-wave flattening or inversion	
Leucocytosis	
Teratogenicity	

[a] *The treatment of lithium toxicity is supportive, ensuring adequate hydration, renal function and electrolyte balance. Anticonvulsants may be necessary for convulsions and haemodialysis may be indicated in cases of renal failure.*

synergistically increase lithium-induced neurotoxicity; this is important, as lithium and antipsychotics are often coadministered in acute mania. Table 2.3 summarizes the side-effects and signs of toxicity of lithium.

RED FLAG

Lithium toxicity can arise rapidly in someone who becomes dehydrated for any reason (e.g. vomiting, diarrhoea, inadequate fluid intake). Always check a random lithium level in someone who takes lithium and is physically unwell.

It follows that the following investigations are needed prior to initiating therapy:

- Full blood count
- Urea and electrolytes
- Calcium
- Thyroid function
- Pregnancy test (in women of childbearing age)
- Electrocardiogram (if cardiac disease or risk factors)

Blood levels are monitored weekly after starting treatment until a therapeutic level has been stable for 2 consecutive weeks. Lithium blood levels should then be monitored every 3 months for the first year, then every 6 months (unless the patient is at high risk for complications from lithium or has poor concordance). Renal function, calcium and thyroid function should be monitored every 6 months or more frequently if there is any evidence of impairment.

Contraindications/cautions: untreated hypothyroidism, heart failure, cardiac arrhythmia.

Valproate, carbamazepine and lamotrigine

Table 2.4 summarizes the side-effects of carbamazepine, valproate and lamotrigine. It is important to check liver

Table 2.4 Side-effects of valproate, carbamazepine and lamotrigine

Valproate[a]	Carbamazepine[b]	Lamotrigine[c]
Increased appetite and weight gain	Nausea and vomiting	Nausea and vomiting
Sedation and dizziness	Skin rashes	Skin rashes (consider
Ankle swelling	Blurred or double vision (diplopia)	withdrawal)
Hair loss	Ataxia, drowsiness, fatigue	Headache
Nausea and vomiting	Hyponatraemia and fluid retention	Aggression, irritability
Tremor	Haematological abnormalities (leucopenia,	Sedation and dizziness
Haematological abnormalities (prolongation of	thrombocytopenia, eosinophilia)	Tremor
bleeding time, thrombocytopenia, leucopenia)	Raised liver enzymes (hepatic or	
Raised liver enzymes (liver damage very uncommon)	cholestatic jaundice, rarely)	

[a] *Serious blood and liver disorders do occur, but are rare.*
[b] *Serious blood and liver disorders do occur, but are rare.*
[c] *Stevens-Johnson syndrome can occur, but it is rare.*

and haematological functions prior to and soon after starting valproate or carbamazepine, due to the risk for serious blood and hepatic disorders.

RED FLAG

Valproate should not be prescribed in women of childbearing age, unless alternative treatments are ineffective or not tolerated, because of its high teratogenic risk (see Chapter 27). If valproate is to be prescribed, ensure the patient is aware of the risk for developmental disorders (approximately a third of births) and congenital malformations (approximately 1 in 10 babies), is using adequate contraception and knows to consult promptly if she does become pregnant.

RED FLAG

Carbamazepine is a potent CYP450 enzyme inducer. Before prescribing new medication for someone taking carbamazepine, check a drug interactions reference (e.g. Appendix 1 in the British National Formulary).

RED FLAG

Lamotrigine can, rarely, be associated with Stevens-Johnson syndrome, particularly in the first 8 weeks of use. Patients should be advised to stop immediately if there is development of a rash, and reintroduction of lamotrigine at a later date should be considered only by a specialist.

ANTIPSYCHOTICS

History and classification

Antipsychotics or neuroleptics (originally known as 'major tranquillizers') appeared in the early 1950s with the introduction of the phenothiazine chlorpromazine. A number of antipsychotics with a similar pharmacodynamic action soon followed (e.g. the butyrophenone haloperidol in the 1960s). Their ability to treat psychotic symptoms had a profound impact on psychiatry, accelerating the movement of patients out of asylums and into the community. However, serious motor side-effects (extrapyramidal side-effects (EPSEs)) soon became apparent with all these drugs.

Clozapine was the first antipsychotic with fewer EPSEs, and thus was termed 'atypical'. It led to the introduction of several other atypical (or 'second generation') antipsychotics, including risperidone, olanzapine and quetiapine. The older antipsychotics such as haloperidol and chlorpromazine became known as 'conventional', 'first generation' or 'typical' antipsychotics. However, this distinction is increasingly viewed as artificial – all antipsychotics can induce EPSEs if given at high enough doses. Clozapine is the only 'true' atypical antipsychotic, in that it has a distinct receptor binding profile and can be effective in two-thirds of the patients for whom other antipsychotics have failed. Table 2.5 lists common antipsychotics.

Table 2.5 Commonly used antipsychotics

First generation	Second generation
Chlorpromazine	Clozapine
Haloperidol[a]	Olanzapine[a]
Sulpiride	Quetiapine
Flupentixol (Depixol)[a]	Risperidone[a]
Zuclopenthixol (Clopixol)[a]	Aripiprazole[a]

[a] *Can be given in long-acting intramuscular injection (depot) form.*

Mechanism of action and side-effects

The primary mechanism of action of all antipsychotics, with the possible exception of clozapine, is antagonism of dopamine D_2 receptors in the mesolimbic dopamine pathway. Clozapine is a comparatively weak D_2 antagonist, but has a high affinity for serotonin type 2 receptors (5-HT_{2A} receptors) and D_4 receptors, among many other receptor targets. Most second generation antipsychotics also block 5-HT_2 receptors.

Unfortunately, blockade of dopamine D_2 receptors occurs throughout the brain, resulting in diverse side-effects. In addition, antipsychotics also cause side-effects by blocking muscarinic, histaminergic and α-adrenergic receptors (as do TCAs). Fig. 2.2 and Table 2.6 summarize both the useful and troublesome clinical effects of D_2-receptor antagonism, as well as the side-effects caused by the blockage of other receptors. Learn this table well; these effects have a big impact on patients' quality of life and concordance (and as such are frequently asked exam questions). See also Table 21.1 for the relative frequency of side-effects for some commonly used antipsychotics.

The risk for metabolic syndrome (obesity, diabetes, hypertension and dyslipidaemia) is particularly high with clozapine and other second generation antipsychotics. Metabolic syndrome is associated with increased cardiovascular mortality, so it is important to monitor and manage the components of this syndrome.

Clozapine is associated with some rare serious side-effects such as agranulocytosis, myocarditis and cardiomyopathy, which means it is reserved for treatment-resistant cases.

HINTS AND TIPS

If you can remember the side-effects of tricyclic antidepressants, you can remember many of the side-effects of antipsychotics, as both are multireceptor blockers. Both groups are anticholinergic (dry mouth, constipation, blurred vision, urinary retention), antiadrenergic (postural hypotension) and antihistaminergic (sedation, weight gain).

HINTS AND TIPS

'Extrapyramidal' symptoms are motor symptoms arising from dysfunction of the striatum (part of the basal ganglia). The striatum provides input to the motor cortex and hence the upper motor neurons (corticospinal and corticobulbar tracts), which

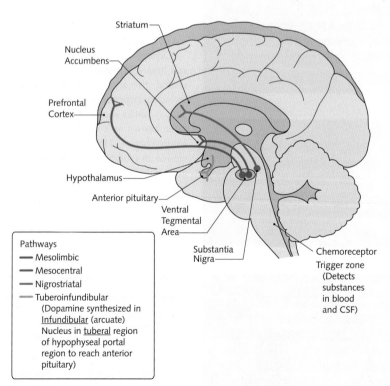

Pathways
- Mesolimbic
- Mesocentral
- Nigrostriatal
- Tuberoinfundibular
  (Dopamine synthesized in Infundibular (arcuate) Nucleus in tuberal region of hypophyseal portal region to reach anterior pituitary)

Fig. 2.2 Dopaminergic pathways.
See Table 2.6 for consequences of D_2 receptor blockade in each of these regions.

Table 2.6 The clinical effects and side-effects of conventional antipsychotics

Dopamine D$_2$-receptor antagonism		
Location of dopamine D$_2$ receptors (see Fig. 2.2)	**Function**	**Clinical effect of dopamine D$_2$-receptor antagonism**
[1] Mesolimbic pathway	Involved in delusions/hallucinations/thought disorders, euphoria and drug dependence	Treatment of psychotic symptoms.
[2] Mesocortical pathway	Mediates cognitive and negative symptoms of schizophrenia	Worsening of negative and cognitive symptoms of schizophrenia.
[3] Nigrostriatal pathway (basal ganglia/striatum)	Controls motor movement	Extrapyramidal side-effects (see Fig. 2.10): • Parkinsonian symptoms • Acute dystonia • Akathisia • Tardive dyskinesia • Neuroleptic malignant syndrome
[4] Tuberoinfundibular pathway	Controls prolactin secretion – dopamine inhibits prolactin release	Hyperprolactinaemia • Galactorrhoea (breast milk production) • Amenorrhoea and infertility • Sexual dysfunction
Chemoreceptor trigger zone	Controls nausea and vomiting	Antiemetic effect: some phenothiazines (e.g. prochlorperazine (Stemetil)) are very effective in treating nausea and vomiting.
Other side-effects		
Anticholinergic: muscarinic receptor blockade		Dry mouth, constipation, urinary retention, blurred vision
α-Adrenergic receptor blockade		Postural hypotension (dizziness, syncope)
Histaminergic receptor blockade		Sedation, weight gain
Cardiac effects		Prolongation of QT-interval, arrhythmias, myocarditis, sudden death
Metabolic effects		Increased risk for metabolic syndrome
Dermatological effects		Photosensitivity, skin rashes (especially chlorpromazine: blue–grey discolouration in the sun)
Other		Lowering of seizure threshold, hepatotoxicity, cholestatic jaundice, pancytopenia, agranulocytosis

travel from cortex to spinal cord (or cranial nerve nuclei). As these tracts pass through the brainstem, they form a bulge, which is termed the *medullary pyramids*. The term 'extrapyramidal' emphasizes that different symptoms arise from disruption to the striatum (e.g. Table 2.7) than from disruption to motor cortex (e.g. hemiparesis following a stroke); however, in both cases, the motor control signals descend via the pyramids.

HINTS AND TIPS

The particular extrapyramidal side-effects (EPSEs) of parkinsonism and dystonia are due to a relative deficiency of dopamine and an excess of acetylcholine induced by dopamine antagonism in the nigrostriatal pathway. This is why anticholinergic drugs are effective treatments (but not for akathisia, which has a different mechanism).

Contraindications

There are no absolute contraindications to ECT. Relative contraindications include:

- Heart disease (recent myocardial infarction, heart failure, ischaemic heart disease)
- Raised intracranial pressure
- Risk for cerebral bleeding (hypertension, recent stroke)
- Poor anaesthetic risk.

ETHICS

Media portrayals of ECT have included its use as a punishment, given without patient consent. In modern practice, a patient with capacity will make his or her own decision about commencing ECT or not. A patient who lacks capacity may be given ECT without his or her consent if it is felt to be in his or her best interests; however, this requires a second opinion from an independent psychiatrist.

Chapter Summary

- Psychotropic medications are classed by the indication for which they were first licensed, but many medications are of benefit in other disorders.
- Antidepressants influence the serotonin, noradrenaline and dopamine systems.
- Many antidepressants are well tolerated.
- Lithium requires regular monitoring of blood levels because high levels are toxic.
- Antipsychotics antagonize dopamine D_2 receptors.
- Antipsychotics often have unpleasant and debilitating side-effects.
- Benzodiazepines and Z-drugs both increase the activity of $GABA_A$ receptors.
- Medications with shorter half-lives are more likely to cause discontinuation symptoms.
- Electroconvulsive therapy is a highly effective and safe treatment for severe mental illness.

Psychological therapy describes the interaction between a therapist and a client that aims to impart beneficial changes in the client's thoughts, feelings and behaviours. Psychological therapy, which is often known as 'psychotherapy' or 'talking therapy,' may be useful in alleviating specific symptoms (e.g. social phobia) or in helping a client improve their overall sense of well-being.

Members of different professional disciplines, including clinical psychologists, psychiatrists, occupational therapists, mental health nurses, art and drama therapists and counsellors, may all practise psychotherapy, provided they have had adequate training and supervision.

PSYCHOTHERAPEUTIC APPROACHES

There are many different approaches to psychotherapy. Research has shown efficacy for many different types of psychotherapies for many conditions. This has led to the idea that the success of psychotherapy might be due to certain common therapeutic factors, as opposed to specific theories or techniques. A comprehensive review of psychotherapy research showed that common factors (occurring in any model of therapy) account for 85% of the therapeutic effect, whereas theoretical orientation only accounts for 15%. Therefore the use of a modality with which the patient can identify, and work may be more important than the theoretical basis of the therapy itself. Common therapeutic factors include client factors (personal strengths, social supports), therapist-client relationship factors (empathy, acceptance, warmth) and the client's expectancy of change.

HINTS AND TIPS

'Self-help' is the umbrella term used to describe the process of self-guided improvement. Often, self-help resources utilize psychological techniques (especially cognitive-behavioural therapy) and educational materials. Self-help may involve books, DVDs, interactive websites and discussion groups (including Internet-based forums). Self-help materials may be provided from, and progress followed and reviewed by, health care professionals (known as 'facilitated' or 'guided' self-help), and can be incredibly useful for some people, either

---

in the management of less severe psychological difficulties or as an adjunct to other forms of treatment. Group-based peer support is a form of self-help delivered to groups of patients with shared symptoms, during which experiences can be shared and progress reviewed by a facilitator.

HINTS AND TIPS

The single factor most commonly associated with a good therapeutic outcome is the strength of the client-therapist relationship (therapeutic alliance), regardless of the modality of therapy. In some cases, it may be beneficial to use a mixture of modalities (e.g. psychodynamic, interpersonal and cognitive-behavioural therapy) uniquely tailored to understanding and treating the patient (known as 'eclectic therapy').

Counselling and supportive psychotherapy

Psychotherapy is sometimes distinguished from counselling, although they exist on a continuum from counselling and supportive psychotherapy (least complex) to psychodynamic psychotherapy and sophisticated cognitive therapy (more complex and requiring more specialist training).

Counselling is usually brief in duration and is recommended for patients with minor mental health or interpersonal difficulties, or for those experiencing stressful life circumstances (e.g. grief counselling for bereavement). Counselling helps patients utilize their own strengths, with the therapist being reflective and empathic. The provision of relevant information and advice, which is undertaken by health care professionals of all specialties, is also considered to be counselling.

In person-centred counselling, the therapist assumes an empathic and reflective role, allowing patients to discover their own insights using the basic principle that the client ultimately knows best. Problem-solving counselling is more directive and focused, as patients are actively assisted in finding solutions to their problems. These types of counselling may provide some benefit for patients with mild

Table 3.5 Main indications for psychological treatments

Psychiatric condition	Main psychological treatment used
Stressful life events, illness, bereavement	Counselling
Depression	Cognitive-behavioural therapy Mindfulness-based cognitive therapy Interpersonal therapy Psychodynamic therapy Group therapy
Anxiety disorders	Cognitive-behavioural therapy Mindfulness-based cognitive therapy Exposure and response prevention (for obsessive-compulsive disorder) Systematic desensitization (for phobias)
Posttraumatic stress disorder	Cognitive-behavioural therapy Eye movement desensitization and reprocessing
Schizophrenia	Cognitive-behavioural therapy Family therapy
Eating disorders	Cognitive-behavioural therapy Focused psychodynamic psychotherapy Interpersonal therapy Family therapy
Emotionally unstable personality disorder	Dialectical behaviour therapy Mentalization-based therapy Psychodynamic therapy Cognitive-behavioural therapy Cognitive analytic therapy Therapeutic communities
Alcohol dependence	Cognitive-behavioural therapy Group therapy Motivational interviewing

● **Chapter Summary**

- Psychological therapies are first-line treatments for mild to moderate mood disorders, stress-related disorders, anxiety disorders, eating disorders and personality disorders.
- The therapeutic relationship is more important than the modality of psychological treatment used.
- Self-help is often sufficient for milder problems.
- Counselling is unstructured, allowing the patient to generate their own solutions to problems.
- Psychodynamic psychotherapy aims to facilitate conscious recognition of unconscious processes causing problematic symptoms.
- Cognitive-behavioural therapy aims to help the patient identify and change the links between how they think, feel, sense and behave.

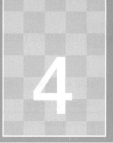

A fundamental principle of medicine is that patients who are capable of doing so are free to make decisions about their treatment, even if those decisions seem imprudent, and this is no different in psychiatry. However, the very nature of mental disorders can affect some patients' ability to make decisions regarding their care and treatment: in these instances, decisions may need to be made without the informed consent or agreement of the patient. Treatment against patients' wishes is usually only considered when the patient would otherwise be at significant risk to themselves (through self-harm, suicide, self-neglect, exploitation) or may place others at risk. Mental health legislation is therefore in place to protect patients and the public.

Differing legal systems within the UK mean that there are differences in mental health legislation across the home nations. This book will focus on mental health legislation applicable in England and Wales.

MENTAL HEALTH ACT 1983 AS AMENDED BY THE MENTAL HEALTH ACT 2007

In England and Wales, the Mental Health Act 1983 as amended by the Mental Health Act 2007 (MHA) provides a legal framework for the care and treatment of individuals with mental disorders. The MHA is divided into a number of parts, each of which is divided into 'Sections' (groups of paragraphs).

Part I: Definitions

The term 'mental disorder' is defined as *any disorder or disability of the mind*. However, the Learning Disability Qualification states that *a person with a learning disability* (intellectual disability) *alone can only be detained for treatment or be made subject to Guardianship if that learning disability* (intellectual disability) *is associated with abnormally aggressive or seriously irresponsible conduct*.

The Appropriate Medical Treatment test stipulates that for long-term powers of compulsion (i.e. longer than 28 days) it is not possible for patients to be compulsorily detained or treated unless 'medical treatment' is available and appropriate. Medical treatment includes not only medication but also psychological treatment, nursing and specialist mental health habilitation and rehabilitation.

Certain officials and bodies are designated to carry out specific duties related to implementation of the MHA. Some of these are summarized in Table 4.1.

Part II: Civil Sections

Part II of the MHA relates to compulsory assessment and treatment, both in hospital and in the community. Table 4.2 summarizes the most important sections in this part.

Normally, the process starts because concerns are raised about an individual's mental health. Following assessment by the appropriate professionals, the patient may be admitted to hospital under Section 2 or 3 of the MHA.

In an emergency, it may not be possible to arrange a review for consideration of a Section 2 or 3. In these cases, there are various options available, depending on circumstances. When any emergency measure is used to detain a patient, this should be reviewed as soon as possible by the appropriate professionals and compulsory measures either revoked, or a Section 2 or 3 granted.

Under Section 135, an Approved Mental Health Professional (AMHP) may apply to a magistrate for a warrant, which allows the police to enter private premises in order to remove someone with a possible mental disorder and take them to a 'place of safety' (usually a police station or hospital) for further assessment. An amendment (2017) also allows the mental health assessment to occur in the private premises if the occupiers consent. Section 136 applies when a police officer has concerns about an individual's mental health in a place that is not the person's dwelling. However, the police officer need not apply for a warrant.

Patients admitted to hospital on an involuntary basis are informed of their detention and their rights. They may apply to have their case reviewed by a Mental Health Review Tribunal or by the Mental Health Act Manager within the hospital, both of whom have the power to remove the detention. Patients may also be discharged from their detention by the Responsible Clinician (RC) or by their nearest relative (unless the right to do this is blocked by the RC).

For patients liable to be detained under Section 3, it may be appropriate to consider the use of a Community Treatment Order (CTO) under Section 17 of the MHA. This can be useful when treatment in the community is an option (i.e. when the associated risks of the mental disorder do not necessitate

Table 4.1 Mental Health Act officials

Official or body	Description
Approved Mental Health Professional (AMHP)	A mental health professional (nurse, social worker, occupational therapist, clinical psychologist) with specialist training in mental health assessment and legislation, approved by the local authority. Duties of an AMHP include assessing patients, and (if appropriate) making an application for Mental Health Act 2007 (MHA) detention.
Section 12 approved doctor	A doctor approved under Section 12 of the Mental Health Act (MHA) as having expertise in the diagnosis and treatment of mental disorders. Section 12 doctors are responsible for the assessment of patients and for recommending MHA detention if appropriate.
Approved Clinician (AC) and Responsible Clinician (RC)	A health care professional (usually a doctor, but can also be a nurse, social worker, occupational therapist, clinical psychologist) who has received specialist training and is responsible for the treatment of individuals with mental disorders detained under the MHA. An AC in charge of the care of a specific patient is known as Responsible Clinician (RC) for that patient. Their responsibility is to oversee the care and treatment of a patient detained under the MHA and to remain responsible for administrative duties of the MHA pertinent to the patient.
Second Opinion Approved Doctor (SOAD)	Appointed by the Care Quality Commission (CQC – see later), the role of the SOAD is to provide an independent second medical opinion regarding treatment in patients subject to prolonged compulsory treatment who are unable to consent to their treatment, or when a patient refuses electroconvulsive therapy (ECT; not applicable in emergency situations, see 'Consent to Treatment').
Nearest Relative (NR)	The spouse, child, parent, sibling or other relative of a patient detained under the MHA. This sometimes varies from 'next of kin.' It is the duty of the AMHP to appoint the nearest relative, although this decision can be appealed in court. AMHPs have a duty to inform the NR of the application for MHA detention. NRs can – in some instances – apply for the patient to be discharged from compulsory measures.
Independent Mental Health Advocates (IMHA)	Advocacy is a process of supporting and enabling people to express their views and concerns, access information and services, defend and promote their rights and responsibilities, and explore choices and options. Most patients detained under the MHA have the right to access an independent mental health advocate.
Care Quality Commission	An independent health and social care regulatory body that oversees the use of the MHA and ensures standards are maintained. All NHS and social care providers involved with the care of patients detained under the MHA must be registered with the CQC.
Mental Health Tribunal (MHT)	MHTs hear appeals against detention under the MHA. Their members include a lawyer, a doctor and a layperson. MHTs have the authority to discharge patients from compulsory measures when they determine that the conditions for detention are not met.
Mental Health Act Managers ('hospital managers')	Represent the hospital responsible for a detained patient. Hospital managers will hear appeals from patients against their detention and review renewals of lengthy detentions. Cases are heard in similar settings to those heard by MHRTs, and Mental Health Act Managers have the authority to discharge patients.

ongoing hospital admission). Conditions such as attending appointments may be enforced. However, specific treatment cannot be forcibly given. A CTO allows the Responsible Clinician to recall the patient to hospital should the patient become non-concordant with treatment or should they become unwell.

HINTS AND TIPS

Note that the term 'informal' applies to hospital patients who not are detained under the Mental Health Act 2007 (i.e. patients who have agreed to voluntary admission).

HINTS AND TIPS

Section 5(2) – doctor's holding power – may be enacted by any hospital doctor provided they are either the responsible clinician or another doctor nominated by them (e.g. a specialist registrar or senior house officer). This means that a psychiatrist need not see suspected mentally ill patients on a medical or surgical ward before they can be detained under this Section.

Table 4.2 Civil sections enabling compulsory admission

Section	Aim	Duration	Application
Section 35 Remand to hospital for report on mental condition	To prepare a report on the mental condition of an individual who is charged with an offence that could lead to imprisonment	28 days, with option to extend to 12 weeks	Crown or Magistrates' Court, on evidence of one doctor, who must be Section 12 approved
Section 36 Remand to hospital for treatment	To treat an individual who is charged with an offence that could lead to imprisonment	28 days, with option to extend to 12 weeks	Crown Court, on evidence of two medical doctors (one of whom must be Section 12 approved)
Section 37 Hospital order	Detention and treatment of an individual convicted of an imprisonable offence (similar to Section 3)	Initially 6 months, with option to extend	Crown or Magistrates' Court, on evidence of two medical doctors (one of whom must be Section 12 approved)
Section 41 Restriction order	Leave and discharge of Section 37 patients may only be granted with approval of the Home Office (recorded as 37/41) – applied to serious persistent offenders	As for Section 37	Crown Court only, on evidence of one medical doctor (who must be Section 12 approved)

Part III: Forensic Sections

Part III of the MHA incorporates Sections 35–55 and relates to mentally ill patients involved in criminal proceedings or under sentence. Table 4.3 summarizes the most important sections in this part. It should be noted that patients who are detained under certain forensic Sections and who are not 'restricted' patients (see Table. 4.3) can be considered for supervised community treatment (CTO) if appropriate.

Part IV: Consent to treatment

This part of the MHA clarifies the extent to which treatments can be imposed on patients subject to compulsory measures. Patients detained under Section 3 or 37 (long-term treatment orders) may be treated with standard psychiatric medication for 3 months with or without their consent. However, after 3 months and in other special cases, an extra Section from a Second Opinion Approved Doctor (SOAD) is required for treatment. Such cases include:

- Psychosurgery and surgical implants of hormones to reduce sex drive: these require the informed consent of a patient with capacity to make such a decision, as well as the approval of a SOAD, under Section 57 of the MHA. Neither of these procedures can be carried out on a patient who lacks capacity to make these decisions.
- Administration of medical treatment in a patient who cannot provide, or refuses to provide, informed consent: this requires the approval of a SOAD, under Section 58 of the MHA.
- ECT: if the patient is 'capable of understanding the nature, purpose and likely effects of the treatment' then electroconvulsive therapy (ECT) cannot be given without his consent. If the patient lacks capacity, then ECT must be certified as 'appropriate' by a SOAD, under Section 58A of the MHA.

In circumstances where urgent treatment is required to save the patient's life or to prevent serious suffering or deterioration, it may be appropriate to use Section 62 to waive the second opinion requirements of Sections 57 and 58 (e.g. emergency ECT for a patient who is not eating or drinking). Section 62 is only used until a second opinion can be obtained.

MENTAL HEALTH (CARE & TREATMENT) (SCOTLAND) ACT 2003

Compulsory measures in Scotland are legislated for by the Mental Health (Care & Treatment) (Scotland) Act 2003. They can be used when a patient is suffering (or thought to be suffering) from a mental disorder (mental illness, intellectual disability, personality disorder), by virtue of which the individual's ability to make decisions about treatment of their mental disorder is significantly impaired, when treatment for the mental disorder (including medication, nursing and psychosocial care) is available, and if there would be considerable risk to the health, safety or welfare of the individual, or to the safety of others, without treatment. The use of compulsory powers must be considered necessary and lesser restrictive options must be deemed inappropriate. The use of the Act is overseen by the Mental Welfare Commission for Scotland. Under civil law, the following orders are frequently used:

Emergency Detention Certificate

An Emergency Detention Certificate (EDC) allows an individual with a mental disorder (or suspected mental disorder) to be detained in hospital for up to 72 hours, where

Mental health service provision

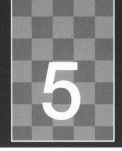

HISTORY

Until the 18th century, the mentally ill in the UK received no formal psychiatric care and those who were not looked after by their families were kept in workhouses and private institutions. In 1845, the Lunatics Act led to the building of an asylum in every county so that those patients with severe mental illness could be cared for in large remote asylum communities. Since the introduction in the 1950s of chlorpromazine, the first effective medication for schizophrenia, there has been a significant decline in the number of patients in psychiatric hospitals. The attempts to reduce the cost of inpatient care, as well as the criticism levelled at asylums regarding the 'institutionalization' of patients and the loss of patient autonomy, led to the closure of the large asylums and the rise of community care. Today, most mentally ill patients are assessed and managed in the community and hospital admission, when indicated, is usually only brief in duration.

PRIMARY CARE

Up to 95% of mental illness is seen and managed exclusively in primary care by general practitioners (GPs), with mild to moderate mood and anxiety disorders and alcohol misuse being the most common conditions. Depression, which is the most common mental illness treated, is frequently associated with symptoms of anxiety as well as physical complaints.

It is important to note that up to half of all mentally ill patients go undetected in primary care. This is because many of these patients present with physical, rather than psychological, symptoms. Also, some patients are reluctant to discuss emotional issues with their doctor, due to feelings of embarrassment or uncertainty about how they will be received.

Some GPs have the option of referring patients with mild symptoms or those going through a life crisis (e.g. bereavement) to a practice counsellor (see Chapter 3). Practice and district nurses may be helpful in screening for, and educating patients about, mental illness.

Primary care liaison teams exist in many areas. These act as a single point of contact for GPs to refer to. Referrals are allocated to psychiatrists, psychologists, community psychiatric nurses (CPNs) or occupational therapists as appropriate. This means the GP does not have to work out which professional is best placed to help the patient before referring; the team can discuss this among themselves.

Some patients will continue to receive intervention at a primary care level and others will require secondary care. The following box lists the common reasons for referral from primary to secondary mental health care.

REASONS FOR REFERRAL TO SECONDARY MENTAL HEALTH SERVICES

- Moderate to severe mental illness (e.g. schizophrenia, bipolar affective disorder, severe depression or anxiety disorder)
- Patients who pose a serious risk for harm to self, others or property
- Uncertainty regarding diagnosis
- Poor response to standard treatment, despite adequate dose and concordance
- Specialist treatment required (e.g. psychological therapy, specialist medication regimens)

SECONDARY CARE

Community mental health teams

In the UK, specialist psychiatric care in the community is mostly coordinated by regional community mental health teams (CMHTs), which consist of a multidisciplinary team of psychiatrists, CPNs, social workers, psychologists, occupational therapists and support workers. Team members usually operate from a base that is easily accessible to the community they serve, although local GP surgeries are also used to see patients. Patients who are unable to come to the CMHT location are often seen at home.

Care programme approach

The approach taken by some secondary care psychiatric services is called the care programme approach (CPA), introduced by the Department of Health in 1991. This approach applies to all patients under specialist psychiatric care and includes patients based in the community, in hospitals and in prisons. The key components of the CPA are:

- The systematic assessment of patients' health and social care needs
- The formation of an agreed care plan that addresses these identified needs

- The allocation of a *care coordinator* (previously called 'key worker') to keep in touch with the patient to monitor and to coordinate the care of these needs. This is usually a CPN, social worker or psychiatrist.
- Regular review meetings, which include all relevant professionals, patients and their carers, to adjust the care plan, if necessary

Patients may be placed on a *standard* or an *enhanced* CPA according to the severity of their needs.

HINTS AND TIPS

The diverse and multiple needs of patients with mental health problems make a multidisciplinary approach indispensable in psychiatry. A multidisciplinary team consists of members with medical, psychological, social and occupational therapy expertise.

Outpatient clinics

Psychiatric outpatient clinics take place in CMHT centres, GP surgeries and hospitals. Types of clinics include psychiatrists' clinics for new referrals and follow-up patients and special purpose clinics (e.g. depot antipsychotic injection clinics, clozapine monitoring clinics). Some areas offer regional assessment services for neurodevelopmental disorders.

Liaison psychiatry

Liaison psychiatrists work in general hospitals. They provide psychiatric opinions for people who attend a general hospital with physical health problems, with or without a preexisting mental health problem. Common referrals are for assessment following self-harm, advice on management of delirium and distinguishing depression from symptoms of physical health disorders. People with intellectual disability can find hospital admissions particularly challenging and therefore some hospitals provide an intellectual disability liaison nurse who can advise on strategies to manage distress and challenging behaviour.

Day hospitals

Day hospitals are nonresidential units that patients attend during the day. They are an alternative to inpatient care for patients who, although needing intensive support, are able to go home in the evening and at weekends. Having a supportive family is helpful in such cases. They may also be used for patients who have just been discharged from hospital, but who still need a high level of support, as a form of 'partial hospitalization.' They are now mainly used for older adults.

Assertive outreach teams

These are like CMHTs and involve a multidisciplinary team but provide a more intensive service, providing more flexible and frequent patient contact. They are targeted at challenging patients who have not engaged well with mainstream mental health services in the past. Patients who use this service often have histories of severe and enduring mental illness, significant social problems and complex needs, and are usually considered relatively high risk in some regard (e.g. self-harm or suicide, violence to others, self-neglect, or vulnerable). The nature of their illness requires more focused and intensive input.

Home treatment teams

There is increasing emphasis on treating patients at home, thus avoiding expensive and disruptive inpatient admissions. A hospital admission can be very challenging for anyone, particularly someone with an acute mental illness. Treatment at home also allows practical problems with housing and activities of daily living to be better identified and addressed. Most regions now have home treatment teams (also called crisis teams) who can provide short periods of support (from a few days to weeks) to people who might otherwise have to be admitted. They can also facilitate earlier discharge than would otherwise be possible. Such teams include similar professionals to a CMHT but generally are available out of hours and can visit patients more often (e.g. multiple times per day, if required). Medication, practical help and psychological therapy can be offered.

Early intervention in psychosis teams

There is some evidence that the longer a psychotic episode goes untreated, the poorer the prognosis, suggesting that early treatment is preferable. However, not all mild or vague symptoms of possible psychosis become a definite psychotic episode, meaning it can be hard to know when to start treatment (e.g. a person who is suspicious of others, but not holding a certain belief of persecution). Specialist teams exist in many regions to manage such cases, offering assessment, medication, psychological strategies and education for patients and families. Teams are open to psychosis secondary to any diagnosis (e.g. schizophrenia, bipolar disorder, substance-induced) and generally accept people aged 14–35 years.

Inpatient units

Occasionally, community care is not possible and hospital admission is necessary. Reasons for admission include the following:

- To provide a safe environment when there is: (1) high risk for harm to self or others or (2) grossly disturbed behaviour.
- A period of inpatient assessment is needed (e.g. of response to treatment or when the diagnosis is uncertain).
- It is necessary to institute treatment in hospital (e.g. electroconvulsive therapy, clozapine therapy – although both of these can be initiated as outpatients if the patient is at low risk for complications).

There are various types of inpatient units. These range from a general adult acute ward for uncomplicated admissions to psychiatric intensive care units (PICUs) for severely disturbed patients who cannot be adequately looked after on an open ward. High security units (also called 'special hospitals' (e.g. Broadmoor, Rampton)) are for mentally ill offenders who pose a significant risk to others. Mother and baby units provide care to women who have recently given birth and eating disorder units provide care to those with severe physical complications resulting from anorexia nervosa.

Rehabilitation units

These units aim to reintegrate patients whose social and living skills have been severely handicapped by the effects of severe mental illness and institutionalization into the community. Admissions are often for months or even years. The approach taken is holistic and uses the 'Recovery Model' (i.e. learning to live well with ongoing symptoms, rather than aim for complete remission of symptoms).

Accommodation

Certain patients, who are unable to live independently due to severe and enduring mental illness, may need *supported accommodation*. Types of supported accommodation range from warden-controlled property to residential homes with trained staff on hand 24 hours a day.

● Chapter Summary

- Most mental health conditions are managed in primary care.
- Patients with severe and enduring mental illness can benefit from input from a community mental health team.
- Many services exist to manage acutely unwell patients at home.
- High-risk patients are likely to need hospital admission.

PRESENTING COMPLAINTS

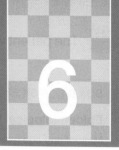

The patient with thoughts of suicide or self-harm

6

CASE SUMMARY

The duty psychiatrist is asked for their opinion on Mr SA, a 28-year-old unemployed, recently divorced man, who was brought in by his landlord. The landlord had called round to discuss payment arrears, only to find the door unlocked and Mr SA asleep on his bed with an empty box of paracetamol tablets and several empty cans of lager littered around the floor. He also found a hastily scribbled suicide note on the bedside table, addressed to Mr SA's children. Mr SA was easily roused but was upset to have been found and initially refused the landlord's pleas that they go to the hospital. Only when he was violently sick did Mr SA finally agree. The doctor in the accident and emergency (A&E) department reports that, other than the smell of alcohol on his breath, Mr SA's medical examination was normal. Blood tests revealed raised paracetamol levels, but these were not sufficiently high to require medical treatment. The A&E doctor is concerned because Mr SA is ambivalent about further acts of self-harm or suicide, saying that his 'life is a failure' and that 'there is nothing worth living for'. Before coming to see the patient, the duty psychiatrist checks Mr SA's past medical and psychiatric history.

(For a discussion of the case study see the end of the chapter).

While many psychiatric illnesses can be associated with self-harm or suicidal intent (both as a presenting feature and a chronic symptom), many patients who self-harm or attempt suicide are not previously known to mental health services. Assessments of these patients are often made by nonpsychiatric staff, so it is vital that all doctors are able to detect and manage any underlying mental illness, and have a sound approach to assessing and managing risk.

DEFINITIONS AND CLINICAL FEATURES

Self-harm is a blanket term used to describe any intentional act done with the knowledge that it is potentially harmful. It can take the form of self-poisoning (e.g. overdosing) or self-injury (e.g. cutting, burning, hitting). The motives for self-harm are vast and include emotional relief, self-punishment, attention seeking, and can even be a form of self-help (albeit maladaptive) by way of channelling an intolerable emotional experience into a discrete physical sensation. *Suicide* is the act of intentionally and successfully ending one's own life. *Attempted suicide* refers to an unsuccessful suicide bid.

HINTS AND TIPS

Self-harm is one of the top five reasons for acute medical admissions for both men and women in the UK. Further, it is estimated that a large number of people do not attend hospital following self-harm.

ASSESSMENT OF PATIENTS WHO HAVE INFLICTED HARM UPON THEMSELVES

Compared with the general population, which has an annual suicide rate of 0.01%, patients who present with self-harm have a 50- to 100-fold greater chance of completing suicide in the following year (resulting in about 1% of people dying by suicide), emphasizing the need for comprehensive risk assessment. It is incredibly difficult to predict suicide reliably, but numerous studies have shown that certain epidemiological and clinical variables are more prevalent among those who have completed suicide (Box 6.1) and it is important to bear these in mind when assessing risk. No patient questionnaire or suicide risk-scoring system has been shown to be better than thorough clinical assessment.

The key areas to assess are:

1. Suicide risk factors
2. Suicidal intent (including circumstances surrounding the act)
3. Mental state examination
4. Current social supports

RED FLAG

Suicidal thoughts and actions are common. In the general population within the last year, around 1 in 20 people will have had suicidal thoughts, around 1 in 200 will have attempted to kill themselves, and around 1 in 10000 will have died by suicide. Suicide is the commonest cause of death in men and women under the age of 35 years, and the 13th commonest cause of years of life lost worldwide.

BOX 6.1   RISK FACTORS FOR SUICIDE

Epidemiological factors:

Male of any age (younger females more likely to self-harm but less likely to complete suicide)

Being lesbian, gay, bisexual or transgender (particularly younger people)

Prisoners (especially remand)

Being unmarried (single, widowed, divorced)

Unemployment

Working in certain occupations (farmer, vet, nurse, doctor)

Low socioeconomic status

Living alone, social isolation

Clinical factors:

Psychiatric illness or personality disorder (see Table 6.1)

Previous self-harm

Alcohol dependence

Physical illness (especially debilitating, chronically painful, or terminal conditions)

Family history of depression, alcohol dependence, or suicide

Recent adverse life-events (especially bereavement)

COMMUNICATION

Suicidal patients often feel distressed and guilty. One of the most important therapeutic aspects of the assessment is to convey empathy and optimism.

Suicide risk factors

Box 6.1 summarizes the most important epidemiological and clinical risk factors for suicide.

Psychiatric illness

About 90% of patients who commit suicide have a diagnosed or retrospectively diagnosable mental disorder; however, only around a quarter of these patients have contact with mental health services in the year before completing suicide. Patients recently released from inpatient psychiatric care are at a significantly elevated risk for suicide, particularly during the first couple of weeks after discharge. Table 6.1 summarizes the most important psychiatric conditions associated with suicide.

COMMUNICATION

Every patient with suicidal ideas should be asked about alcohol or substance misuse, no matter how unlikely it seems. Taking a nonjudgemental stance is likely to enhance the therapeutic relationship and help the patient feel understood.

Physical illness

Many disabling or unpleasant medical conditions can be associated with self-harm and suicide. Often, a patient may have comorbid depression that will respond to treatment. However, a minority of patients have no mental illness and make a capacitous decision to die. The most common examples are:

- Chronic illnesses which cause a lot of functional impairment or pain (e.g. chronic obstructive pulmonary disease, asthma, stroke, epilepsy)
- Life-limiting illnesses (e.g. cancer, Huntington disease)

Recent adverse life events

Stressful life events are more common in the 6 months prior to a suicide attempt, and include relationship break-ups, health problems, legal/financial difficulties, or problems at home or within the family.

Suicidal intent

Suicidal intent, which is commonly defined as the seriousness or intensity of the wish of a patient to terminate their life, is suggested by the following:

The attempt was planned in advance

A lethal suicide attempt typically involves days or weeks of planning. It is rarely an impulsive, spur-of-the-moment idea (the exception is the psychotic patient who impulsively responds to hallucinations or delusions). Planning is strongly suggested by the evidence of final acts. These include the writing of a will or suicide note.

Precautions were taken to avoid discovery or rescue

For example, a patient might check into a hotel room in a distant town or ensure that no friends or family will be visiting over the ensuing hours or days.

A dangerous method was used

Violent methods (hanging, jumping from heights, firearm use) are suggestive of lethal intent. That said, use of an apparently ineffective method (e.g. taking six paracetamol tablets) might reflect lack of knowledge of the lethal dose

Table 6.1 Association between psychiatric disorders and suicide

Psychiatric disorder	Risk relative to general population	Comments
Personality disorders	Approximately 40-fold	Highest in borderline personality disorder. Also, strong association with antisocial and narcissistic personality disorders. Often have comorbid depression or substance misuse.
Unipolar depression	20-fold	Risk greatest in patients with anxiety/agitation or severe insomnia and higher in patients having received inpatient treatment in the past. Risk greatest in first 3 months of diagnosis.
Substance use	Cocaine dependence 17-fold Alcohol dependence 12-fold Opioid dependence 7-fold Amphetamine dependence 5-fold	Highest risk when comorbid depression.
Schizophrenia	13-fold	Highest risk is young, intelligent, unemployed males with good insight and recurrent illness.
Eating disorders	Anorexia nervosa 8-fold Bulimia lower risk than anorexia	Mortality in anorexia nervosa is also increased due to complications of malnutrition.
Bipolar affective disorder	6-fold	More common in depressive phase but can also happen in manic or mixed affective episodes.
Anxiety disorders	3-fold	Increased risk in GAD, panic disorder and PTSD even without comorbid depression. OCD not associated with increased risk.

GAD; Generalized anxiety disorder; OCD, obsessive-compulsive disorder; PTSD, posttraumatic stress disorder.

needed, rather than a lack of intent to die. Therefore it should be ascertained whether the method used was seen as dangerous from the patient's perspective.

No help was sought after the act

Patients who immediately regret their action and seek help are less at risk than those who do not seek help and wait to die. The person communicated with is often of significance – they may be someone whose behaviour the patient is seeking to influence by their act of self-harm, and/or they may be someone who provides support to the patient.

Mental state examination

This should ideally be conducted in a calm, quiet and confidential setting, preferably when the patient has had a chance to rest and is not under the influence of drugs or alcohol. Check specifically for:

- **Current mood state:** does the patient appear to be suffering from a depressive illness? Assess for features of hopelessness, worthlessness or agitation (all of which are associated with a higher risk for completed suicide).
- **Other psychiatric illness:** does the patient appear to be preoccupied, delusional or responding to hallucinations? Is there evidence of eating disorder, substance abuse or cognitive impairment?

- **Current suicidality:** is the act now regretted, or is there strong intent to die? What does the patient plan to do if discharged?
- **Protective factors:** what aspects of the patient's life (family, children and dependents) would guard against further acts? Lack of protective factors, or dismissal of their importance, is a worrying sign.

The following questions might be helpful when asking about suicidal ideation:

- Have you been feeling that life isn't worth living?
- Do you sometimes feel like you would like to end it all?
- Have you given some thought as to how you might do it?
- How close are you to going through with your plans?
- Is there anything that might stop you from attempting suicide?

HINTS AND TIPS

Patients who are tired, emotionally upset or intoxicated may appear to be at greater risk for imminent self-harm. Allowing some time to sober up and reflect can be of great therapeutic value. However, this will always be a matter of clinical judgment.

PATIENT MANAGEMENT FOLLOWING SELF-HARM OR ATTEMPTED SUICIDE

Management planning should follow assessment of risk factors and mental state. It is important to remember that self-harm and suicidality are not discrete illnesses; instead they are symptoms reflecting a complex interplay of mental disorders, personality types and social circumstances. Rather than taking the form of a prescribed care pathway, management of the suicidal or self-harming patient requires clinical judgement, taking into consideration the needs of the individual patient and the availability of local resources. This can often be anxiety-provoking for health care workers.

Formulation of a management plan should be made after a thorough review of any available past history, including care programmes or crisis plans if relevant. It is always desirable to obtain a collateral history from a family member or close friend. A good plan should include both short- and long-term management strategies.

Immediate management considerations include the following:

- Is the patient in need of inpatient psychiatric care to ensure their safety? If so, can this be achieved on a voluntary basis, or is the use of mental health legislation required?
- Would the patient benefit from the input of home treatment, outreach or crisis teams (see Chapter 5)?
- Does the patient have existing social supports that could be called upon?
- Reducing access to means of self-harm: does the patient have a collection of tablets or rope remaining in their home they could dispose of? Should their prescription medication be dispensed weekly (or more frequently)?

Longer-term management involves the modification of factors that could increase the risk for further acts of self-harm or suicidality, and may include:

- Treatment of psychiatric illness (medication, self-help, psychological therapies, community mental health team, outpatient appointments, GP follow-up).
- Avoidance of substance use (highlighting association with suicide to patient, encouraging patient to attend voluntary organisations and/or addictions services)
- Optimizing social functioning (social work, Citizens Advice Bureau, community groups and activities, encouragement of family support, voluntary support agencies).

- Crisis planning (relaxation or distraction techniques, telephone counselling services, information on accessing emergency psychiatric services).

DISCUSSION OF CASE STUDY

Self-harm risk assessment

Mr SA's epidemiological risk factors are that he is a young man, recently divorced, unemployed and lives alone in social isolation. His clinical risk factors are that he may have alcohol problems and has recently experienced adverse life events (divorce, financial difficulties). The evidence of final acts (suicide note) and the failure of Mr SA to seek help after the act suggest strong suicide intent. The fact that he would not have been discovered but for the landlord's timely arrival indicates a degree of forward planning, although his leaving the door unlocked and his willingness to go to hospital after vomiting suggest some ambivalence. Mr SA had consumed a significant quantity of alcohol at the time of the overdose, which could have clouded his judgement and increased his impulsivity. On mental state examination, Mr SA has ongoing suicidal ideation and cognitive features of worthlessness and hopelessness, which are associated with suicide.

Further management

The duty psychiatrist should ask about all the epidemiological and clinical risk factors, specifically about: past or current mental illness (is Mr SA known to mental health services?); previous episodes of self-harm; alcohol or substance dependence; physical illness; family history of depression, alcohol dependence or suicide; and recent adverse life events. The duty psychiatrist will also be interested in Mr SA's current social support in order to try and help him formulate the most appropriate management plan.

As this is a complex risk assessment, the duty psychiatrist will probably have to reassess the patient himself, especially as regards detecting mental illness on mental state examination. The psychiatrist might ask the A&E doctor to keep Mr SA overnight, so that a mental state examination can be performed in the morning when he is refreshed and no longer under the influence of alcohol. A hospital admission or follow-up by a high-intensity support mental health team (e.g. crisis team) seems to be the most likely outcome.

Chapter Summary

Self-harm is a very common presentation with many different causes.

Self-harm increases the risk for completed suicide, but the vast majority of people who self-harm will not die by suicide.

Assess risk for suicide in all those who have self-harmed, by identifying:

- risk factors for suicide (epidemiological and clinical),
- degree of suicidal intent,
- evidence of mental disorder,
- use of alcohol or other substances and
- social support and protective factors.

Management is very specific to the individual but should include crisis planning for all.

The patient with impairment of consciousness, memory or cognition

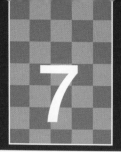

7

Cognitive impairment is common and important, but often underdiagnosed and underinvestigated. It is associated with a high morbidity and mortality, and you are likely to frequently encounter people with cognitive impairment in most specialties of medical practice.

DEFINITIONS AND CLINICAL FEATURES

Consciousness

To be conscious is to be aware, both of the environment and of oneself as a subjective being. It is a global cognitive function. It is a poorly understood, complex phenomenon with multiple vaguely defined terms for its abnormalities. It is best to avoid terms such as 'confused,' 'obtunded,' 'clouding of consciousness' and 'stupor' as they are not well defined and mean different things to different specialties. Clinically, the key question is whether someone has a normal or altered conscious level. This is assessed at a practical level by observing arousal level (hyperaroused or lowered) (Fig. 7.1).

Cognition

This chapter considers 'cognition' in its broadest sense as meaning all the mental activities that allow us to perceive, integrate and conceptualize the world around us. These include the global functions of consciousness, attention and orientation and the specific domains of memory, executive function, language, praxis and perception. The term 'cognition' is also used more narrowly in cognitive psychology and cognitive therapy where individual thoughts or ideas are also referred to as 'cognitions'.

Impairments in cognition can be generalized (multiple domains) or specific (one domain only). An altered level of consciousness is generally associated with a generalized impairment in all aspects of cognition, as it is difficult to concentrate on any tasks when feeling very agitated or drowsy.

A large number of specific cognitive impairments exist (Table 7.1). These can be isolated impairments, for example, if they are developmental or secondary to a small stroke or occur together in disorders of generalized cognitive impairment such as dementia.

Memory

Memory is one of the commonest cognitive domains to be impaired. There are two main ways to categorize memory: the duration of storage (working or long-term) or the type of information stored (implicit or explicit). Explicit

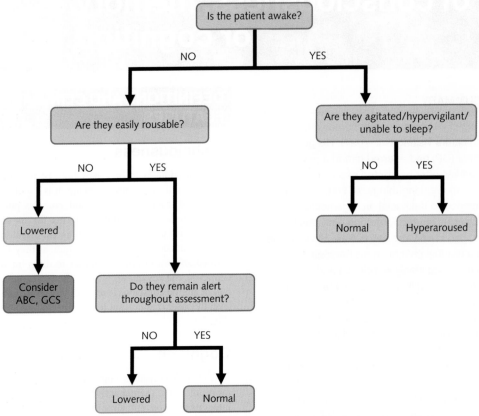

Fig. 7.1 Assessment of conscious level. *ABC,* Airway, Breathing, Circulation; *GCS,* Glasgow Coma Scale.

Table 7.1 Specific cognitive impairments

Cognitive domain	Term(s) for impairment	Description
Language	Dysphasia/aphasia	Loss of language abilities despite intact sensory and motor function (e.g. difficulty in understanding commands or other words (receptive dysphasia) or difficulty using words with correct meaning (expressive dysphasia)). Not being able to name items correctly despite knowing what they are (nominal dysphasia) is a subtype of expressive dysphasia
Praxis	Dyspraxia/apraxia	Loss of ability to carry out skilled motor movements despite intact motor function (e.g. inability to put a letter in an envelope, use a tinopener, button up a shirt)
Perception	Dysgnosia/agnosia	Loss of ability to interpret sensory information despite intact sensory organ function (e.g. not able to recognize faces as familiar)
Memory	Amnesia	Loss of ability to learn or recall new information (e.g. not able to recall time or recent events, not able to learn new skills)
Executive function (umbrella term for many abilities)	Many terms, including: Disinhibition, perseveration, apathy, dysexecutive syndrome	Loss of ability to plan and sequence complex activities, or to manipulate abstract information (e.g. not able to plan the preparation of a meal, not able to return to a task once distracted)

memory (sometimes called *declarative memory*) includes all stored material of which the individual is consciously aware and can thus 'declare' to others. Implicit memory (sometimes called *procedural memory*) includes all material that is stored without the individual's conscious awareness (e.g. the ability to speak a language or ride a bicycle).

Explicit memory is the most common type of memory to be disrupted. It can be further subdivided into *semantic* and *episodic* memory. Semantic memory is knowledge of facts (e.g. Edinburgh is the capital of Scotland). Episodic memory is knowledge of autobiographical events (e.g. remembering a trip to Edinburgh when you were 10 years old). See Table 7.2 for the characteristics of different durations of explicit memory and how to test them.

Retrograde amnesia results in the patient being unable to retrieve memories, although the ability to store new memories may remain unaffected. Retrograde amnesia usually results from damage to the frontal or temporal cortex.

> **HINTS AND TIPS**
>
> Implicit memory (procedural memory) is typically preserved despite severe disruptions to explicit (declarative) memory, probably due to its independent neural location. Implicit memory is associated with basal ganglia circuitry. Explicit memory is associated with the hippocampal, diencephalic and cortical structures.

> **COMMUNICATION**
>
> There are different ways of classifying memory, and different terms have similar or overlapping meanings. For example, some clinicians use the term 'short-term memory' to mean recent long-term memory whereas others mean working memory. When speaking to colleagues it can be useful to define the type of memory referred to by the name of the test used to measure it.

Amnesia refers to the loss of the ability to store new memories or retrieve memories that have previously been stored. Anterograde amnesia is when the patient is unable to store new memories (impaired learning of new material), although the ability to retrieve memories stored before the event or onset of disorder may remain unimpaired. Anterograde amnesia usually results from damage to the medial temporal lobes, especially the hippocampal formation.

COMMON COGNITIVE DISORDERS

Delirium

Delirium can be thought of as acute brain failure. It is a syndrome manifesting as acute or fluctuating cognitive impairment associated with altered consciousness and impaired attention. If someone is newly disorientated and is drowsy or agitated, they are very likely to have delirium. Psychotic features such as hallucinations or persecutory delusions are often present but are not essential to make the diagnosis. Delirium often fluctuates, so a patient may appear normal on the morning ward round but cognitively impaired and agitated in the evening.

Delirium is a final common pathway of severe injury to the brain or body and is a marker of severity of illness (e.g. the 'C' in the CURB65 score for severity of community-acquired pneumonia). It is usually multifactorial and often arises from illnesses that do not directly affect the brain (Box 7.1). It has a high mortality, with around a third of people with delirium dying during the presentation. It is therefore a medical emergency and the cause should be thoroughly investigated and treated. It is particularly common in those with 'at risk' brains, such as those with pre-existing dementia. In individuals with vulnerable brains a relatively

Table 7.2 Explicit memory types, disorders and tests

Explicit memory type	Capacity duration	Key brain regions	Tests
Working/short-term	7 ± 2 items 15–30 s	Frontal cortex	Recall of unrelated words (e.g. 'lemon, key, ball')
Long-term (recent)	Unlimited Minutes to months	Hippocampus Mamillary bodies	Anterograde: delayed recall of an address or objects Retrograde: questions about recent events (e.g. what did you have for breakfast?)
Long-term (remote)	Unlimited Lifetime	Frontal and temporal cortex	Questions about past important events. Ask about personal events (episodic; e.g. what school did you attend?) and general knowledge (semantic; e.g. which US president was assassinated in the 1960s?)

BOX 7.1   CAUSES OF DELIRIUM (ANYTHING THAT DISRUPTS HOMEOSTASIS)

Environmental change or stress

- Hospital admission, particularly intensive care
- Urinary catheterisation
- Use of physical restraint
- Major surgery
- Sleep deprivation

Drugs (use or discontinuation)

Prescribed (plus many more)

- Anticholinergics
- Benzodiazepines
- Opiates
- Antiparkinsonian drugs
- Steroids

Recreational

- Alcohol (delirium tremens, see Chapter 8)
- Opiates
- Cannabis
- Amphetamines

Poisons

- Heavy metals (lead, mercury, manganese)
- Carbon monoxide

Systemic illness

Infections and sepsis

Hypoxia

- Respiratory failure
- Heart failure
- Myocardial infarction

Metabolic and endocrine

- Dehydration
- Electrolyte disturbances
- Renal impairment
- Hepatic encephalopathy
- Porphyria
- Hypoglycaemia
- Hyper- and hypothyroidism
- Hyper- and hypoparathyroidism
- Hyper- and hypoadrenocorticism (Cushing syndrome, Addison disease)
- Hypopituitarism

Nutritional

- Thiamine (Wernicke encephalopathy), vitamin B_{12}, folic acid or niacin deficiency

Trauma

- Any fracture, but frequently hip fracture

Intracranial causes

Space-occupying lesions

- Tumours, cysts, abscesses, haematomas

Head injury (especially concussion)

Infection

- Meningitis
- Encephalitis

Epilepsy

Cerebrovascular disorders

- Transient ischaemic attack
- Cerebral thrombosis or embolism
- Intracerebral or subarachnoid haemorrhage
- Hypertensive encephalopathy
- Vasculitis (e.g. from systemic lupus erythematosus)

minor insult can result in delirium (e.g. dehydration or a new medication). Delirium is also a risk factor for development or worsening of dementia. Delirium usually resolves when the cause is treated, but sometimes can be prolonged for weeks or months. The terms 'acute confusional state' and 'encephalopathy' have roughly the same meaning as delirium. Prominent symptoms of delirium are described further below. There are three main subtypes: hyperactive, hypoactive and mixed.

HINTS AND TIPS

Key risk factors for delirium are an abnormal brain (e.g. dementia, previous serious head injury, alcohol misuse), age (children, adults over 65 years), polypharmacy and sensory impairment.

HINTS AND TIPS

The four key diagnostic features of delirium are: (1) impaired consciousness, (2) impaired attention and (3) impaired cognition, all with (4) acute or fluctuating onset. Supportive diagnostic features are perceptual and thought disturbance, sleep-wake cycle disturbance and mood disturbance.

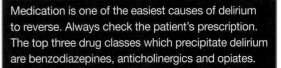

Impaired consciousness

Patients may have a reduced level of consciousness ranging from drowsiness to coma (hypoactive delirium), or they can be hypervigilant and agitated (hyperactive delirium).

Impaired attention

Ability to sustain attention is reduced and patients are easily distractible. Assess attention using tests such as serial sevens or months of the year backwards.

Impaired cognitive function

Short-term memory and recent memory are impaired with relative preservation of remote memory. Patients with delirium are almost always disorientated to time and often to place. Orientation to self is seldom lost. Language abnormalities such as rambling, incoherent speech and an impaired ability to understand are common.

Perceptual and thought disturbance

Patients may have perceptual disturbances ranging from misinterpretations (e.g. a door slamming is mistaken for an explosion) to illusions (e.g. a crack in the wall is perceived as a snake) to hallucinations (especially visual and, to a lesser extent, auditory). Transient persecutory delusions and delusions of misidentification may occur.

Sleep–wake cycle disturbance

Sleep is characteristically disturbed and can range from daytime drowsiness and night-time hyperactivity to a complete reversal of the normal cycle. Nightmares experienced by patients with delirium may continue as hallucinations after awakening.

Mood disturbance

Emotional disturbances such as depression, euphoria, anxiety, anger, fear and apathy are common.

> **RED FLAG**
>
> A physical illness should always be sought when a patient presents with visual hallucinations in isolation because patients with schizophrenia or psychotic mood disorders usually also experience auditory hallucinations.

> **RED FLAG**
>
> Delirium is a medical emergency. Around a third of people with delirium die during an episode of delirium. Thoroughly assess for and treat the probable cause.

> **RED FLAG**
>
> Medication is one of the easiest causes of delirium to reverse. Always check the patient's prescription. The top three drug classes which precipitate delirium are benzodiazepines, anticholinergics and opiates.

Dementia

Dementia is a syndrome of acquired progressive generalized cognitive impairment associated with functional decline. Conscious level is nearly always normal. Symptoms should be present for 6 months before a diagnosis can be confirmed. The following text describes the general categories of impairment in dementia.

Functional impairment

Functional impairment must be present to make a diagnosis of dementia. Functional impairment means difficulties with basic or instrumental activities of daily living (ADL). Basic ADLs refer to self-care tasks such as eating, dressing, washing, toileting, continence and mobility (being able to make crucial movements such as from bed to chair to toilet). Instrumental ADLs refer to tasks which are not crucial to life, but which allow someone to live independently, such as cooking, shopping and housework. As well as being diagnostically important, someone's ability to perform ADLs determines what level of support they need (home carers or 24-hour residential care).

Memory impairment

Impairment of memory is a common feature of dementia. Recent memory is first affected (e.g. forgetting where objects are placed, conversations and events of the previous day). With disease progression, all aspects of memory are affected, although highly personal information (name, previous occupation, etc.) is usually retained until late in the disease. Note that memory is essential for orientation to person, place and time and this will also be gradually affected (e.g. patients may lose their way in their own house).

Other cognitive symptoms (aphasia, apraxia, agnosia, impaired executive functioning)

See Table 7.1.

Behavioural and psychological symptoms of dementia

'Behavioural and psychological symptoms of dementia' (BPSD) is an umbrella term for noncognitive symptoms associated with dementia, including changes in behaviour, mood and psychosis. Behavioural symptoms are very common and include pacing, shouting, sexual disinhibition, aggression and apathy. Depression and anxiety may occur in up to 50% of all those with dementia. Delusions, especially persecutory, may occur in up to 40% of patients. Hallucinations in all sensory modalities (visual is more common) occur in up to 30% of patients. BPSD can be similar to symptoms of delirium, but generally has a more gradual onset and conscious level is normal. See Table 7.3 for more ways to differentiate BPSD from delirium.

Neurological symptoms

Between 10% and 20% of patients will experience seizures. Primitive reflexes (e.g. grasp, snout, suck) and myoclonic jerks may also be evident.

COMMUNICATION

When seeing a new patient with a likely diagnosis of dementia, always take a collateral history as patients may have poor insight and recall of their difficulties.

Distinguishing the type of dementia

Dementia can result from a primary neurodegenerative process or be secondary to substance use or another medical condition. Early onset dementia begins before age 65 years. A small number of cases are due to treatable, potentially reversible causes (Box 7.2). However, the most common causes of dementia are neurodegeneration and/or vascular disease. Table 7.4 describes the distinguishing clinical features of the various types of dementias although clinically, it is often difficult to tell what form of dementia is present and definitive diagnosis can normally only be made by postmortem examination. It is important to establish the likely underlying type of dementia because:

- A secondary dementia-causing process (e.g. brain tumour) may be detected and possibly treated.
- The progress of certain types of dementia may be slowed with specific medication (e.g. cholinesterase inhibitors in Alzheimer dementia).
- Certain drugs may be contraindicated in some dementias (e.g. antipsychotics can cause a catastrophic parkinsonian reaction in patients with dementia with Lewy bodies).
- The prognoses of the various dementias differ; this may have practical implications for patients and their families as regards final arrangements (e.g. wills).
- The patient's relatives may enquire about genetic counselling (e.g. Huntington disease, early-onset Alzheimer dementia).

In a minority of cases the distinction will be obvious, based on other symptoms produced by the disease process (e.g. jerky movements of the face and body (chorea)) and a positive family history would be suggestive of Huntington disease. In the majority of cases, the different dementias may be distinguished to some degree based on a detailed history from the patient and an informant, physical examination, relevant investigations and follow-up over time. However, the definitive diagnosis of a dementia subtype can only be established with absolute certainty on detailed microscopic examination of the brain at autopsy, and even then, a conclusive diagnosis may not be possible.

Table 7.3 Factors differentiating delirium from dementia

Feature	Delirium	Dementia
Onset	Acute	Gradual
Duration	Hours to weeks	Months to years
Attention	Impaired	Normal
Course	Fluctuating	Progressive deterioration
Consciousness	Altered	Normal
Context	New illness/medication	Health unchanged
Perceptual disturbance	Common	Occurs in late stages
Sleep–wake cycle	Disrupted	Usually normal
Orientation	Usually impaired for time and unfamiliar people/places	Impaired in late stages
Speech	Incoherent, rapid or slow	Word finding difficulties.
Things you may think	'Why aren't they listening?', 'Why won't they wake up properly?', or 'They need to calm down'	'Why do they keep telling me about the past?', 'Why do they keep asking me the same question?'

BOX 7.2   DISEASES THAT MAY CAUSE DEMENTIA

Neurodegenerative

- Alzheimer disease
- Frontotemporal dementia (includes Pick disease)
- Dementia with Lewy bodies (DLB)
- Parkinson disease
- Huntington disease
- Progressive supranuclear palsy

Cerebrovascular disease

- Vascular dementia
- Mixed Alzheimer and vascular dementia

Space-occupying lesions

- Tumours, cysts, abscesses, haematomas

Trauma

- Head injury
- Dementia pugilistica
  (sometimes called 'punch-drunk syndrome')

Infection

- Creutzfeldt–Jakob disease
  (including 'new variant CJD')
- HIV-related dementia
- Neurosyphilis
- Viral encephalitis
- Chronic bacterial and fungal meningitides

Metabolic and endocrine

- Chronic renal impairment
  (also called 'dialysis dementia')
- Liver failure
- Wilson disease
- Hyper- and hypothyroidism
- Hyper- and hypoparathyroidism
- Cushing syndrome and Addison disease

Nutritional

- Thiamine, vitamin B_{12}, folic acid or niacin
  deficiency (pellagra)

Drugs and toxins

- Alcohol (see Chapter 8), benzodiazepines,
  barbiturates, solvents

Chronic hypoxia

Inflammatory disorders

- Multiple sclerosis
- Systemic lupus erythematosus

Normal pressure hydrocephalus

Table 7.4 Distinguishing clinical features of the commonest types of dementia

Dementia type	Distinguishing clinical features
Alzheimer dementia (62%)	Gradual onset with progressive cognitive decline Early memory loss
Vascular dementia (multi-infarct dementia) (17%)	Focal neurological signs and symptoms Evidence of cerebrovascular disease or stroke May be uneven or stepwise deterioration in cognitive function
Mixed (10%)	Features of both Alzheimer and vascular dementia

Lewy body dementia (4%)	Core:
	  Day-to-day (or shorter) fluctuations in cognitive performance
	  Recurrent visual hallucinations
	  Motor signs of parkinsonism (rigidity, bradykinesia, tremor) (not drug-induced)
	Supporting:
	  REM sleep behaviour disorder
	  Recurrent falls and syncope
	  Transient disturbances of consciousness
	  Extreme sensitivity to antipsychotics (induces parkinsonism)

Frontotemporal dementia (including Pick disease) (2%)	*Behavioural variant:*
	  Early decline in social and personal conduct (disinhibition, tactlessness)
	  Dietary changes (preference for sweet food)
	  Early emotional blunting and loss of insight
	Primary progressive aphasia (nonfluent and semantic variants):
	  Attenuated speech output, echolalia, perseveration, mutism
	  Loss of semantic knowledge and naming
	  Relative sparing of other cognitive functions

Parkinson disease with dementia (2%)	Diagnosis of Parkinson disease (motor symptoms over a year prior to cognitive symptoms) Dementia features very similar to those of Lewy body dementia

Percentages are prevalence of dementia subtypes in UK population (Dementia UK report, 2007).

To aid the clinical distinction of dementia, some authors differentiate cortical, subcortical and mixed dementias based on the predominance of cortical or subcortical dysfunction, or a mixture of the two (see Table 7.5 for the features of cortical and subcortical dementias). Unfortunately,

Table 7.5 Features of cortical and subcortical dementias

Characteristic	Cortical dementia	Subcortical dementia
Language	Aphasia early	Normal
Speech	Normal until late	Dysarthric
Praxis	Apraxia	Normal
Agnosia	Present	Usually absent
Calculation	Early impairment	Normal until late
Motor system	Usually normal posture/tone	Stooped or extended posture, increased tone
Extra movements	None (may have myoclonus in Alzheimer disease)	Tremor, chorea, tics

Cortical:
Alzheimer disease and the frontotemporal dementias (including Pick disease)

Subcortical:
Parkinson disease, dementia with Lewy bodies, Huntington disease, progressive supranuclear palsy, Wilson disease, normal pressure hydrocephalus, multiple sclerosis, HIV-related dementia

Mixed:
Vascular dementias, infection-induced dementias (Creutzfeldt–Jakob disease, neurosyphilis and chronic meningitis)

there is often a considerable overlap of symptoms in advanced dementia of whatever type.

HINTS AND TIPS

At this point you might find it helpful to read up on the aetiology and neuropathology of the various neurodegenerative dementias in Chapter 19.

DIFFERENTIAL DIAGNOSIS

There are four key questions when a patient presents with possible cognitive impairment:

- Is there objective evidence of cognitive impairment on a standardized test?
- If so, is it acute, chronic, or acute-on-chronic? (this may require a collateral history)
- Is the patient's conscious level normal or abnormal?
- What impact is the cognitive impairment having on the patient's functioning?

See Fig. 7.2 for a diagnostic algorithm and Box 7.3 for a summary of differential diagnosis.

Acute, acute-on-chronic or fluctuating cognitive impairment: delirium

See Common cognitive disorders section earlier for clinical features of delirium.

Chronic cognitive impairment

Key questions when a patient presents with chronic cognitive impairment:

- Which cognitive domains are impaired? (one or many?)
- Is the impairment stable, fluctuating or progressive?
- Is the cognitive impairment causing functional impairment?
- Are there any other associated symptoms? (e.g. mood change, personality change, perceptual disturbance).

Chronic impairment in multiple cognitive domains is due most often to dementia, mild cognitive impairment or depression (see Box 7.3 for more differentials). Sometimes a patient has an isolated impairment (see Table 7.1 for examples), most often due to a head injury or stroke. Causes of isolated amnesia (amnesic syndrome) are considered in more detail at the end of the section.

RED FLAG

Lewy body dementia and multi-infarct dementia are the only dementias that feature transient episodes of impaired consciousness as a typical feature. All other dementias do not feature an impairment of consciousness unless complicated by a delirium.

Dementia

See Common cognitive disorders section, above, for clinical features.

Older adults presenting with both physical health problems and generalized cognitive impairment are very common, and it is imperative that you understand how to differentiate between dementia and delirium. Table 7.3 summarizes the factors differentiating delirium from dementia – learn it well.

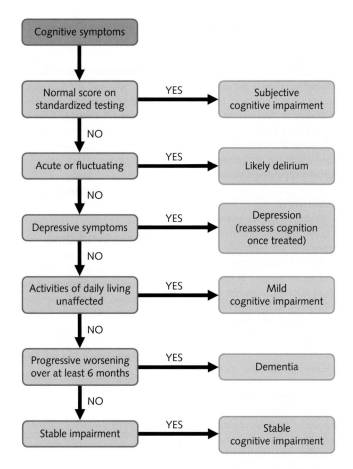

Note: Other differentials of cognitive impairment include intellectual disability, psychotic illness, amnesic syndrome, dissociative disorders, factitious disorder and malingering (see Box 7.3)

Fig. 7.2 Diagnostic algorithm for cognitive symptoms.

BOX 7.3   DIFFERENTIAL DIAGNOSIS OF COGNITIVE IMPAIRMENT

Delirium
Dementia
Mild cognitive impairment
Subjective cognitive impairment
Stable cognitive impairment post insult (e.g. stroke, hypoxic brain injury, traumatic brain injury)
Depression ('pseudodementia')
Psychotic disorders
Mood disorders
Intellectual disability
Dissociative disorders
Factitious disorder and malingering
Amnesic syndrome

HINTS AND TIPS

Dementia and delirium are by far the most common causes of generalized cognitive impairment. A key question in differentiating them is the duration of impairment: is it acute, chronic or acute-on-chronic? The patient may not be able to tell you, but their notes or a collateral history from a relative or GP can be invaluable.

Mild cognitive impairment

Mild cognitive impairment is objective cognitive impairment (confirmed with a standardized test) that does not interfere notably with activities of daily living. Mild cognitive impairment is a risk state for dementia, with around 10% to 15% of patients developing dementia each year. However, in some cases the impairment remains stable or even improves. All the processes that cause dementia can also cause mild cognitive impairment, so it is normally investigated in the same way.

Subjective cognitive impairment

Subjective cognitive impairment is when a patient complains of cognitive problems but scores normally on standardized tests. It can reflect anxiety or depression, but can also represent early deterioration in a highly educated individual that is unidentifiable using standard tests. People with subjective memory impairment are at increased risk for later developing mild cognitive impairment or dementia.

Stable cognitive impairment

Some 'one off' insults to the brain can impair one or more aspects of cognition but not cause progressive deterioration (e.g. following a stroke, hypoxic brain injury, traumatic brain injury or viral encephalitis). Improvement post-insult can occur over several months, so it is important not to make a firm diagnosis of stable chronic impairment too soon. Often someone who has had one cerebrovascular event continues to have further episodes, so an initially stable post-stroke cognitive impairment can evolve into vascular dementia.

Depression

Depressive 'pseudodementia' is a term sometimes used when patients present with clinical features resembling a dementia that result from an underlying depression. Both depression and dementia can be associated with a gradual onset of low mood, anorexia, sleep disturbance and generalized cognitive and functional impairment, and they can be very difficult to distinguish. If there is uncertainty, treatment for depression is trialled and cognition rechecked after mood has improved. Unfortunately, depression presenting with cognitive impairment is a risk factor for later developing dementia.

Psychosis

Patients with schizophrenia often have multiple cognitive deficits, particularly relating to memory, but unlike dementia, the age of onset is earlier and psychotic symptoms are present from the start. An acute psychotic state may resemble a delirium due to disturbed behaviour, vivid hallucinations, distractibility and thought disorder. However, patients generally remain orientated and symptoms do not fluctuate to the same degree as in delirium.

Intellectual disability

Patients with intellectual disability have an IQ below 70 with an impaired ability to adapt to their social environment. Unlike dementia, intellectual disability manifests in the developmental period (before age 18 years) and the level of cognitive functioning tends to be stable over time, not progressively deteriorating (see Chapter 29). However, intellectual disability can be comorbid with dementia or de-

lirium: around 50% of people with Down Syndrome will develop Alzheimer dementia, often early-onset.

Dissociative disorders

Memory loss and altered conscious levels can occur in the dissociative disorders (e.g. dissociative amnesia, fugue and stupor; see Chapter 14, Table 14.1). These usually occur in younger adults; however, there is no evidence of a physical cause and they are usually precipitated by a psychosocial stressor.

Factitious disorder and malingering

See Chapter 15.

Amnesic syndrome

While dementia is the most common cause of chronic memory dysfunction overall, certain brain diseases can cause a severe disruption of memory with minimal or no deterioration in other cognitive functions. This is termed 'amnesic syndrome' and usually results from damage to the hypothalamic–diencephalic system or the hippocampal region (see Box 7.4 for the causes of amnesic syndrome). The amnesic syndrome is characterized by all of the following:

- Anterograde and retrograde amnesia. The impairment of memory for past events is in reverse order of their occurrence (i.e. recent memories are the most affected).
- There is no impairment of attention or consciousness or global intellectual functioning. There is also no defect in working memory as tested by digit span.

BOX 7.4   CAUSES OF AMNESIC SYNDROME

Diencephalic damage

Vitamin B1 (thiamine) deficiency (i.e. Korsakoff syndrome):
  Chronic alcohol abuse
  Gastric carcinoma
  Severe malnutrition
  Hyperemesis gravidarum
  Bilateral thalamic infarction
  Multiple sclerosis
  Post subarachnoid haemorrhage
  Third ventricle tumours/cysts

Hippocampal damage
  Bilateral posterior cerebral artery occlusion
  Carbon monoxide poisoning
  Closed head injury
  Herpes simplex virus encephalitis
  Transient global amnesia

- There is strong evidence of a brain disease known to cause the amnesic syndrome.

Although there is no impairment of global cognitive functioning, patients with the amnesic syndrome are usually disorientated in time due to their inability to learn new material (anterograde amnesia). Other associated features are confabulation (filling of gaps in memory with details which are fictitious, but often plausible), lack of insight and apathy.

The commonest cause of amnesic syndrome is thiamine deficiency resulting in Wernicke encephalopathy followed by Korsakoff syndrome. See Chapter 8 for details.

HINTS AND TIPS

Due to their unimpaired intellectual functioning, maintained communication and language skills, tendency to confabulate and lack of insight, patients with an amnesic syndrome can present as problem-free. Therefore, as in dementia, a collateral history is crucial.

ASSESSMENT

History

The following questions may be helpful in eliciting symptoms of cognitive impairment:

To the patient:

- Do you find yourself forgetting familiar people's names?
- Do you get lost more easily than you used to?
- Are you able to handle money confidently?
- Do you feel being forgetful is stopping you from doing anything?

To the informant:

- Are they repetitive in conversation?
- Has their personality changed?
- Are they having difficulty with aspects of their day-to-day life?
- Do you have any concerns about their safety?

Examination

Cognitive examination

The key when assessing cognition is to use a standardized test and avoid vague descriptions such as 'alert and orientated'. Many patients maintain a good social veneer, making it surprisingly easy to miss cognitive impairment if it is not formally assessed. There is a wide range of tests available of varying comprehensiveness, length and generalizability across cultures. The one you choose depends on the time available and degree of concern about a patient's cognition. In the UK, it is recommended that all hospital inpatients aged more than 65 years have their cognition screened whether or not they appear impaired. Table 7.6 lists the advantages and disadvantages of some widely used screening tests. There are many more cognitive tests which may be useful for specific disorders (e.g. the Wisconsin card test to assess frontal lobe function). Assessment of conscious level is described in Fig. 7.1.

HINTS AND TIPS

Try to ensure the result of a cognitive assessment reflects cognitive abilities rather than other difficulties as far as possible: check for medications which may be influencing cognition, ensure the patient has their glasses and/or hearing aid, is not hungry, needing the toilet or exhausted.

Table 7.6 Standardized tests of cognition: advantages and disadvantages

Test	Acronym	Time to perform (min)	Advantages	Disadvantages
Abbreviated Mental Test	AMT	3	Fast	Not sensitive to mild to moderate impairment
Montreal Cognitive Test	MoCA	10	Tests all cognitive domains Sensitive to mild impairment	Influenced by premorbid IQ, language and culture Tester needs to practice prior to administration
Addenbrooke's Cognitive Examination – III	ACE-III	20	Tests all cognitive domains Sensitive to mild impairment	Lengthy Influenced by premorbid IQ, language and culture

In the past, the MMSE (mini mental state exam) was commonly used but is less so now because of both licensing restrictions and availability of more comprehensive tests.

Physical examination

A physical examination, including a neurological examination, is important in everyone with cognitive impairment as it may provide evidence of:

- Reversible causes of impairment such as hypothyroidism or a space occupying lesion
- Risk factors for dementia (e.g. hypertension or atrial fibrillation).
- Differential diagnosis of dementia (e.g. a hemiparesis or visual field defect suggestive of a stroke and hence increased risk for vascular dementia)
- Complications of impairment such as self-neglect or injuries from falls
- Factors that may influence future prescribing decisions (e.g. bradycardia should lead to caution with cholinesterase inhibitors)

Investigations

The main aim of investigation in cognitive impairment is to exclude reversible causes (Table 7.7). In delirium, additional investigations for acute illness are likely to be appropriate, including an electrocardiogram (ECG) and a septic screen in the presence of infective symptoms or pyrexia.

Although some types of dementia have characteristic radiological findings (Table 7.8), these differences are not yet robust enough to be diagnostic. In some rarer forms of dementia, genetic testing may be useful (Huntington disease and early onset Alzheimer; see Chapter 19). If the diagnosis

Table 7.7 Investigations recommended in chronic cognitive impairment

Investigation	Potentially treatable cause
Vitamin B12/folate level	Nutrient deficiency/malabsorption
Thyroid function tests, calcium, glucose, urea and electrolytes (U&E)	Hypothyroidism, hypercalcaemia, Cushing, or Addison disease
CT/MRI head scan	Subdural haematoma, tumour, normal pressure hydrocephalus

The above investigations are recommended by NICE (2006) as a minimum for excluding reversible causes of dementia in the UK. Other investigations may also be appropriate depending on features in the history or examination (e.g. HIV or syphilis serology, heavy metal screen, autoantibodies).

CT, Computed tomography; MRI, magnetic resonance imaging.

Table 7.8 Typical CT appearances for the main forms of dementia

Condition	CT appearance
Normal ageing	Progressive cortical atrophy and increasing ventricular size
Alzheimer disease	Generalized cerebral atrophy. Widened sulci. Dilated ventricles. Thinning of the width of the medial temporal lobe (in temporal lobe-oriented CT scans)
Vascular dementia	Single/multiple areas of infarction. Cerebral atrophy. Dilated ventricles
Frontotemporal dementia (including Pick disease)	Greater relative atrophy of frontal and temporal lobes. Knife-blade atrophy (appearance of atrophied gyri)
Huntington disease	Dilated ventricles. Atrophy of caudate nuclei (loss of shouldering)
Creutzfeldt–Jakob disease (CJD)	Usually appears normal
nvCJD (new variant CJD)	nvCJD has a characteristic MRI picture: a bilaterally evident high signal in the pulvinar (post-thalamic) region

Note that an MRI scan is generally preferable to a CT scan for aiding in the diagnosis of dementia because more detailed images can be obtained. CT findings are provided here because MRI is less commonly available.

CT, Computed tomography; MRI, magnetic resonance imaging.

is in doubt or atypical, a more detailed cognitive assessment by a neuropsychologist may be of benefit (usually accessed via a 'memory clinic').

DISCUSSION OF CASE STUDY

Mr DD first presented with memory loss for recent events. His personality gradually changed (withdrawn, prone to verbal aggression) and he also developed numerous other cognitive deficits: aphasia (rambling incoherently), agnosia (unable to recognize his pipe), apraxia (unable to dress himself) and impaired executive functioning (unable to make a cup of coffee). This 6-year deterioration in cognitive and functional abilities associated with a normal level of consciousness suggests the diagnosis of dementia.

Mr DD then developed a delirium as evidenced by the rapid onset of a fluctuating conscious level, disturbed sleep–wake cycle, psychomotor agitation and apparent perceptual disturbances (visual hallucinations). It is crucial that the cause of the delirium is diagnosed and treated. In this case, it could be pneumonia as Mr DD had developed a productive cough.

Now go on to Chapter 19 to read about delirium and dementia and their management.

Chapter Summary

- Cognitive impairment is common and associated with high morbidity and mortality, but is often under-recognized.
- Delirium is a syndrome of impaired consciousness, impaired attention and impaired cognition, all with acute or fluctuating onset.
- Dementia is a syndrome of acquired, gradually progressive, generalized cognitive impairment associated with functional decline.
- Always assess cognition using a standardized cognitive test.
- A collateral history is often crucial to establish the temporal pattern of cognitive difficulties and degree of functional impairment.
- Always screen for treatable causes of delirium and dementia.

CASE SUMMARY

Mr AD, aged 42 years, presented to his general practitioner (GP) smelling of alcohol and complaining of depression, anxiety, relationship difficulties and erectile dysfunction. He admitted to drinking up to a bottle and a half of whisky per day. He reported drinking increasing amounts over the past year as the same amount no longer gave him the same feeling of well-being. Recently, he noticed that he had to drink in order to avoid shaking, sweating, vomiting and feeling 'on edge'. These symptoms meant having to take two glasses of whisky before breakfast, just to feel better. Mr AD admitted that he had neglected his family and work because of his drinking. Whereas in the past, he would vary what and when he drank, he now tended to drink exactly the same thing at the same time each day, irrespective of his mood or the occasion. He found himself craving alcohol and felt unable to walk home past the pub without going in. He continued to drink although he knew it was harming his liver. He was also concerned about his mental health because, on more than one occasion, he thought he saw a witch, about the same height as the kitchen kettle, walking around the room. He decided to contact his GP after he was charged with drink-driving by the police. Mr AD had no previous psychiatric history or family history of psychiatric illness and was not taking any medication.

(For a discussion of the case study see the end of the chapter).

Psychoactive substances have been used for centuries, and their use is seen in many cultures as entirely acceptable. They have many beneficial effects including relief of pain and distress; without them, life would be grim for some. However, psychoactive substances may cause symptoms and behaviour changes which are damaging to the individual or those around them, particularly when the substance is used regularly or to excess. Initial use of a substance can lead to a cycle of further use even when the person wishes to stop, as many recreational substances are associated with dependence, and withdrawal can be unpleasant and, with a minority of substances, fatal.

DEFINITIONS AND CLINICAL FEATURES

The term 'psychoactive' refers to any substance that has an effect on the central nervous system. This includes recreational drugs, alcohol, nicotine, caffeine, prescribed or over-the-counter medication and poisons or toxins.

This section will introduce five concepts in relation to psychoactive substance use: intoxication, hazardous use, harmful use, dependence and withdrawal. Fig. 8.1 provides an overview of these and some other substance-related disorders.

Substance intoxication

Substance intoxication describes a transient, substance-specific condition that occurs following the use of a psychoactive substance. Symptoms can include disturbances of consciousness, perception, mood, behaviour and physiological functions. Severity of intoxication is normally proportional to dose or levels.

HINTS AND TIPS

Hazardous use of a substance

'Hazardous use' is a widely used term introduced by the World Health Organization and National Institute for Health and Care Excellence but is not in ICD-10. Hazardous use of a substance is defined as a quantity or pattern of substance use that places the user at risk for adverse consequences, without dependence. For example, drinking alcohol above the recommended limits (see Fig 8.2) is hazardous use, whether or not the person feels they have come to any harm.

Harmful use of substance

Harmful use of a substance is defined as a quantity or pattern of substance use that actually causes adverse consequences, without dependence. It may result in difficulties within interpersonal relationships (e.g. domestic violence, erectile dysfunction); problems meeting work or educational obligations (e.g. absenteeism); impaired physical health (e.g. alcohol-related liver disease, trauma); worsening of mental health problems (e.g. low mood or anxiety); or legal difficulties (e.g. arrest for disorderly conduct, stealing to fund habit, drink-driving).

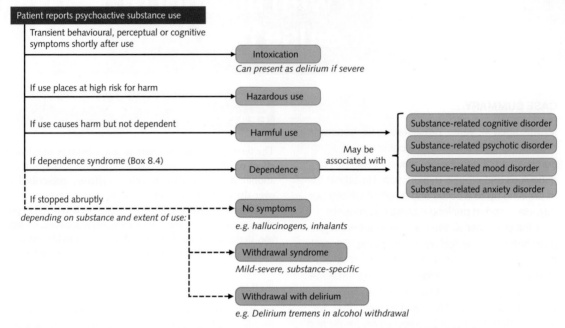

Notes on classification: This diagram is primarily based on ICD-10. Hazardous use is a widely used term introduced by the WHO but is not in ICD-10. ICD-10 does not specify substance-induced mood or anxiety disorder, but these are included in the current draft of ICD-11 (not yet published). ICD-10 refers to substance-induced 'amnestic disorder' (see Chapter 7) rather than cognitive disorder.

Fig. 8.1 Diagnostic algorithm for a person presenting with psychoactive substance use.

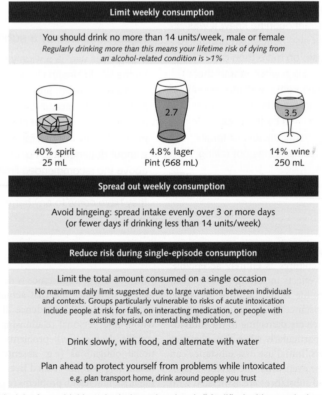

Fig. 8.2 How to keep health risks from drinking alcohol to a low level. (Modified with permission from UK Chief Medical Officers' Low Risk Drinking Guidelines, 2016.)

COMMUNICATION

Remember the 'four Ls' (love, livelihood, liver, law) as a framework for assessing harm arising from substance use.

Substance dependence

HINTS AND TIPS

The confusion regarding use of the term 'addiction' led the World Health Organization (1964) to recommend that the term be abandoned in scientific literature in favour of the term 'dependence'.

COMMUNICATION

Substance 'misuse' is a general term used to refer to substance use without legal or medical guidelines. It includes both harmful or dependent use of substances. Substance 'abuse' has the same meaning but is usually avoided because it has negative connotations.

Substance dependence describes a syndrome that incorporates physiological, psychological and behavioural elements (Box 8.1). If patients exhibit either tolerance or withdrawal, they may be specified as having physiological dependence. However, patients can meet the criteria for the dependence syndrome without having developed tolerance or withdrawal. The dependence syndrome (ICD-10 criteria) is diagnosed if three or more of the criteria in Box 8.1 have been present together at some time during the previous year.

HINTS AND TIPS

Patients are physiologically dependent on a psychoactive substance when they exhibit signs of tolerance and/or withdrawal.

Substance withdrawal

Substance withdrawal describes a substance-specific syndrome that occurs on reduction or cessation of a psychoactive substance that has generally been used repeatedly, in high doses, for a prolonged period. It is one of the criteria of the dependence syndrome.

BOX 8.1 ICD-10 CRITERIA FOR DEPENDENCE ON A SUBSTANCE

1. A strong *desire or compulsion* to take the substance
2. *Difficulties in controlling* substance-taking behaviour (onset, termination, levels of use)
3. Physiological *withdrawal* state when substance use has reduced or ceased; or continued use of the substance to relieve or avoid withdrawal symptoms
4. *Tolerance* where increased quantities of the substance are required to produce the same effect originally produced by lower amounts
5. *Priority* given to substance with neglect of other interests and activities due to time spent acquiring and taking substance, or recovering from its effects
6. *Persistence despite harm* where use of the substance is continued despite a clear awareness of its harmful consequences (physical or mental)

ALCOHOL-RELATED DISORDERS

Many people who drink alcohol come to no apparent harm. However, drinking even a small amount of alcohol without overt harm at the time increases the risk for many subsequent illnesses (e.g. cancer, stroke, heart disease, liver disease) and also death through accidents (e.g. head injuries, fractures, facial injuries). This increase in mortality far outweighs the potential health benefits of moderate consumption (which are limited to a small reduction in risk for ischaemic heart disease in women over 55 years old who drink around 5 units per week). The Chief Medical Officer (2016) advised that 'there is no safe level of alcohol consumption'. However, for many people alcohol is a large part of their social lives and they may feel the benefits of consumption outweigh the risks (similar decisions are made by those who choose to partake in high-risk sports). For those who choose to drink alcohol, a number of steps can be taken to keep the associated harms to a low level: see Fig. 8.2 and Box 8.8.

HINTS AND TIPS

One unit of alcohol = 8 g/10 mL of pure alcohol *(note this varies between countries)*
One unit is approximately equivalent to the amount of alcohol metabolized in 1 hour. For example, if

you drink a large glass of wine (usually containing around three units) it will typically be at least 3 hours before blood alcohol concentration returns to zero.

Alcohol metabolism follows zero-order kinetics; it cannot be speeded up (e.g. by drinking coffee).

You can calculate units by multiplying alcohol by volume (ABV) in percent by volume in litres: ABV × vol = units (e.g. a pint (568 mL) of 5.3% lager would contain 5.3 × 0.568 = 3 units

---

COMMUNICATION

The Chief Medical Officer's advice on alcohol consumption can be summarized as:

- There's no safe level at which to drink alcohol
- Drinking at most 14 units/week keeps risks low (but some people will be harmed by less)
- Don't drink all 14 units in one night

Acute intoxication

Ingestion of alcohol results in transient psychological, behavioural and neurological changes, the severity of which are roughly correlated to the alcohol concentration in the blood and brain. Initially, this may produce an enhanced sense of well being, greater confidence and relief of anxiety, which may lead to individuals becoming disinhibited, talkative and flirtatious. As blood levels increase, some drinkers may exhibit inappropriate sexual or aggressive behaviour whereas others might become sullen and withdrawn, with labile mood and possibly self-injurious behaviour. As levels rise further, drinkers can suffer incoordination, slurred speech, ataxia, amnesia (see later) and impaired reaction times, and at very high concentrations, a lowered level of consciousness, respiratory depression, coma and death.

HINTS AND TIPS

Extreme alcohol intoxication states can cause impaired concentration, inability to sustain attention and global cognitive impairment, and can meet diagnostic criteria for delirium (see Chapter 7). However, this should not be confused with delirium tremens, associated with alcohol withdrawal.

RED FLAG

Alcohol intoxication can cause dangerous disinhibition, increasing a person's likelihood of having and acting upon thoughts of self-harm or suicide. Seven out of ten men who complete suicide are intoxicated.

Alcohol intoxication can be a potentially life-threatening condition due to the risk for respiratory depression, aspiration of vomit, hypoglycaemia, hypothermia and trauma (e.g. head injury, fractures or blood loss following accidents or assaults).

HINTS AND TIPS

Patients may report drinking alcohol in order to sleep better. This is counterproductive. It is true that alcohol reduces sleep latency and leads to increased slow-wave (deep) sleep during the first half of the night. However, alcohol also inhibits the time to onset and duration of REM sleep, causing disruption to sleep architecture during the second half of the night and overall reduced quality sleep.

Harmful use of alcohol

Harmful use of alcohol is when drinking causes physical, psychological or social harm to the patient or others around them. People who harmfully drink are not dependent on alcohol; if features of dependence are present, the patient has alcohol dependence syndrome (Box 8.1). Box 8.2 lists the adverse physical, psychological and social consequences of drinking.

COMMUNICATION

It is frequently useful to explain that, although a patient may not be suffering from alcohol dependence, they are drinking at harmful levels, and are likely to benefit from support to reduce their consumption.

Alcohol dependence

After a significant time of heavy, regular drinking, users may develop dependence (Box 8.1). Alcohol dependence does not just mean physical dependence (although that is an important part of it), but describes a heterogeneous collection of symptoms, signs and behaviours which are determined by biological, psychological and sociocultural factors. There is a

BOX 8.2 COMPLICATIONS OF EXCESSIVE ALCOHOL USE

Mental health

- Substance-related disorders (Fig. 8.1)
- Self-harm or suicidal behaviour

Social

- Absenteeism from, or poor performance at, work or education
- Victim of theft (e.g. wallet, phone, keys)
- Unprotected sex with risk for sexually transmitted disease or unplanned pregnancy
- Legal problems (increased risk for violent crime, drink-driving, alcohol-related disorderly conduct, child abuse)
- Interpersonal problems (arguments with friends or family due to alcohol)
- Financial problems (expense of drinking, unemployment)
- Homelessness

Physical health

- *Nervous system*
  Intoxication delirium
  Withdrawal delirium (delirium tremens)
  Withdrawal seizures
  Cerebellar degeneration
  Haemorrhagic stroke
  Peripheral and optic neuropathy
  Wernicke–Korsakoff syndrome
  Alcohol-related cognitive impairment
- *Gastrointestinal system*
  Alcoholic liver disease (fatty liver, alcoholic hepatitis, alcoholic cirrhosis)
  Acute and chronic pancreatitis
  Peptic ulceration and gastritis

Cancers: oropharynx, larynx, oesophagus, liver, breast, colon and pancreas.

- *Cardiovascular system*
  Hypertension
  Arrhythmias
  Ischaemic heart disease (in heavy drinkers)
  Alcoholic cardiomyopathy
- *Immune system*
  Increased risk for infections (especially meningitis and pneumonia)
- *Metabolic and endocrine system*
  Hypoglycaemia
  Hyperlipidaemia/hypertriglyceridemia
  Hyperuricaemia (gout)
  Hypomagnesaemia, hypophosphatemia, hyponatraemia
  Alcohol-induced pseudo–Cushing syndrome
- *Haematological system*
  Red cell macrocytosis
  Anaemia
  Neutropenia
  Thrombocytopenia
- *Musculoskeletal system*
  Acute and chronic myopathy
  Osteoporosis
- *Reproductive system*
  Intrauterine growth retardation
  Fetal alcohol syndrome
  Erectile dysfunction
  Infertility
- *Increased incidence of trauma (fractures, head injury, soft tissue injury following accidents or assaults).*

range in the severity of dependence; one dependent drinker may experience a mild tremor and anxiety while at work ('the fear') whereas another may shake so much after waking that he is unable to drink a cup of tea in the morning without spilling it.

Alcohol withdrawal (including delirium)

The development of withdrawal symptoms upon discontinuation of substance use is part of the dependence syndrome. Box 8.3 summarizes the continuum of clinical features of alcohol withdrawal, from uncomplicated withdrawal to life-threatening delirium tremens ('the DTs'). However, 'uncomplicated' does not mean not serious. All withdrawal states are potentially life-threatening, if they are associated with autonomic hyperactivity or perceptual disturbances which may cause a person to engage in risky behaviour.

RED FLAG

Always check whether previous episodes of alcohol withdrawal have been complicated by medical problems (such as delirium tremens or seizures) or psychiatric problems (such as suicidality). These points will be important in determining where detoxification takes place.

BOX 8.3   CLINICAL FEATURES OF ALCOHOL WITHDRAWAL

Uncomplicated alcohol withdrawal syndrome

- Symptoms develop 4–12 hours after drinking cessation
- Tremulousness ('the shakes')
- Sweating
- Nausea and vomiting
- Mood disturbance (anxiety, depression, 'feeling edgy')
- Sensitivity to sound (hyperacusis)
- Autonomic hyperactivity (tachycardia, hypertension, mydriasis, pyrexia)
- Sleep disturbance
- Psychomotor agitation

With perceptual disturbances

- Illusions or hallucinations (typically visual, auditory, or tactile)

With withdrawal seizures

- Develop 6–48 hours after drinking cessation
- Occurs in 5%–15% of all alcohol-dependent drinkers
- Generalized and tonic–clonic
- Predisposing factors: previous history of withdrawal fits, concurrent epilepsy, low potassium or magnesium

Withdrawal delirium (delirium tremens)

- Develops 1–7 days after drinking cessation (mean = 48 hours)
- Altered consciousness and marked cognitive impairment (i.e. delirium; see Chapters 7 and 19)
- Vivid hallucinations and illusions in any sensory modality (patients often interact with or are horrified by them; Lilliputian visual hallucinations, i.e. miniature humans/animals; formication, i.e. sensation of insects crawling on the skin)
- Marked tremor
- Autonomic arousal (heavy sweating, raised pulse and blood pressure, fever)
- Paranoid delusions (often associated with intense fear)
- Mortality (5% to 15% of people with delirium tremens die from cardiovascular collapse, hypothermia/hyperthermia, infection)
- Predisposing factors such as physical illness (hepatitis, pancreatitis, pneumonia)

Withdrawal often precipitates Wernicke encephalopathy

- Triad of ataxia, ophthalmoplegia and acute cognitive impairment
- Risk for long-term cognitive impairment (Korsakoff syndrome)

ALCOHOL-RELATED COGNITIVE DISORDERS

Blackouts

Episodes of anterograde amnesia ('blackouts') can occur during acute alcohol intoxication. Memory loss may be patchy, or for a discrete block of time during which nothing can be remembered. Blackouts are common and have been experienced by two-thirds of dependent drinkers and one-third of young men in the general population. Blackouts refer to amnesia, not collapsing or 'passing out' at the end of the night. They are evidence of hazardous use of alcohol as they place an individual at great vulnerability.

Wernicke–Korsakoff syndrome

Both Wernicke encephalopathy and Korsakoff syndrome occur because of thiamine (vitamin B_1) deficiency. Although the two disorders were initially described separately it is now clear they represent a continuum, with Wernicke encephalopathy occurring during acute brain damage due to thiamine deficiency and Korsakoff being the chronic state that emerges later. Any disorder that is associated with low thiamine can cause Wernicke–Korsakoff syndrome, but heavy drinkers are at particular risk. This is because of nutritional deficiency secondary to poor dietary intake and impaired absorption.

Wernicke encephalopathy is characterized by the classical clinical triad of delirium, ophthalmoplegia (mainly nystagmus, sixth nerve palsy or conjugate gaze palsy), and ataxia (which can be impossible to distinguish from intoxication). All three triad components are found in only a minority of cases; the presence of any of them should prompt treatment. Early treatment with parenteral thiamine (Pabrinex) can reduce the likelihood of progression to Korsakoff syndrome. Korsakoff syndrome is characterized by extensive anterograde and retrograde amnesia, frontal lobe dysfunction and psychotic symptoms occurring in the absence of delirium. See Chapter 20 for more details of treatment.

alcohol or substance use problems

COMMUNICATION

You cannot completely exclude the use of substances, or gauge the severity of established misuse, without a collateral history (or in some cases even with one). A urine or oral toxicology screen are useful in establishing recent use of common recreational substances.

ASSESSMENT

History

The CAGE and AUDIT questionnaires (see later) can be helpful in screening for alcohol dependence. A thorough clinical history should pay particular attention to all substances used, the pattern of use, the route of use, features of dependence, periods of abstinence or controlled use, reasons for relapse, previous treatments, and consequences of substance use (relationships, employment, physical health, criminality). History of psychiatric illness and substance misuse, as well as family history of substance misuse should be explored. Mental state examination is important to establish psychiatric comorbidity or sequelae, current suicidality, and insight into current substance misuse (e.g. whether the patient considers it to be a problem and what they would consider to be helpful).

RED FLAG

Taking multiple substances at once is a major risk factor for drug related death, with recreational, prescribed and over the counter drugs all implicated. The top four drugs involved in overdose are all depressants: heroin, diazepam, alcohol, methadone. Always ask about polydrug use, and whether the person has ever unintentionally overdosed. All patients prescribed opioid substitution treatment should be offered a take home naloxone kit, and training in how to recognize and treat an overdose.

The CAGE questionnaire is a simple tool to screen for alcohol dependence. If patients answer yes to two or more questions, regard the screen as positive and go on to check if they meet criteria for the alcohol dependence syndrome:

1. Have you ever felt you ought to **C**ut down on your drinking?
2. Have people ever **A**nnoyed you by criticizing your drinking?
3. Have you ever felt **G**uilty about your drinking?
4. Have you ever needed an '**E**ye-opener' (a drink first thing in the morning to steady your nerves or get rid of a hangover)?

The Alcohol Use Disorders Identification Test (AUDIT) is a 10-item screening questionnaire for problem drinking developed by the WHO. It takes 3 minutes to complete and score, and is recommended by NICE (2011). Severity of dependence can be rated using the 'Severity of Alcohol Dependence Questionnaire' (SADQ).

RED FLAG

Always ask about driving and the patient's responsibilities for caring for children. These are common areas of risk to others caused by alcohol or other substance use.

RED FLAG

General Medical Council guidance states that use of illegal substances and misuse of alcohol are fitness to practice issues. This applies to medical students as well as qualified doctors and is intended to be supportive rather than punitive, aiming to protect patient safety while facilitating the doctor or student to engage in treatment and recovery. If you are misusing substances, contact your general practitioner and seek support from your medical school. If you suspect a peer or senior colleague is misusing substances in a way which may influence patient care, speak to a senior doctor or your medical school.

Examination

The physical examination requires an awareness of both the acute and chronic effects of alcohol or substance use and should focus on:

- Evidence of acute use or intoxication (e.g. pupil constriction with opioid use; incoordination and slurred speech with alcohol use)
- Signs of withdrawal (e.g. tremulousness, sweating, nausea and vomiting, tachycardia and pupil dilatation with opioid withdrawal)
- Immediate and short-term medical complications of substance use (e.g. head injury following alcohol intoxication; infection caused by intravenous drug use (always inspect injection sites))

- Long-term medical complications (e.g. alcohol-related liver disease, hepatitis B or C or HIV infection with intravenous drug use)

Investigations

There is no investigation that is absolutely indicative of substance dependence. A urine or saliva drug-screening test is essential whenever the use of psychoactive substances is suspected. Saliva testing is more dignified than urine testing, and is now most commonly used. Hair testing is occasionally used to get an accurate picture of drug use over longer time periods. However, toxicology testing generally is only set up to detect a limited number of well-known drugs (and testing laboratories will often not yet be set up to detect drugs which are new to the black market). Breath alcohol level (via a breathalyser) only detects recent alcohol use; however, a high reading in the absence of signs of intoxication suggests some degree of tolerance, which is likely to be indicative of chronic heavy drinking.

Investigations are also useful to identify possible longer-term complications of alcohol (see Table 8.1) and include a full blood count (mean corpuscular volume, or MCV, may be elevated), urea and electrolytes, liver function tests (gamma glutamyl transpeptidase may be raised; elevated aminotransferases (ALT or AST) indicate liver injury and a high AST:ALT ratio suggests alcohol is the cause), clotting screen (prolonged prothrombin time is a sensitive marker of liver function) and electrocardiogram.

HINTS AND TIPS

If a patient is drinking too much alcohol, check their liver function. If a patient has abnormal liver function tests (LFT), take an alcohol history. Alcohol can cause abnormalities in any LFT.

If the patient has injected drugs ensure serology for blood-borne viruses has been performed (hepatitis B and C, HIV) subsequent to the most recent injection (and consider the need to repeat testing after potential seroconversion). Signpost the patient to a needle exchange where they will also get access to a wide variety of harm-reduction information and education, including sexual health issues.

If the patient is suffering from a withdrawal delirium, brain imaging may be necessary to exclude an alternative cause or additional complication (e.g. infection, head injury, stroke).

HINTS AND TIPS

All patients, especially people presenting for the first time with psychotic symptoms, should have a urine or saliva drug-screening test. It is important to collect the sample as soon as possible because the half-lives (and hence detection windows) of some drugs are short. Urine dip-sticks are the fastest way to get a result.

DISCUSSION OF CASE STUDY

Mr AD has an alcohol dependence syndrome as evidenced by his tolerance, withdrawal symptoms, relief of withdrawal by drinking, strong desire to consume alcohol, and continued drinking despite awareness of harmful consequences. He has physical (sexual, possibly other systems), social (relationship problems, neglect of family and work), legal (drink-driving offence) and mental health (depression, anxiety, hallucinations) complications of his alcohol use. The first priority is treating the alcohol dependence. Following detoxification, it is important to reassess his mental health to ensure that his depression, anxiety and hallucinations are not indicative of a primary psychiatric disorder. The visual hallucinations may be suggestive of a withdrawal syndrome or be one of the perceptual disturbances sometimes caused by heavy alcohol use (alcoholic hallucinosis), although the latter is much less likely.

Now go on to Chapter 20 to read about the alcohol and substance disorders and their management.

● Chapter Summary

Problematic psychoactive substance use can be classified as:
- Substance use disorders including
  - intoxication, hazardous use, harmful use, dependent use, withdrawal states
- Substance-induced psychiatric disorders
  - including cognitive impairment, psychosis, depressive episode, manic episode, anxiety

Substance use is often comorbid with primary psychiatric disorders

Intoxication by and withdrawal from psychoactive substances can be life-threatening

When assessing substance misuse, don't forget to assess for impact on physical health and psychosocial function

FURTHER READING

Clinical Opiate Withdrawal Scale (COWS) https://www.drugabuse.gov/sites/default/files/files/ClinicalOpiateWithdrawalScale.pdf

Alcohol Use Disorders Identification Test (AUDIT) https://www.drugabuse.gov/sites/default/files/files/AUDIT.pdf

The patient with psychotic symptoms

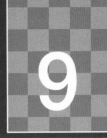

CASE SUMMARY

Mr PP, aged 23 years, was assessed by his general practitioner (GP) because his family had become concerned about his behaviour. Over the last 6 months his college attendance had been uncharacteristically poor and he had terminated his part-time work. He had also become increasingly reclusive, spending more time alone in his flat, refusing to answer the door or see his friends. After some inappropriate suspiciousness, he allowed the GP into his flat and then disclosed that government scientists had started to perform experiments on him over the last year. These involved the insertion of an electrode into his brain that detected gamma rays transmitted from government headquarters, which issued him with commands and 'planted' strange ideas in his head. When the GP asked how he knew this, he replied that he heard the 'men's voices' as 'clear as day' and that they continually commented on what he was thinking. He explained that his suspicion that 'all was not right' was confirmed when he heard the neighbour's dog barking in the middle of the night; at that point he knew 'for certain' that he was being interfered with. Prompted by the GP, Mr PP also mentioned that a man in his local pub knew of his plight and had sent him a 'covert signal' when he overheard the man conversing about the dangers of nuclear experiments. He also admitted to 'receiving coded information' from the radio whenever it was turned on. Mr PP found his experiences very disturbing and had been considering suicide to escape his situation. The GP found no evidence of abnormal mood, incoherence of speech or disturbed motor function. Mr PP denied use of recreational drugs and appeared physically well. After the GP discussed the case with a psychiatrist, Mr PP was admitted to a psychiatric hospital for a period of assessment and to manage his risk to himself. Mr PP agreed to a voluntary admission, as he was now afraid of staying alone at home.

(For a discussion of the case study see the end of the chapter).

The patient with psychotic symptoms can present in many varied ways. It is often very difficult to elicit and describe specific symptoms when a patient is speaking or behaving in a grossly disorganized fashion. Therefore it is important to approach the assessment in a logical and systematic fashion as well as to have a good understanding of the psychopathology involved.

DEFINITIONS AND CLINICAL FEATURES

The term 'psychosis' refers to a mental state in which reality is grossly distorted, resulting in symptoms such as delusions, hallucinations and thought disorder. However, patients with schizophrenia and other psychotic disorders often have other symptoms too (e.g. psychomotor abnormalities, mood/affect disturbance, cognitive deficits and disorganized behaviour).

There are many classifications that attempt to describe all the symptoms seen in schizophrenia and psychosis, but it is useful to approach psychotic psychopathology using five somewhat interrelated parameters:

1. Perception
2. Abnormal beliefs
3. Thought disorder
4. Negative symptoms
5. Psychomotor function

Perceptual disturbance

Perception is the process of making sense of the physical information we receive from our sensory modalities.

Hallucinations are perceptions occurring in the absence of an external physical stimulus, which have the following important characteristics:

- To the patient, the nature of a hallucination is the same as a normal sensory experience (i.e. it appears real). Therefore patients often have little insight into their abnormal experience.
- They are experienced as external sensations from any one of the sensory modalities (e.g. hearing, vision, smell, taste, touch) and should be distinguished from ideas, thoughts, images or fantasies which originate in the patient's own mind.
- They occur without an external stimulus and are not merely distortions of an existing physical stimulus (see Illusions).

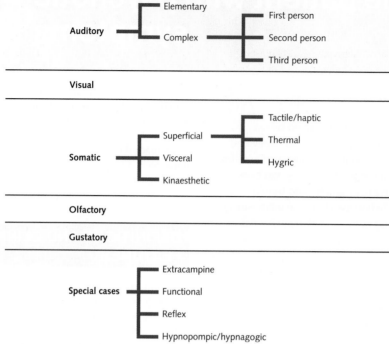

Fig. 9.1 Outline of classification of hallucinations.

According to which sense organ they appear to arise from, hallucinations are classified as auditory, visual, olfactory, gustatory or somatic. Special forms of hallucinations will also be discussed. See Fig. 9.1 for an outline of the classification of hallucinations.

Illusions are misperceptions of real external stimuli (e.g. in a dark room, a dressing gown hanging on a bedroom wall is perceived as a person). Illusions often occur in healthy people and are usually associated with inattention or intense emotional state (e.g. situational anxiety).

A *pseudohallucination* is a perceptual experience which differs from a hallucination in that it appears to arise in the subjective inner space of the mind, not through one of the external sensory organs. Although experienced in internal space pseudohallucinations are not under conscious control (e.g. someone hearing a voice inside their own head telling them to harm themselves or someone experiencing distressing flashbacks in posttraumatic stress disorder). These are not viewed as true psychotic experiences. Note that some psychiatrists define pseudohallucinations to mean hallucinations that patients recognize as false perceptions (i.e. they have insight into the fact that they are hallucinating). The former definition is probably more widely used.

Auditory hallucinations

These are hallucinations of the hearing modality and are the most common type of hallucinations in clinical psychiatry. Elementary hallucinations are simple, unstructured sounds (e.g. whirring, buzzing, whistling or single words); this type of hallucination occurs most commonly in acute organic states (e.g. epilepsy, migraine, delirium). Complex hallucinations occur as spoken phrases, sentences or even dialogue that are classified as:

- *Audible thoughts* (*first person*): patients hear their own thoughts spoken out loud as they think them. When patients experience their thoughts as echoed by a voice after they have thought them, it is termed thought echo.
- *Second person auditory hallucinations*: patients hear a voice or voices talking directly to them. Second person hallucinations can be persecutory, highly critical, complimentary or can issue commands to the patient (command hallucinations). Second person hallucinations are often associated with mood disorders with psychotic symptoms and so will be critical or persecutory in a depressed patient or complimentary in a manic patient (i.e. mood-congruent hallucinations).
- *Third person auditory hallucinations*: patients hear a voice or voices speaking about them, referring to them in the third person. This may take the form of two or more voices arguing or discussing the patient among themselves or one or more voices giving a running commentary on the patient's thoughts or actions.

HINTS AND TIPS

Particular types of auditory hallucination are highly suggestive of schizophrenia and known as 'first-rank symptoms'. See Box 9.7 for a list.

Visual hallucinations

These are hallucinations of the visual modality. They occur most commonly in organic brain disturbances (delirium, occipital lobe tumours, epilepsy, dementia) and in the context of psychoactive substance use (lysergic acid diethylamide, mescaline, petrol/glue-sniffing, alcoholic hallucinosis). An autoscopic hallucination is the experience of seeing an image of oneself in external space. Charles Bonnet syndrome describes the condition where patients experience complex visual hallucinations associated with no other psychiatric symptoms or impairment in consciousness; it usually occurs in older adults and is associated with loss of vision. Lilliputian hallucinations are hallucinations of miniature people or animals and are associated with alcohol withdrawal.

Somatic hallucinations

These are hallucinations of bodily sensation and include superficial, visceral and kinaesthetic hallucinations.

Superficial hallucinations describe sensations on or just below the skin and may be:

- *Tactile* (*haptic*): experience of the skin being touched, pricked or pinched. Formication is the unpleasant sensation of insects crawling on or just below the skin; it is commonly associated with long-term cocaine use (cocaine bugs) and alcohol withdrawal.
- *Thermal*: false perception of heat or cold.
- *Hygric*: false perception of a fluid (e.g. 'I can feel water sloshing in my brain').

Visceral hallucinations describe false perceptions of the internal organs. Patients may be distressed by deep sensations of their organs throbbing, stretching, distending or vibrating.

Kinaesthetic hallucinations are false perceptions of joint or muscle sense. Patients may describe their limbs vibrating or being twisted. The fleeting but distressing sensation of free falling just as one is about to fall asleep is an example that most people have experienced (see Hypnagogic hallucinations later in this chapter).

Olfactory and gustatory hallucinations

These are the false perceptions of smell and taste. They commonly occur together because the two senses are closely related. A classic example is mood-congruent hallucinations of rotting flesh or burning in depression. However, in patients with new olfactory or gustatory hallucinations, it is important to rule out epilepsy (especially of the temporal lobe) and other organic brain diseases.

RED FLAG BOX

If a patient presents with visual, olfactory, or elementary hallucinations, consider the possibility of brain disorders such as delirium, migraine, epilepsy or cancer before attributing these symptoms to a primary psychiatric disorder.

Special forms of hallucination

Hypnagogic hallucinations are false perceptions in any modality (usually auditory or visual) that occur as a person goes to sleep; whereas, *hypnopompic hallucinations* occur as a person awakens. These occur commonly and do not indicate mental disorder.

Extracampine hallucinations are false perceptions that occur outside the limits of a person's normal sensory field (e.g. a patient describes hearing voices from 100 miles away). Patients often give delusional explanations for this phenomenon.

A *functional hallucination* occurs when a normal sensory stimulus is required to precipitate a hallucination in that same sensory modality (e.g. voices that are only heard when the doorbell rings). A *reflex hallucination* occurs when a normal sensory stimulus in one modality precipitates a hallucination in another (e.g. voices that are only heard whenever the lights are switched on).

Abnormal beliefs

Abnormal beliefs include primary and secondary delusions and overvalued ideas.

Delusions

A delusion is an unshakeable false belief that is not accepted by other members of the patient's culture. It is important to understand the following characteristics of delusional thinking:

- To the patient, there is no difference between a delusional belief and a true belief; they are the same experience. Therefore only an external observer can diagnose a delusion. A delusion is to ideation what an hallucination is to perception: both have the quality of reality to the person experiencing them.
- The delusion is false because of faulty reasoning. A man's delusional belief that his wife is having an affair may actually be true (she may indeed be unfaithful), but it remains a delusion because the reason he gives for this belief is undoubtedly false (e.g. she 'must' be having an affair because she is part of a top-secret sexual conspiracy to prove that he is a homosexual).
- A delusion is out of keeping with the patient's social and cultural background. It is crucial to establish that the belief is not one likely to be held by that person's subcultural group (e.g. a belief in the imminent second coming of Christ may be appropriate for a member of a religious group, but not for a formerly atheist, middle-aged businessman).

It is diagnostically significant to classify delusions as:

- Primary or secondary
- Mood congruent or mood incongruent

- Bizarre or non-bizarre
- According to the content of the delusion

Primary delusions (autochthonous delusions) do not occur in response to any previous psychopathological state; their genesis is not understandable. They may be preceded by a delusional atmosphere (mood) where patients have a sense that the world around them has been subtly altered, often in a sinister or threatening way. In this state a fully formed delusion has not yet developed and patients appear perplexed and apprehensive. Note that when a delusion occurs after a delusional atmosphere it is still regarded as primary; the delusional atmosphere is probably a precursor to the fully developed primary delusion. A delusional perception is also a primary delusion and occurs when a delusional meaning is attached to a normal perception (e.g. a patient believed he was a terrorist target because he heard an aeroplane flying in the distance). Primary delusions occur typically in schizophrenia and other primary psychotic disorders. *Secondary delusions* are the consequences of pre-existing psychopathological states, usually mood disorders (see Chapters 10 and 11). Many interrelated delusions that are centred on a common theme are termed systematized delusions.

In mood-congruent delusions, the contents of the delusions are appropriate to the patient's mood and are commonly seen in depression or mania with psychotic features.

Bizarre delusions are those which are extremely implausible (e.g. the belief that aliens have planted radioactive detonators in the patient's brain). They are considered to be characteristic of schizophrenia.

Table 9.1 lists the classification of delusions by their content. It is important that you can label a delusion according to its content, so take some time to familiarize yourself with this table.

HINTS AND TIPS

Note that the term 'paranoid' refers to any delusions or ideas that are unduly self-referent, typically feelings of persecution, grandeur or reference. It should not be used synonymously with the term 'persecutory'; (i.e. when a patient has a false belief that people are trying to harm him), do not say that he is paranoid, rather say that he has a persecutory delusion.

Finally, beliefs that were previously held with delusional intensity but then become held with less conviction are termed partial delusions. This occurs when patients are recovering.

COMMUNICATION

Direct questioning about perceptual experience may alienate a nonpsychotic patient and raise undue suspicion in a psychotic patient. To maintain rapport with patients, begin these questions with a primer such as: 'I am now going to ask you some questions which may seem a little strange, but are routine questions which I ask all patients'.

Overvalued ideas

An overvalued idea is a plausible belief that a patient becomes preoccupied with to an unreasonable extent. The key feature is that the pursuit of this idea causes considerable distress to the patient or those living around them (i.e. it is overvalued). Patients who hold overvalued ideas have usually had them for many years and typically have abnormalities of personality. They are distinguished from delusions by the lack of a gross abnormality in reasoning; these patients can often give fairly logical reasons for their beliefs. They differ from obsessions in that they are not experienced as recurrent intrusive thoughts. However, one will frequently encounter beliefs that span definitions. Typical disorders that feature overvalued ideas are anorexia nervosa, hypochondriacal disorder, dysmorphophobia, paranoid personality disorder and morbid jealousy (this can also take the form of a delusion). See Table 13.1 for tips on how to distinguish different types of abnormal thoughts.

Thought disorder

Thought disorder is when someone's speech is so disorganized that it is difficult to follow what is meant. Many patients with delusions are able to communicate in a clear and coherent manner; although their beliefs may be false, their speech is organized (thus delusions are an abnormality of thought content, not thought form). However, there is a subgroup of psychotic patients who speak in such a disorganized way that it becomes difficult to understand what they are saying. The coherency of patients with disorganized thinking varies from being mostly understandable in patients exhibiting circumstantial thinking to being completely incomprehensible in patients with a word salad phenomenon (see Fig. 9.2).

Describing the disturbance of a patient's thought form is one of the most challenging tasks facing clinicians. This problem is compounded by two factors: it is impossible to know what patients are actually thinking (i.e. thought form has to be inferred from their speech and behaviour); the unfortunate situation has arisen where various authors in psychiatry have described a different conceptual view of thought disorder, which has resulted in conflicting and confusing classification systems. It is not essential to be able to identify all the subgroups of thought disorder, but it is important that you are able to say when thought form is or is not disordered. To describe the nature of the thought

Table 9.1 Classification of delusions by content

Classification	Content
Persecutory delusions	False belief that one is being harmed, threatened, cheated, harassed or is a victim of a conspiracy
Grandiose delusions	False belief that one is exceptionally powerful (including having 'mystical powers'), talented or important
Delusions of reference	False belief that certain objects, people or events have intense personal significance and refer specifically to oneself (e.g. believing that a television newsreader is talking directly about one)
Religious delusions	False belief pertaining to a religious theme, often grandiose in nature (e.g. believing that one is a special messenger from God)
Delusions of love (erotomania)	False belief that another person is in love with one (commoner in women). In one form, termed 'de Clérambault syndrome', a woman (usually) believes that a man, frequently older and of higher status, is in love with her
Delusion of infidelity (morbid jealousy, Othello syndrome)	False belief that one's lover has been unfaithful. Note that morbid jealousy may also take the form of an overvalued idea, that is, nonpsychotic jealousy
Delusions of misidentification	Capgras syndrome: belief that a familiar person has been replaced by an exact double – an impostor Fregoli syndrome: belief that a complete stranger is actually a familiar person already known to one
Nihilistic delusions (see Cotard syndrome, Chapter 11.)	False belief that oneself, others or the world is nonexistent or about to end. In severe cases, negation is carried to the extreme with patients claiming that nothing, including themselves, exists
Somatic delusions	False belief concerning one's body and its functioning (e.g. that one's bowels are rotting). Also called 'hypochondriacal delusions' (to be distinguished from the overvalued ideas seen in hypochondriacal disorder)
Delusions of infestation (Ekbom syndrome)	False belief that one is infested with small but visible organisms. May also occur secondary to tactile hallucinations (e.g. formication; see Chapter 8)
Delusions of control (passivity or 'made' experiences) Note: these are all first-rank symptoms of schizophrenia	False belief that one's thoughts, feelings, actions or impulses are controlled or 'made' by an external agency (e.g. believing that one was 'made' to break a window by demons) Delusions of thought control include: 'Thought insertion': belief that thoughts or ideas are being implanted in one's head by an external agency 'Thought withdrawal': belief that one's thoughts or ideas are being extracted from one's head by an external agency 'Thought broadcasting': belief that one's thoughts are being diffused or broadcast to others such that they know what one is thinking

disorder you should have a clear understanding of the individual definitions you intend to use. To help describe thought disorder, it is particularly helpful if you document and are able to cite examples of the patient's speech in their own words.

HINTS AND TIPS

Many people have mildly disordered communication styles, particularly when tired or stressed. Perhaps you can think of someone you know who is often mildly circumstantial in their story telling? To count as thought disorder, the patient's thinking style should significantly impair effective communication.

The following are important signs of disorganized thinking:

Circumstantial and tangential thinking
See Chapter 10.

Flight of ideas
See Chapter 10.

Loosening of association (derailment/knight's move thinking)
This is when the patient's train of thought shifts suddenly from one very loosely or unrelated idea to the next. In its worst form, speech becomes a mixture of incoherent words and phrases and is termed 'word salad'. Loosening of association is characteristic of schizophrenia. Note that some

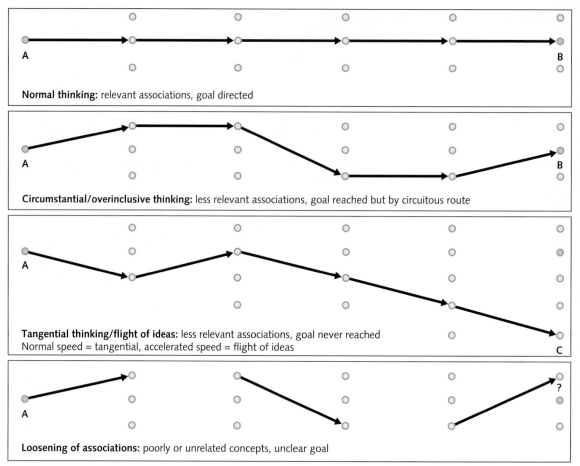

Fig. 9.2 Thought disorder: simplified representation.

psychiatrists, but not all, use the term 'formal thought disorder' synonymously with loosening of association.

Special forms of thought disorder

Thought blocking occurs when patients experience a sudden cessation to their flow of thought, often in mid-sentence (observed as sudden breaks in speech). Patients have no recall of what they were saying or thinking and thus continue talking about a different topic.

Neologisms are new words created by the patient, often combining syllables of other known words. Patients can also use recognized words idiosyncratically by attributing them with an unrecognized but related meaning (*metonyms*).

Perseveration is when an initially correct response is inappropriately repeated (e.g. unnecessarily repeating a previously expressed word or phrase). Palilalia describes the repetition of the last word of a sentence; logoclonia describes the repetition of the last syllable of the last word. Perseveration is highly suggestive of organic brain disease.

Echolalia is when patients senselessly repeat words or phrases spoken around them by others (i.e. like a parrot).

Irrelevant answers is when patients give answers that are completely unrelated to the original question.

Negative symptoms

Positive symptoms are those that are present when they should not be and include delusions, hallucinations and thought disorder. In contrast, negative symptoms are abilities that are absent when they should be present and include marked apathy, poverty of thought and speech, blunting of affect, social isolation, poor self-care and cognitive impairment. Patients can have positive and negative symptoms simultaneously or, as often happens, develop a negative presentation after initially presenting with predominantly positive symptoms. Remember that patients with a depressed mood or those experiencing significant side-effects from psychotropic medication may also present with what appear to be negative symptoms, which often presents a diagnostic challenge.

Psychomotor function

Although a relatively rare phenomenon in industrialized countries, some patients with psychosis will present with abnormalities of motor function. Motor system dysfunction in schizophrenia is usually due to the extrapyramidal side-effects of neuroleptic medication (see Chapter 2). However, patients with psychosis can occasionally present

Table 9.2 Motor symptoms in schizophrenia

Catatonic rigidity	Maintaining a fixed position and rigidly resisting all attempts to be moved
Catatonic posturing	Adopting an unusual or bizarre position that is then maintained for some time
Catatonic negativism	A seemingly motiveless resistance to all instructions or attempts to be moved; patients may do the opposite of what is asked
Catatonic waxy flexibility (cerea flexibilitas)	Patients can be 'moulded' like wax into a position that is then maintained
Catatonic excitement	Agitated, excited and seemingly purposeless motor activity, not influenced by external stimuli
Catatonic stupor	A presentation of 'akinesis' (lack of voluntary movement), 'mutism' and 'extreme unresponsiveness' in an otherwise alert patient (there may be slight clouding of consciousness)
Echopraxia	Patients senselessly repeat or imitate the actions of those around them. Associated with 'echolalia'; also occurs in patients with frontal lobe damage
Mannerisms	Apparently goal-directed movements (e.g. waving, saluting) that are performed repeatedly or at socially inappropriate times
Stereotypies	A complex, identically repeated movement that does not appear to be goal-directed (e.g. rocking to and fro, gyrating)
Tics	Sudden, involuntary, rapid, recurrent, nonrhythmic motor movements or vocalizations

with striking motor signs that are not caused by psychiatric medication or a known organic brain disease. Although undoubtedly associated with the patient's abnormal mental state, the cause of this psychomotor dysfunction is far from clarified. The term 'catatonia' literally means extreme muscular tone or rigidity; however, it commonly describes any excessive or decreased motor activity that is apparently purposeless and includes abnormalities of movement, tone or position. Note that catatonic symptoms are not diagnostic of schizophrenia; they may also be caused by brain diseases, metabolic abnormalities or psychoactive substances, and can also occur in mood disorders. Table 9.2 describes the common motor symptoms seen in schizophrenia.

DIFFERENTIAL DIAGNOSIS

Psychotic symptoms are nonspecific and are associated with many primary psychiatric illnesses. They can also present secondary to a general medical condition or psychoactive substance use. See Box 9.1 for the differential diagnosis for psychotic symptoms.

Psychotic disorders

Schizophrenia

There are no pathognomonic or singularly defining symptoms of schizophrenia; it is a syndrome characterized by a heterogeneous cluster of symptoms and signs. The International Statistical Classification of Diseases and Related Health Problems, 10th edition (ICD-10) has set out diagnostic guidelines based on the most commonly occurring symptom groups, which have been discussed in

> **BOX 9.1   DIFFERENTIAL DIAGNOSIS OF PSYCHOSIS**
>
> Psychotic disorders
> - Schizophrenia
> - Schizophrenia-like psychotic disorders
> - Schizoaffective disorder
> - Delusional disorder
>
> Mood disorders
> - Manic episode with psychotic features
> - Depressive episode, severe, with psychotic features
>
> Secondary to a general medical condition
> Secondary to psychoactive substance use
> Dementia/delirium
> Personality disorder (schizotypal, borderline, schizoid, paranoid)
> Neurodevelopmental disorder (autistic spectrum)

the preceding section (Box. 9.2). It is also important to establish that there has been a clear and marked deterioration in the patient's social and work functioning.

In the past, psychiatrists used Schneider's first-rank symptoms to make the diagnosis of schizophrenia. Kurt Schneider suggested that the presence of one or more first-rank symptoms in the absence of organic disease was of pragmatic value in making the diagnosis of schizophrenia. First-rank symptoms are still referred to, so you should familiarize yourself with them; they are presented in Box 9.3.

93

BOX 9.2   ICD-10 DIAGNOSTIC GUIDELINES FOR SCHIZOPHRENIA

One or more of the following symptoms:

a. Thought echo, insertion, withdrawal or broadcast
b. Delusions of control or passivity; delusional perception
c. Hallucinatory voices giving a running commentary; discussing the patient among themselves or 'originating' from some part of the body
d. Bizarre delusions

OR

Two or more of the following symptoms:

e. Other hallucinations that either occur every day for weeks or that are associated with fleeting delusions or sustained overvalued ideas
f. Thought disorganization (loosening of association, incoherence, neologisms)
g. Catatonic symptoms
h. Negative symptoms
i. Change in personal behaviour (loss of interest, aimlessness, social withdrawal)

Symptoms should be present for most of the time during at least 1 month

Schizophrenia should not be diagnosed in the presence of organic brain disease or during drug intoxication or withdrawal

BOX 9.3   SCHNEIDER'S FIRST-RANK SYMPTOMS OF SCHIZOPHRENIA

- Delusional perception
- Delusions of thought control: insertion, withdrawal, broadcast
- Delusions of control: passivity experiences of affect (feelings), impulse, volition and somatic passivity (influence controlling the body)
- Hallucinations: audible thoughts (first person or thought echo), voices arguing or discussing the patient, voices giving a running commentary

HINTS AND TIPS

Memory aid: if you add 'bizarre delusions' and 'hallucinations coming from a part of the body' to Schneider's first-rank symptoms you will have the a to d criteria of the ICD-10 diagnostic guidelines for schizophrenia.

Schizophrenia subtypes

Due to the differing presentations of schizophrenia, researchers have tried to identify schizophrenia subtypes. The importance of these subtypes is that they vary in their prognosis and treatment response. The ICD-10 has coded the following subtypes, which are not necessarily exclusive:

- *Paranoid schizophrenia*: dominated by the presence of delusions and hallucinations (positive symptoms). Negative and catatonic symptoms as well as thought disorganization are not prominent. The prognosis is usually better and the onset of illness later (typically 18–25 years) than the other subtypes.
- *Hebephrenic (disorganized) schizophrenia*: characterized by thought disorganization, disturbed behaviour and inappropriate or flat affect. Delusions and hallucination are fleeting or not prominent. Onset of illness is earlier (15 to 25 years of age) and the prognosis poorer than paranoid schizophrenia.
- *Catatonic schizophrenia*: a rare form characterized by one or more catatonic symptoms (see Table. 9.2).
- *Residual schizophrenia*: 1 year of predominantly chronic negative symptoms which must have been preceded by at least one clear-cut psychotic episode in the past.

Schizophrenia-like psychotic disorders

Some psychotic episodes with schizophrenia-like symptoms seem to have an abrupt onset (without a prodromal phase), precipitated by an acute life stress, or to have a shorter duration of symptoms than that usually observed in schizophrenia. The ICD-10 codes these as acute and transient psychotic disorders. The Diagnostic and Statistical Manual of Mental Disorders, 5th Edition, on the other hand, suggests diagnoses of schizophreniform disorder and brief psychotic disorder. Often these diagnoses are superseded by a later diagnosis of schizophrenia as the clinical picture evolves.

Schizoaffective disorder

Schizoaffective disorder describes the presentation of both schizophrenic and mood (depressed or manic) symptoms that present in the same episode of illness, either simultaneously or within a few days of each other. The mood symptoms should meet the criteria for either a depressive or manic episode. Patients should also have at least one, preferably two, of the typical symptoms of schizophrenia (i.e. symptoms (a) to (d) as specified in the ICD-10 schizophrenia diagnostic guidelines; see Box. 9.2). Depending on the particular mood symptoms displayed, this disorder can be coded in the ICD-10 as schizoaffective disorder, manic type or schizoaffective disorder, depressed type.

HINTS AND TIPS

When psychiatrists talk about the typical symptoms of schizophrenia, they are generally referring to points (a) to (d) of the ICD-10 criteria for schizophrenia (or Schneider's first-rank symptoms; e.g. delusions of control, running commentary hallucinations, etc).

Delusional disorder

In this disorder, the development of a single or set of delusions for the period of at least 3 months is the most prominent or only symptom. It usually has onset in middle age and may persist throughout the patient's life. Delusions can be persecutory, grandiose and hypochondriacal. Typically, schizophrenic delusions, such as delusions of thought control or passivity, exclude this diagnosis. Hallucinations, if present, tend to be only fleeting and are not typically schizophrenic in nature; brief depressive symptoms may also be evident. Affect, speech and behaviour are all normal and these patients usually have well-preserved personal and social skills. Rarely, patients may present with an induced delusional disorder (*folie à deux*), which occurs when a nonpsychotic patient with close emotional ties to another person suffering from delusions (usually a dominant figure) begins to share those delusional ideas themselves. The delusions in the non-psychotic patient tend to resolve when the two are separated.

Mood (affective) disorders

Manic episode with psychotic features
See Chapter 10.

Depressive episode, severe with psychotic features
See Chapter 11.

Psychotic episodes secondary to a general medical condition or psychoactive substance use

A medical or psychoactive substance cause of psychosis should always be sought for and ruled out. Box 9.4 lists the medical and substance-related causes of psychotic episodes. The medical condition or substance use should predate the development of the psychosis and symptoms should resolve with treatment of the condition or abstinence from the offending substance (although sometimes exposure to a recreational substance can precipitate a psychotic illness which never resolves). Absence of

---

BOX 9.4 MEDICAL AND SUBSTANCE-RELATED CAUSES OF PSYCHOTIC SYMPTOMS

Medical conditions:
- Cerebral neoplasm, infarcts, trauma, infection, inflammation (including HIV, CJD, neurosyphilis, herpes encephalitis)
- Endocrinological (thyroid, parathyroid, adrenal disorders)
- Epilepsy (especially temporal lobe epilepsy)
- Huntington disease
- Systemic lupus erythematosus
- Vitamin B_{12}, niacin (pellagra) and thiamine deficiency (Wernicke encephalopathy)
- Acute intermittent porphyria

Substances:
- Alcohol
- Cannabis
- Novel psychoactive substances
- Amphetamines
- Cocaine
- Hallucinogens
- Inhalants/solvents

Prescribed:
- Antiparkinsonian drugs
- Corticosteroids
- Anticholinergics

CJD, Creutzfeldt-Jakob disease; HIV, human immunodeficiency virus.

---

previous psychotic episodes and absence of a family history of schizophrenia also supports this diagnosis.

Delirium and dementia

Visual hallucinations and delusions are common in delirium and may also occur in dementia, particularly diffuse Lewy body dementia (see Chapter 19).

Personality disorder

In general, schizophrenia presents with a clear change in behaviour and functioning, sometimes with a prodrome, whereas patients with a personality or neurodevelopmental disorder have never achieved a normal baseline. Schizotypal (personality) disorder is characterized by eccentric behaviour and peculiarities of thinking and appearance. Although there are no clear psychotic symptoms evident and its course resembles that of a personality disorder, the ICD-10 actually describes schizotypal disorder in the chapter on psychotic disorders. This is because it is more prevalent among relatives of patients with schizophrenia and, occasionally, it progresses to overt schizophrenia. Borderline, paranoid and schizoid personality disorders also share similar features to schizophrenia without displaying clear-cut psychotic symptoms. Personality disorders are discussed in greater detail in Chapter 17.

Neurodevelopmental disorder

Social difficulties and rigid thinking are found in both autistic spectrum disorders and schizophrenia. See Chapter 18.

ALGORITHM FOR THE DIAGNOSIS OF PSYCHOTIC DISORDERS

See Fig. 9.3.

ASSESSMENT

History

The following questions may be helpful in eliciting psychotic phenomena on mental state examination:

Hallucinations

- Do you ever hear strange noises or voices when there is no one else about?
- Do you ever hear your own thoughts spoken aloud such that someone standing next to you might possibly hear them? (audible thoughts; first person auditory hallucinations)
- Do you ever hear your thoughts echoed just after you have thought them? (thought echo)
- Do these voices talk directly to you or give you commands? (second person auditory hallucinations)
- Do these voices ever talk about you with each other or make comments about what you are doing? (third person auditory hallucinations/running commentary)

Delusions

- Are you afraid that someone is trying to harm or poison you? (persecutory delusions)
- Have you noticed that people are doing or saying things that have a special meaning for you? (delusions of reference)
- Do you have any special abilities or powers? (grandiose delusions)
- Does it seem as though you are being controlled or influenced by some external force? (delusions of control)
- Are thoughts that don't belong to you being put into your head? (thought insertion)

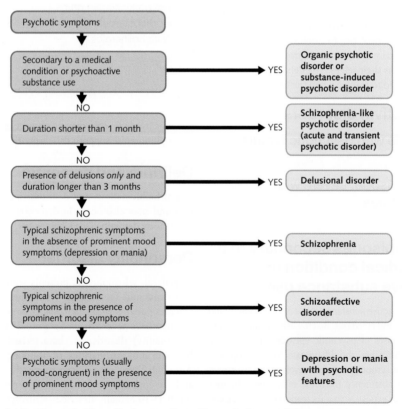

Fig. 9.3 Algorithm for the diagnosis of a patient presenting with psychotic symptoms.

It is important to obtain collateral information from the patient's GP, family and any other mental health professionals involved in their care to establish premorbid personality and functioning, as well as pattern of deterioration.

Examination

A basic physical examination including a thorough neurological and endocrine system examination should be performed on all patients with psychotic symptoms.

Investigations

Blood investigations are performed to:
- Exclude possible medical or substance-related causes of psychosis.
- Establish baseline values before administering antipsychotics and other psychotropic drugs.
- Assess renal and liver functioning which may affect elimination of drugs that are likely to be taken long-term and possibly in depot form.
- If the patient presents with a first episode of psychosis, a good basic screen comprises full blood count, erythrocyte sedimentation rate, urea and electrolytes, thyroid function, liver function tests, glucose, lipids, serum calcium, and serology for any suspected infections.
- A urine drug screen should always be done because recreational drugs both cause and exacerbate psychosis.
- An electrocardiogram should be done in patients with cardiac problems as many antipsychotics prolong the QT interval and have the potential to cause lethal ventricular arrhythmia.
- The use of a routine electroencephalogram, computed tomography (CT) or magnetic resonance imaging brain scan to help exclude an organic psychosis (e.g. temporal lobe epilepsy, brain tumour) varies between psychiatric units; they should always be considered in atypical cases, cases with treatment resistance or if there are cognitive or neurological abnormalities.

DISCUSSION OF CASE STUDY

Mr PP meets the ICD-10 criteria for schizophrenia, paranoid subtype. He has had a marked deterioration in his social and work functioning. He has delusions of persecution (believing he was a victim of government experiments), thought control (believing that ideas were being planted in his head – thought insertion) and reference (believing that the man in the pub was referring specifically to him). His claim that he knew these things after hearing the neighbour's dog bark suggests delusional perception. He also has second person command hallucinations and third person running commentary hallucinations. 'Receiving coded information' from the radio might be a hallucination or a delusion of reference depending on how Mr PP described this experience subjectively. Mr PP's description that 'all was not right' could indicate the presence of a delusional atmosphere, prior to the development of the full-blown delusions.

It is imperative that a substance-induced psychotic disorder or psychotic disorder secondary to a medical condition is excluded. It would be important to ascertain the duration of Mr PP's psychotic symptoms. It seems as though he has had schizophrenic symptoms for over a month. If the duration of symptoms had been less than a month, it would be advisable to diagnose a schizophrenia-like psychotic disorder (e.g. acute and transient psychotic disorder). It is important to rule out a mood disorder with psychotic features. The presence of a mood episode associated with simultaneous schizophrenic symptoms would suggest a schizoaffective episode. Prominent hallucinations militate against a diagnosis of delusional disorder.

Now go on to Chapter 21 to read more about the psychotic disorders and their management.

Chapter Summary

Psychosis is when the experience of reality is grossly distorted.
Psychotic symptoms comprise delusions, hallucinations and thought disorder.
- A delusion is a fixed, false, belief which arises through faulty reasoning, is not altered by evidence to the contrary, and is outside cultural norms.
- A hallucination is a perception in the absence of a stimulus.
- Thought disorder is speech so disorganized that communication is impaired.

When assessing someone with psychotic symptoms, explore
- the nature and content of their abnormal experiences (their signs and symptoms)
- how these symptoms are affecting them, and their current and past social circumstances (functional impact)
- their physical health and use of recreational substances
- obtain a collateral history from someone who knows them well (as lack of insight can prevent the patient giving a full history)

The key differentials for someone presenting with psychotic symptoms are: schizophrenia, mania with psychotic symptoms, drug-induced psychosis and psychosis secondary to a general medical condition.

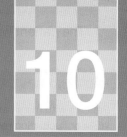
CASE SUMMARY

Feeling that she was no longer able to cope, Mrs EM consulted her general practitioner (GP) about a Mental Health Act assessment for her husband, Mr EM, a 37-year-old freelance writer. He had no psychiatric history other than a period of depression 2 years ago. He had progressively needed less sleep over the past 2 weeks and had not slept at all for 48 hours. Recently, he had started taking on increasing amounts of work and seemed to thrive on this due to an 'inexhaustible source of boundless energy'. He told his wife and all his friends that he had a new lease of life, as he was 'happier than ever'. Mrs EM became concerned when he developed lofty ideas that he was a world expert in his field, remaining convinced of this even when she tried to reason with him, and would talk incessantly for hours about elaborate and complicated writing schemes. Mr EM's behaviour had become markedly uncharacteristic over the past day or two, when he started making sexually inappropriate comments to his neighbour's wife and presented her with reams of poetry which he had spent the night writing. When Mrs EM suggested that he visit the GP, Mr EM became verbally aggressive saying that she was trying to bring him down because she was threatened by his 'irresistible sex appeal and wit'. Mrs EM was unable to reason with him and noticed that he struggled to keep to the point of the conversation, often bringing up issues that seemed completely irrelevant. The GP noted that, other than a recent bout of flu, Mr EM had no medical problems and was not using any prescribed medication. He denied using drugs or alcohol.

(For a discussion of the case study see the end of the chapter).

Just as spells of feeling sad and miserable are quite normal to the human experience, so too are periods where we feel elated, excited and full of energy. Although an irritable or elevated mood is not in itself pathological, it can be when grossly and persistently so, and when associated with another psychopathology.

DEFINITIONS AND CLINICAL FEATURES

In Chapter 11 we will observe how a disturbance in mood in addition to various other cognitive, biological and psychotic symptoms all contribute to the recognition of a depressive episode. A similar approach is taken to hypomanic and manic episodes; these occur on the opposite pole of the mood disorder spectrum to depression.

Core symptoms

The International Statistical Classification of Diseases and Related Health Problems, 10th edition (ICD-10) classification system specifies two core symptoms of a manic or hypomanic episode:

- Sustained elated, irritable or expansive mood
- Excessive activity or feelings of energy

When manic and depressive symptoms rapidly alternate (e.g. within the same day), this is termed a *mixed affective episode*.

Mood

The hallmark of a hypomanic or manic episode is an elevated or irritable mood. Patients often enjoy the experience of elevated mood and might describe themselves as feeling: 'high', 'on top of the world', 'fantastic' or 'euphoric'. This mood has an infectious quality, although those who know the patient well clearly see it as a deviation from normal. However, some patients tend to become extremely irritable or suspicious when manic and do not enjoy the experience at all. They have a low frustration tolerance and any thwarting of their plans can lead to a rapid escalation in anger or even delusions of persecution.

Increased energy

This initially results in an increase in goal-directed activity and, when coupled with impaired judgement, can have disastrous consequences (e.g. patients may instigate numerous risky business ventures, go on excessive spending sprees, or engage in reckless promiscuity that is unusual for them). However, in severe episodes actions can become repetitive, stereotyped and apparently purposeless, even progressing to a *manic stupor* in the extremely unwell. If left untreated, excessive overactivity can lead to physical exhaustion, dehydration and sometimes even death. On mental state examination, increased energy can be seen as *psychomotor excitation*: the patient is unable to sit still, frequently standing up, pacing around the room and gesticulating expansively.

Biological symptoms

Decreased need for sleep

This is a very important early warning sign of mania or hypomania. Sleep disturbance can range from only needing a few hours of sleep a night to a manic patient going for days on end with no sleep at all. Crucially, it is not associated with fatigue.

Cognitive symptoms

Elevated sense of self-esteem or grandiosity

Hypomanic patients may overestimate their abilities and social or financial status. In severe cases, manic patients may have delusions of grandeur (see later).

Poor concentration

Manic patients may find it difficult to maintain their focus on any one thing as they struggle to filter out irrelevant external stimuli (background noise, other objects or people in the room), making them, as a consequence, highly distractible.

Accelerated thinking and speech

Manic patients may subjectively experience their thoughts or ideas racing even faster than they can articulate them. When patients have an irrepressible need to express these thoughts verbally, making them difficult to interrupt, it is termed *pressure of speech*. When thoughts are rapidly associating in this way in a stream of connected (but not always relevant) concepts it is termed *flight of ideas*. Some hypomanic patients express themselves by incessant letter writing, poetry, doodling or artwork.

Impaired judgement and insight

This is typical of manic illness and sometimes results in costly indiscretions that patients may later regret. Lack of insight into their illness can be a difficult barrier to overcome when trying to engage patients in essential treatment.

Psychotic symptoms

Psychotic symptoms are far more common in manic than in depressive episodes and include disorders of *thought form, thought content* and *perception*.

Disordered thought form

Disordered thought form (see Chapter 9 and Fig. 9.2) commonly occurs in schizophrenia but is regularly seen in manic episodes with psychotic features and to a lesser degree in psychotic forms of unipolar depression. The most common thought form disorders in mania are circumstantiality, tangentiality and flight of ideas. However, signs of thought disorder most typical for schizophrenia can also be seen in manic episodes (e.g. loosening of association, neologisms and thought blocking).

Circumstantiality and tangentiality

Circumstantial (over-inclusive) speech means speech that is delayed in reaching its final goal because of the over-inclusion of details and unnecessary asides and diversions; however, the speaker, if allowed to finish, does eventually connect the original starting point to the desired destination. Circumstantiality need not be pathological – most families have at least one person who takes forever to finish a story! Tangential speech, on the other hand, is more indicative of psychopathology and sees the speaker diverting from the initial train of thought but never returning to the original point, jumping tangentially from one topic to the next.

Flight of ideas

As described earlier, flight of ideas occurs when thinking is markedly accelerated, resulting in a stream of connected concepts. The link between concepts can be as in normal communication where one idea follows directly on from the next or can be links that are not relevant to an overall goal. For example, links made through wordplay such as a pun or clang association; or through some vague idea which is not part of the original goal of speech (e.g. 'I need to go to bed now. Have you ever smelt my bed of roses? Ah, but a rose by any other name would smell just as sweet!'). Even though manic patients may appear to be talking gibberish, a written transcript of their speech will usually reveal that their ideas are related in some, albeit obscure, way.

As patients become increasingly manic, their associations tend to loosen as they find it increasingly difficult to link their thoughts. Eventually they approach the incoherent thought disorder sometimes seen in schizophrenia (see Chapter 9).

Abnormal beliefs

Patients with elated mood will typically present with *grandiose delusions* in which they believe they have special importance or unusual powers. *Persecutory delusions* are also common, especially in patients with an irritable mood, and often feature them believing that others are trying to take advantage of their exalted status. When the content of delusions matches the mood of the patient, the delusions are termed *mood-congruent*. Very often, patients with elevated mood may have overvalued ideas as opposed to true delusions, which are important to distinguish, as the former are not regarded as psychotic in nature (see Chapter 9).

Perceptual disturbance

Some hypomanic patients may describe subtle distortions of perception. These are not psychotic symptoms and mainly include altered intensity of perception such that sounds seem louder (hyperacusis) or colours seem brighter and more vivid (visual hyperaesthesia). Psychotic perceptual features develop when manic patients experience hallucinations. This is usually in the form of voices encouraging or exciting them.

HINTS AND TIPS

Always screen for psychotic symptoms in patients suffering from a manic episode. The prevalence is very high – two-thirds report experiencing psychotic symptoms during such an episode. Interestingly, only one third report psychotic symptoms during a depressive episode.

DIFFERENTIAL DIAGNOSIS

Like depression, an elevated or irritable mood can be secondary to a medical condition, psychoactive substance use or other psychiatric disorder. These will have to be excluded before a primary mood disorder can be diagnosed. Box 10.1 shows the differential diagnosis for patients presenting with elevated or irritable mood.

BOX 10.1 DIFFERENTIAL DIAGNOSIS FOR PATIENT PRESENTING WITH ELEVATED OR IRRITABLE MOOD

Mood disorders
- Hypomania, mania, mixed affective episode (isolated episode or part of bipolar affective disorder)
- Cyclothymia
- Depression (may present with irritable mood)

Secondary to a general medical condition

Secondary to psychoactive substance use

Psychotic disorders
- Schizoaffective disorder (may be similar to mania with psychotic features)
- Schizophrenia

Personality disorder (with prominent traits of disinhibition, negative affect or dissocial features)

Neurodevelopmental disorder (attention deficit hyperactivity disorder)

Delirium/dementia

Mood (affective) disorders

Hypomanic, manic and mixed affective episodes

The ICD-10 specifies three degrees of severity of a manic episode: *hypomania, mania without psychotic symptoms* and *mania with psychotic symptoms*. All of these share the above-mentioned general characteristics, most notably: an elevated or irritable mood and an increase in the quantity and speed of mental and physical activity. If psychotic symptoms are present, the episode is by definition mania. In those without psychotic symptoms, the distinction between mania and hypomania can be hard to judge and hinges on the degree of functional impairment (Fig. 10.1) If the person is experiencing rapidly alternating (e.g. within a few hours of each other) manic and depressive symptoms they are diagnosed with a *mixed affective episode*.

Bipolar affective disorder

Most patients who present with a hypomanic, manic or mixed affective episode will have experienced a previous episode of mood disturbance (depression, hypomania, mania or mixed). In this case they should be diagnosed with bipolar affective disorder. Most patients who experience hypomanic or manic episodes also experience depressive episodes, hence, the commonly used term: 'manic-depression'. However, patients who only suffer from manic or hypomanic episodes with no intervening depressive episodes are also classified as having bipolar affective disorder, even though their mood does not swing to the depressive pole. It is good practice to record the

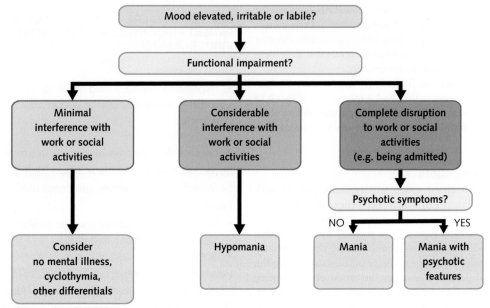

Fig. 10.1 Distinguishing mania from hypomania.

nature of the current episode in a patient with bipolar affective disorder (e.g. '*bipolar affective disorder, current episode manic without psychotic features*').

Cyclothymic disorder

Cyclothymic disorder (or cyclothymia) is analogous to dysthymia (see Chapter 11) in that it usually begins in early adulthood and follows a chronic course with intermittent periods of wellness in between. It is characterized by an instability of mood over at least 2 years resulting in alternating periods of mild elation and mild depression, none of which are sufficiently severe or long enough to meet the criteria for either a hypomanic or a depressive episode.

Depression

There are three common scenarios where a patient with a primary depressive disorder may present with an elevated or irritable mood. An 'agitated depression' can present with a prominent irritable mood, which, when coupled with psychomotor agitation, can be difficult to distinguish from a manic episode; depressed patients who are responding to antidepressants or electroconvulsive therapy may experience a transient period of elevated mood; and a patient with a recently resolved depressive disorder might misidentify euthymia for hypomania.

Manic episodes secondary to a general medical condition or psychoactive substance use

A medical or psychoactive substance cause of mania should always be sought for and ruled out. Box 10.2 lists the medical

---

BOX 10.2   MEDICAL AND SUBSTANCE CAUSES OF MANIA

Medical conditions:

- Cerebral neoplasms, infarcts, trauma, infection (including HIV), autoimmune encephalitis
- Cushing disease
- Huntington disease
- Hyperthyroidism
- Multiple sclerosis
- Renal failure
- Systemic lupus erythematosus
- Temporal lobe epilepsy
- Vitamin B12 and niacin (pellagra) deficiency

Substances:

- Amphetamines
- Cocaine
- Hallucinogens
- Novel psychoactive substances

Prescribed:

- Anabolic steroids
- Antidepressants
- Corticosteroids
- Dopaminergic agents (e.g. L-dopa, selegiline, bromocriptine)

and substance-related causes of mania. The medical condition or substance use should predate the development of the mood disorder and symptoms should resolve with treatment of the condition or abstinence from the offending substance. Absence of previous manic episodes and lack of a family history of bipolar affective disorder also supports this diagnosis.

Schizophreniform disorders

Schizoaffective disorder

See Chapter 9. This can be very difficult to distinguish from a manic episode with psychotic features.

Schizophrenia

Patients with schizophrenia can present with an excited, suspicious or agitated mood and therefore can be difficult to distinguish from manic patients with psychotic symptoms. Table 10.1 compares relevant features that might act as clues to the correct diagnosis.

Personality/neurodevelopmental disorders

Patients with disorders of personality or neurodevelopment often report features similar to hypomania, e.g. impulsivity, displays of temper and lability of mood in personality disorder with prominent features of negative affect, disinhibition or dissocial features or in attention deficit hyperactivity disorder. However, personality and neurodevelopmental disorders involve stable and enduring behaviour patterns, unlike the more discrete episodes of bipolar affective disorder, which are characterized by a distinct, demarcated deterioration in psychosocial functioning. Further, mood instability in personality disorder or neurodevelopmental disorder tends to fluctuate more rapidly (e.g. from hour to hour). See Chapters 17 and 18.

Delirium/dementia

Insomnia, agitation and psychotic symptoms in an older adult can be a presentation of hyperactive delirium or of behavioural and psychological symptoms of dementia. See Chapter 19.

ASSESSMENT

History

The following questions might be helpful in eliciting the key symptoms of mania/hypomania:

- Have you been feeling particularly happy or on top of the world lately?

Table 10.1 Psychopathological distinctions between mania and schizophrenia (these are guidelines only; typically schizophrenic symptoms can occur in mania and vice versa)

Psychopathology	Mania	Schizophrenia
Thought form	Circumstantiality, tangentiality, flight of ideas	Loosening of association, neologisms, thought blocking
Delusions	Most often mood-congruent (grandiose delusions or persecutory delusions)	Delusions unrelated to mood, bizarre delusions, delusions of passivity (e.g. thought insertion, withdrawal, broadcast)
Speech	Pressured speech, difficult to interrupt	Speech is often hesitant or halting
Biological symptoms	Significantly reduced need for sleep, increased physical and mental energy	Sleep less disturbed, less hyperactive
Psychomotor function	Agitation	Agitation, catatonic symptoms or negative symptoms

- Do you sometimes feel as though you have too much energy compared with people around you?
- Do you find yourself needing less sleep but not getting tired?
- Have you had any new interests or exciting ideas lately?
- Have you noticed your thoughts racing in your head?
- Do you have any special abilities or powers?

Examination

A basic physical examination, including a thorough neurological and endocrine system examination, should be performed on all patients with elevated mood.

Investigations

As for the depressive disorders (see Chapter 11), social, psychological and physical investigations are normally performed on manic patients to establish the diagnosis and to rule out an organic or substance-related cause (see Box 10.2). A urine drug screen is essential in anyone presenting with a first episode of elated mood.

ALGORITHM FOR THE DIAGNOSIS OF MOOD DISORDERS

See Fig. 10.2.

DISCUSSION OF CASE STUDY

Mr EM appears to be suffering from a *manic episode with psychotic features*. He has an elated mood and has developed the grandiose delusion that he is a world expert (mood-congruent psychotic symptom); note also the rapid switch to irritable mood when confronted. Biological symptoms include the reduced need for sleep and increased mental and physical energy with overactivity. Cognitive symptoms include elevated sense of self-importance, poor concentration, accelerated thinking with pressure of speech and impaired judgement and insight. The episode is classified as manic because of the severe impairment in social and probably work functioning, and because of the psychotic features.

Although Mr EM denied using drugs or alcohol, intoxication with substances (e.g. a novel psychoactive substance) is an important differential. A urine drug screen could exclude amphetamines and a collateral history might help to identify any existing pattern of substance use. However, the long duration of symptoms (2 weeks) is less suggestive of substance-induced manic symptoms, which would typically resolve over a few days.

The past psychiatric history is extremely important in this case. A previous mood episode (hypomanic, manic, depressive, mixed) is required in order to make the diagnosis of bipolar affective disorder. Mr EM had a period of depression 2 years prior to developing this manic episode, suggesting the diagnosis is: *bipolar affective disorder, current episode manic with psychotic features*. Previous psychotic episodes would add schizoaffective disorder and schizophrenia to the differential diagnosis. Now go on to Chapter 22 to read about the mood disorders and their management.

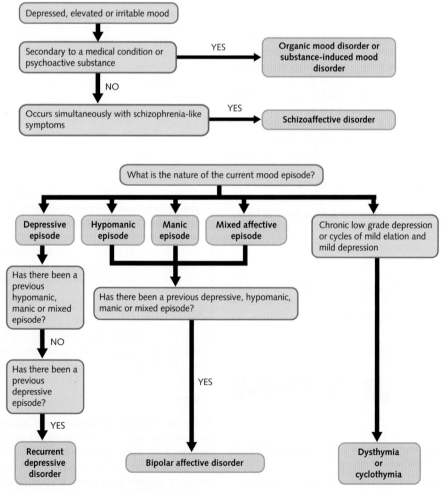

Fig. 10.2 Algorithm for the diagnosis of mood disorders.

- A manic episode is a sustained period (at least a week) of extremely elated or irritable mood associated with increased activity and energy.
- A hypomanic episode has the same symptoms as a manic episode but without marked impairment in functioning.
- A mixed affective episode is the rapid alternation between symptoms of mania and depression over a sustained period (at least 2 weeks).
- Psychotic symptoms can occur in mania, generally mood-congruent.
- Bipolar affective disorder is diagnosed when episodes of mood disorder recur.
- The key differential diagnoses for an episode of elated mood are a substance use disorder or psychotic disorder.
- When assessing someone with elated mood, ask about the four domains of: core symptoms, biological symptoms, cognitive symptoms and psychotic symptoms.

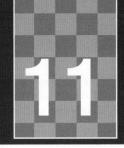
CASE SUMMARY

Mrs LM, a 32-year-old married housewife with two children aged 4 and 6 years, presented to her general practitioner stating that she was persistently unhappy and had been crying repeatedly over the past few weeks. She had no previous psychiatric history or significant medical history and her only regular medication was oral contraception. She had moved to the area 3 years earlier when her husband was promoted and, at first, appeared to have integrated well into the neighbourhood by involving herself in the organization of a toddlers' group. Unfortunately, the group had dissolved a few months ago when her co-organizer and only close confidante had moved away. Deprived of her most important social outlet, Mrs LM found herself increasingly dominated by her young children. Although usually an outgoing person, she noticed that her motivation to keep in touch with other mothers from the group had started to dwindle. At the same time, she started feeling persistently weary even though her work schedule had not increased, and often awakened 2–3 hours earlier in the morning. Although her appetite had not increased, she had turned to food for 'comfort' and had gained over 14 pounds. in weight. Mrs LM also candidly admitted that she was drinking more alcohol than usual. She described feeling incompetent because she was always miserable and had become too tired to look after the children. She felt guilty for burdening her husband and started crying when talking about her loss of interest in sex and her feelings of unattractiveness. Mrs LM maintained that no aspect of her life gave her pleasure and when asked specifically by her doctor, admitted that she had started to wonder whether her children and husband would be better off without her.

(For a discussion of the case study see the end of the chapter).

Feeling sad or upset is a normal part of the human condition; thus a patient presenting with emotional suffering does not necessarily warrant a psychiatric diagnosis or require treatment. However, psychiatrists agree that when patients present with a certain number of key depressive features, they are probably suffering from some form of psychopathology that will require, and usually respond to, specific kinds of treatment.

DEFINITIONS AND CLINICAL FEATURES

Core symptoms

Whereas feelings describe a short-lived emotional experience, mood refers to a patient's sustained, subjectively experienced emotional state over a period of time. Patients may describe a depressed mood in a number of ways, such as feeling sad, dejected, despondent, 'down in the dumps', miserable, 'low in spirits' or 'heavy-hearted'. They are unable to just lift themselves out of this mood and its severity is often out of proportion to the stressors in their surrounding social environment.

HINTS AND TIPS

At least 2 weeks of daily low mood, loss of interest or pleasure, and fatigability are the three core symptoms of depression.

The term 'affect' has two uses in psychiatry. It can be used synonymously with mood or emotion, as in the affective (mood) disorders. However, it is most often used to describe the transient natural fluctuations of emotional state that occur from moment to moment. For example, you might notice a patient is tearful when discussing the death of their mother but smiles when discussing their holiday plans. The range and appropriateness of a patient's affect is documented as part of the mental state exam. People with depression may have a reduced range of affect, with a monotonous voice and minimal facial expression (see Chapter 1).

The International Statistical Classification of Diseases and Related Health Problems, 10th edition (ICD-10) classification system specifies three core symptoms of depression:

- Depressed mood, which varies little from day to day and is unresponsive to circumstances (although diurnal variation may be present, with mood worse in the mornings)
- Markedly reduced interest in almost all activities, associated with the loss of ability to derive pleasure from activities that were formerly enjoyed (partial or complete anhedonia)
- Lack of energy or increased fatigability on minimal exertion leading to diminished activity (anergia)

A range of other symptoms are also associated with a depressive episode. They can be considered under the subheadings biological, cognitive and psychotic symptoms.

HINTS AND TIPS

Remember the distinction between the terms 'mood' and 'affect'; they are not the same. One way to remember the difference is that mood is like the climate and affect like the weather.

HINTS AND TIPS

Know the biological symptoms of depression; they are often asked for in exams. The key ones relate to sleep and appetite.

Biological (somatic) symptoms

In the past, psychiatrists distinguished between 'endogenous' or 'reactive' depression. 'Endogenous' depression (also called somatic, melancholic, vital or biological depression) was assumed to occur in the absence of an external environmental cause and have a 'biological' clinical picture. This is opposed to so-called 'reactive' or 'neurotic' depression where it is assumed that the patient is, to some degree, understandably depressed, reacting to adverse psychosocial circumstances. However, most depression is a mixture of the two, and an 'understandable depression' does not require any less treatment than a 'spontaneous depression'. 'Biological' symptoms are still important to enquire about as, if present, they suggest a more severe depression; however, they are no longer viewed as providing information on aetiology.

Early morning wakening

Although patients may get off to sleep at their normal time, they wake at least 2 hours earlier than they would usually, and then find it impossible to get back to sleep again. Further disturbances of sleep in depression include: difficulty falling asleep (initial insomnia), frequent awakening during the night and excessive sleeping (hypersomnia). Although all of these contribute to the diagnosis of depression, only early morning wakening is a biological symptom.

Depression worse in the morning

Diurnal variation of mood means that a patient's abnormal mood is more pronounced at a specific time of day. A depressive mood consistently and specifically worse in the morning is an important biological symptom.

Marked loss of appetite with weight loss

Although some depressed patients have an increased appetite and turn to 'comfort eating', only a dramatic reduction in appetite with weight loss (5% of body weight in last month) is regarded as a biological symptom. Note that the reversed biological features of overeating and oversleeping are sometimes referred to as atypical depressive symptoms.

Psychomotor retardation or agitation

The term 'psychomotor' is used to describe a patient's motor activity as a consequence of their concurrent mental processes. Psychomotor changes in depression can include retardation (slow, monotonous speech, long pauses before answering questions, or muteness; leaden body movements and limited facial expression (i.e. blunted affect)) or conversely, agitation (inability to sit still; fidgeting, pacing or hand-wringing; rubbing or scratching skin or clothes). Note that psychomotor changes must be severe enough to be observable by others, not just the subjective experience of the patient.

Loss of libido

Sensitive questioning will often reveal a reduction in sex drive that may lead to guilt when the sufferer feels unable to satisfy their partner.

Cognitive symptoms

Cognition has two meanings in psychiatry: it refers broadly to brain processing functions (e.g. concentrating, learning, making decisions) and also more specifically to the thoughts patients have about themselves and the world, which are conclusions arrived at by cognition (e.g. I failed my maths exam, therefore I will fail all exams; (see Chapter 3)).

Reduced concentration and memory

Depressed patients report difficulty in sustaining attention while doing previously manageable tasks. They often appear easily distracted and may complain of memory difficulties. They may feel indecisive.

- Obsessions or compulsions must be present for at least 2 successive weeks and are a source of distress or interfere with the patient's functioning
- They are acknowledged as coming from the patient's own mind
- The obsessions are unpleasantly repetitive
- At least one thought or act is resisted unsuccessfully (note that in chronic cases some symptoms may no longer be resisted)
- A compulsive act is not in itself pleasurable (excluding the relief of anxiety)

definition of obsessions and compulsions. Also, when repetitive thoughts occur in the context of other mental disorders, the contents of these thoughts are limited exclusively to the type of disorder concerned (e.g. morbid fear of fatness in anorexia nervosa, ruminative thoughts of worthlessness in depression, fear of dreaded objects in phobias). Table 13.3 lists the differential diagnoses and key distinguishing features of patients presenting with obsessive-compulsive symptomatology. OCD can also be comorbid with other psychiatric conditions, particularly depression and, less commonly, schizophrenia. Fig. 13.1

suggests a diagnosis algorithm that may be useful in differentiating OCD from other psychiatric conditions (see also Fig. 12.3).

HINTS AND TIPS

A key differential for an obsession is a delusion. They can be distinguished by checking whether the patient knows the thought is false and a product of their own mind (an obsession) or believes it to be true and representing external reality (a delusion).

You should always consider depression in patients with obsessions or compulsions because:

- Over 20% of depressed patients have obsessive-compulsive symptoms, which occur at or after the onset of depression. They invariably resolve with treatment of the depression.
- Over two-thirds of patients with OCD experience a depressive episode in their lifetime. Obsessions and compulsions are present before and persist after the treatment of depression.
- OCD is a disabling illness and patients often have chronic mild depressive symptoms that do not fully meet the criteria for a depressive episode. These symptoms usually resolve when the OCD is treated and the patient's quality of life improves.

Table 13.3 Differential diagnosis for patients presenting with obsessions or compulsions

Diagnosis	Diagnostic features
Obsessions and compulsions	
Obsessive-compulsive disorder	At least 2 weeks of genuine obsessions and compulsions (see Box 13.2)
Eating disorders[a] (see Chapter 16)	Morbid fear of fatness (over-valued idea) Thoughts and actions are not recognized by patient as excessive or unreasonable and are not resisted (ego-syntonic) Thoughts do not necessarily provoke, nor do actions reduce, distress
Obsessive-compulsive (anankastic) personality disorder (see Chapter 17)	Enduring behaviour pattern of rigidity, doubt, perfectionism and pedantry Ego-syntonic No true obsessions or compulsions
Autism spectrum disorder (see Chapter 18)	Restricted, stereotyped interests, typically related to physical aspects of objects or to classification and collecting. Pleasurable, not viewed as unreasonable, not resisted. Repetitive behaviours (e.g. rocking or hand-flapping) are performed to gain or reduce sensory input, not to reduce anxiety following an obsessional thought. Associated features are impairments in communication and social understanding.
Mainly obsessions	
Depressive disorder (see Chapter 11)	Obsessive-compulsive symptoms occur simultaneously with, or after the onset of, depression and resolve with treatment Obsessions are mood-congruent (e.g. ruminative thoughts of worthlessness)

Continued

Table 13.3 Differentiating diagnosis for patients presenting with obsessions or compulsions—cont'd

Diagnosis	Diagnostic features
Other anxiety disorders (see Chapter 12)	Phobias: provoking stimulus comes from external object or situation rather than patient's own mind Generalized anxiety disorder: excessive concerns about real-life circumstances Absence of genuine obsessions or compulsions
Hypochondriacal disorder (see Chapter 15)	Obsessions only related to the fear of having a serious disease or bodily disfigurement
Schizophrenia (see Chapter 9)	Thought insertion: patients believe that thoughts are not from their own mind Delusion: patients to do not attempt to resist thought Presence of other schizophrenic symptoms Lack of insight
Mainly compulsions	
Habit and impulse-control disorders: pathological gambling, kleptomania, trichotillomania	Repetitious impulses and behaviour (gambling, stealing, pulling out hair) with no other unrelated obsessions/compulsions Concordant with the patient's own wishes (therefore ego-syntonic)
Gilles de la Tourette syndrome (see Chapter 18)[b]	Motor and vocal tics, echolalia, coprolalia

[a] There is a higher incidence of true obsessive-compulsive disorder in patients with anorexia nervosa.
[b] 35%–50% of patients with Gilles de la Tourette syndrome meet the diagnostic criteria for obsessive-compulsive disorder, whereas only 5%–7% of patients with obsessive-compulsive disorder have Tourette syndrome

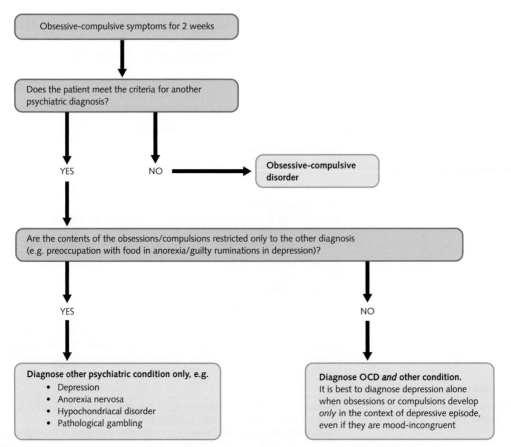

Fig. 13.1 Algorithm for the diagnosis of obsessions and compulsions.

BOX 13.2   ICD-10 DIAGNOSTIC GUIDELINES FOR OBSESSIVE-COMPULSIVE DISORDER

- Obsessions or compulsions must be present for at least 2 successive weeks and are a source of distress or interfere with the patient's functioning
- They are acknowledged as coming from the patient's own mind
- The obsessions are unpleasantly repetitive
- At least one thought or act is resisted unsuccessfully (note that in chronic cases some symptoms may no longer be resisted)
- A compulsive act is not in itself pleasurable (excluding the relief of anxiety)

suggests a diagnosis algorithm that may be useful in differentiating OCD from other psychiatric conditions (see also Fig. 12.3).

HINTS AND TIPS

A key differential for an obsession is a delusion. They can be distinguished by checking whether the patient knows the thought is false and a product of their own mind (an obsession) or believes it to be true and representing external reality (a delusion).

definition of obsessions and compulsions. Also, when repetitive thoughts occur in the context of other mental disorders, the contents of these thoughts are limited exclusively to the type of disorder concerned (e.g. morbid fear of fatness in anorexia nervosa, ruminative thoughts of worthlessness in depression, fear of dreaded objects in phobias). Table 13.3 lists the differential diagnoses and key distinguishing features of patients presenting with obsessive-compulsive symptomatology. OCD can also be comorbid with other psychiatric conditions, particularly depression and, less commonly, schizophrenia. Fig. 13.1

You should always consider depression in patients with obsessions or compulsions because:

- Over 20% of depressed patients have obsessive-compulsive symptoms, which occur at or after the onset of depression. They invariably resolve with treatment of the depression.
- Over two-thirds of patients with OCD experience a depressive episode in their lifetime. Obsessions and compulsions are present before and persist after the treatment of depression.
- OCD is a disabling illness and patients often have chronic mild depressive symptoms that do not fully meet the criteria for a depressive episode. These symptoms usually resolve when the OCD is treated and the patient's quality of life improves.

Table 13.3 Differential diagnosis for patients presenting with obsessions or compulsions

Diagnosis	Diagnostic features
Obsessions and compulsions	
Obsessive-compulsive disorder	At least 2 weeks of genuine obsessions and compulsions (see Box 13.2)
Eating disorders[a] (see Chapter 16)	Morbid fear of fatness (over-valued idea) Thoughts and actions are not recognized by patient as excessive or unreasonable and are not resisted (ego-syntonic) Thoughts do not necessarily provoke, nor do actions reduce, distress
Obsessive-compulsive (anankastic) personality disorder (see Chapter 17)	Enduring behaviour pattern of rigidity, doubt, perfectionism and pedantry Ego-syntonic No true obsessions or compulsions
Autism spectrum disorder (see Chapter 18)	Restricted, stereotyped interests, typically related to physical aspects of objects or to classification and collecting. Pleasurable, not viewed as unreasonable, not resisted. Repetitive behaviours (e.g. rocking or hand-flapping) are performed to gain or reduce sensory input, not to reduce anxiety following an obsessional thought. Associated features are impairments in communication and social understanding.
Mainly obsessions	
Depressive disorder (see Chapter 11)	Obsessive-compulsive symptoms occur simultaneously with, or after the onset of, depression and resolve with treatment Obsessions are mood-congruent (e.g. ruminative thoughts of worthlessness)

Continued

amenorrhoea, lethargy, bradycardia and lanugo (fine downy hair on torso). Her extremely low BMI, moderate bradycardia and history of almost collapsing while exercising place her at moderate to high physical risk. She requires a complete physical examination, and same day bloods and ECG to assess for any acute life-threatening complications.

She will require urgent treatment to stabilize then increase weight.

Now go on to Chapter 24 to read about the eating disorders and their management.

● **Chapter Summary**

- The key psychopathology in eating disorders is the overvalued idea of being overweight.
- Anorexia nervosa is associated with a significantly reduced body mass index (BMI), bulimia with a normal BMI.
- Purging behaviours are common in both disorders, including vomiting and laxative misuse.
- Restrictive behaviours are common in anorexia nervosa, including over-exercise and fasting.
- Anorexia nervosa can be associated with life-threatening physical complications, and it is important to perform a full physical examination (including muscle power), blood tests and electrocardiogram at presentation and frequently during treatment.

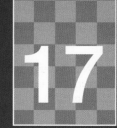
CASE SUMMARY

The on-call psychiatrist was asked to assess Miss BP, a 27-year-old woman who had been known to mental health services since the age of 17 years with symptoms that had been fairly consistent. She lived with her mother, who had contacted services because Miss BP was threatening to jump in front of a bus. Her father had sexually abused her as a child and she had a long history of self-harm that included cutting and repeated overdoses. Her mother was inclined to challenge her promiscuous behaviour and binge drinking, which led to many heated arguments. At interview, Miss BP told the psychiatrist that she was feeling 'more depressed than ever' because her mother had suggested that she move into her own house. With gentle questioning, it transpired that she was afraid that her mother would stop caring for her if she moved out. The psychiatrist, who had known Miss BP for years, recognized that this behaviour was not unusual for her and was able to help her to see another perspective to her mother's suggestion. Miss BP's mood quickly lifted and her suicidal ideation resolved.

(For a discussion of the case study see the end of the chapter).

The description and management of what has been arbitrarily designated 'personality disorder' is one of the most controversial subjects in psychiatry. They overlap substantially with the concept of neurodevelopmental disorders (see Chapter 18) but are currently considered separately. Classification changes are underfoot, with the draft version of the International Statistical Classification of Diseases and Related Health Problems, 11th edition (ICD-11; not yet published) proposing substantial changes. People use the term 'personality' with varying meanings, even within the psychological and psychiatric specialties. Amid the lack of consensus on what defines personality, there is little doubt that some people seem to experience and interact with the world in a manner markedly different to other individuals in their culture. Personality disorders are important: they are common, associated with significant distress to the sufferer and often with great cost to health care and social and criminal justice agencies.

DEFINITIONS AND CLINICAL FEATURES

Personality traits are enduring patterns of perceiving, thinking about, and relating to both self and the environment, exhibited in a wide range of social and personal contexts. A *personality disorder* is when an individual has traits that are persistently inflexible and maladaptive, are stable over time, appeared in adolescence or early adulthood and that cause significant personal distress or functional impairment to the person or those around them.

Patients with a personality disorder tend not to regard their patterns of behaviour as inherently abnormal. Instead, they usually present to health care services with a wide range of problems related or consequent to their abnormal personality traits (e.g. self-harm, feelings of depression or anxiety, violence or disorderly conduct, posttraumatic stress disorder, eating disorders, dissociative or somatoform disorders). Having a major psychiatric illness such as schizophrenia does not preclude patients from also having a personality disorder.

A diagnosis of personality disorder can be stigmatizing. It is important to consider whether making the diagnosis is useful, for example if it will direct the patient towards appropriate therapy or direct them away from potential iatrogenic harm.

CLASSIFICATION

Personality disorders can be classified into two groups according to their aetiology. The first group includes 'acquired' personality disorders where the disorder clearly develops after, and is directly related to, a recognizable 'insult'. *Organic personality disorder* results when this 'insult' is some form of brain damage or disease (e.g. a brain tumour or stroke). A common example is seen in patients with frontal lobe lesions, which can be characterized by social disinhibition (e.g. stealing, sexual inappropriateness) and abnormalities of emotional expression (e.g. shallow cheerfulness, aggression, apathy). Patients can also develop enduring personality changes after experiencing a catastrophic event (e.g. concentration camp or hostage situation leading to posttraumatic stress disorder) or after the development of a severe psychiatric illness. In such cases, a mental illness rather than personality disorder should be diagnosed.

The second group includes what is referred to in the ICD-10 as *specific personality disorders* (these are far more

147

prevalent and therefore simply referred to as 'personality disorders'; this is the term that will be used for the rest of this chapter). In this group of personality disorders, it is difficult to find a direct causal relationship between personality traits and any one specific insult, although genetic and environmental factors have been implicated (see Chapter 28). The onset of personality disorders is in adolescence or early adulthood and any change in symptoms tends to occur very gradually over a long period of time.

Personality disorders can be further classified according to clinical presentation, specifically regarding which particular maladaptive personality traits are present. In this regard, there are two approaches: the *dimensional* and *categorical* classifications:

The *dimensional approach* hypothesizes that the personality traits of patients with personality disorder differ from the normal population only in terms of degree. Maladaptive personality traits can therefore be seen as existing on a continuum that merges into normality. The dimensional approach is used predominantly in the research of personality

disorders and is measured by personality inventories (e.g. Minnesota Multiphasic Personality Inventory – MMPI). The ICD-10 and the Diagnostic and Statistical Manual of Mental Disorders, 5th Edition (DSM-5) use the *categorical approach*, which assumes the existence of distinct types of personality disorder and therefore classifies patients into discrete categories as summarized in Table 17.1. Despite the widespread use of the categorical approach in clinical practice, it seldom conforms to reality as there is a considerable overlap of traits and most individuals do not fit perfectly into these described categories. People are often best described as having a 'mixed personality disorder', listing the specific traits that are causing difficulties.

In an attempt to simplify further the classification of personality disorders, the DSM-5 has designated three personality clusters based on general similarities. Cluster A describes individuals who appear odd or eccentric and includes paranoid, schizoid and schizotypal personality disorders. Cluster B describes individuals who appear dramatic, emotional or erratic and includes borderline (closest

Table. 17.1 Categorical classification of personality disorders (DSM-5)

Cluster A: 'odd or eccentric'	
Paranoid personality disorder	Suspects others are exploiting, harming or deceiving them; doubts about spouse's fidelity; bears grudges; tenacious sense of personal rights; litigious
Schizoid personality disorder	Emotional coldness; neither enjoys nor desires close or sexual relationships; prefers solitary activities; takes pleasure in few activities; indifferent to praise or criticism
Schizotypal personality disorder	Eccentric behaviour; odd beliefs or magical thinking; unusual perceptual experiences (e.g. 'sensing' another's presence); ideas of reference; suspicious or paranoid ideas; vague or circumstantial thinking; social withdrawal
Cluster B: 'dramatic, emotional, erratic'	
Borderline (emotionally unstable) personality disorder	Unstable, intense relationships (fluctuating between extremes of idealization and devaluation); unstable self-image; impulsivity (sex, binge eating, substance abuse, spending money); chronic feelings of emptiness; repetitive suicidal or self-harm behaviour; fluctuations in mood; frantic efforts to avoid (real or imagined) abandonment; transient paranoid ideation; pseudohallucinations; dissociation
Antisocial (dissocial) personality disorder	Repeated unlawful or aggressive behaviour; deceitfulness; lying; reckless irresponsibility; lack of remorse or incapacity to experience guilt
Histrionic personality disorder	Dramatic, exaggerated expressions of emotion; attention seeking; seductive behaviour; labile shallow emotions
Narcissistic personality disorder	Grandiose sense of self-importance, need for admiration
Cluster C: 'anxious or fearful'	
Dependent personality disorder	Excessive need to be cared for; submissive, clinging behaviour; needs others to assume responsibility for major life areas; fear of separation
Avoidant (anxious) personality disorder	Hypersensitivity to critical remarks or rejection; inhibited in social situations; fears of inadequacy
Obsessive-compulsive (anankastic) personality disorder	Preoccupation with orderliness, perfectionism and control; devoted to work at expense of leisure; pedantic, rigid and stubborn; overly cautious

Note that the ICD-10 includes all the personality disorders described in the DSM-5 clusters above, except for schizotypal and narcissistic personality disorder. However, schizotypal disorder (similar to the DSM-5's schizotypal personality disorder) is included in the ICD-10's section on psychotic disorders. Note also that the draft ICD-11 classification of personality disorder includes some substantial changes. DSM-5, Diagnostic and Statistical Manual of Mental Disorders, 5th Edition; ICD-10, International Statistical Classification of Diseases and Related Health Problems, 10th edition.

ICD-10 equivalent: emotionally unstable), antisocial (closest ICD-10 equivalent: dissocial), histrionic and narcissistic personality disorders. Cluster C describes individuals who appear anxious or fearful and includes avoidant, dependent and obsessive-compulsive (anankastic) personality disorders. A hybrid categorical-dimensional approach is being taken by the current draft of the ICD-11, which splits personality disorders into mild, moderate and severe and refers to five 'prominent traits' (anankastic, detached, disinhibited, dissocial, negative affect) rather than 10 individual disorders. Someone may be considered to have one or more prominent traits, potentially improving the accuracy of the personality description.

HINTS AND TIPS

Everybody has a personality that, no matter how 'normal', can have dysfunctional traits (e.g. anger, anxiety, idealization/devaluation, obsessive-compulsive behaviour). These traits often become much more prominent at times of psychological stress, such as mental or physical illness, pain and discomfort, work-related stress and even tiredness and hunger. It is important to remember that personality disorders occur in many settings, remain stable over time and cause significant personal distress or functional impairment.

HINTS AND TIPS

The term 'borderline personality disorder' is derived from the early 20th century psychoanalysts, who described a group of patients who were 'on the borderline' between the neuroses and the psychoses.

COMMUNICATION

Confusingly, the different classification systems use slightly different terms for essentially the same type of personality disorder. Borderline personality disorder (DSM-5) is very similar to emotionally unstable personality disorder, borderline type in ICD-10. Similarly, antisocial personality disorder (DSM-5) is very similar to dissocial personality disorder in ICD-10. The terms are often used interchangeably – don't be confused if both appear in someone's notes!

ASSESSMENT

History

As with other mental illnesses, giving a patient a label of personality disorder gives those involved with their care only a limited amount of information. In fact, the clinical classification of personality disorders is often unreliable, and although psychiatrists usually agree that a patient has a personality disorder, there are often differing points of view regarding the subtype of the disorder. Patients with a possible personality disorder often present at times of crisis and distress, and therefore diagnosis at the first interview can be difficult because of the quantity of background and collateral information required and because diagnosis requires the features to persist over time.

A practical approach includes making a comprehensive assessment of:

- Sources of distress (thoughts, emotions, behaviour and relationships) to self and others
- Any comorbid mental illness
- Specific impairments of functioning at work, home or in social circumstances

It is usually possible to establish some idea of a patient's personality by taking a detailed history of their life, focusing on the areas of education, work, criminality, relationships and sexual behaviour. When patients are not able to describe aspects of their personality, it can be useful to ask how those close to them might describe them. It is also useful – with consent – to obtain collateral information from the patient's family, employer and general practitioner, all of whom might be able to provide information to help distinguish between transient and enduring patterns of behaviour.

It is important to recognize that patients with a personality disorder may exhibit strong emotional reactions (transference and countertransference – see Chapter 3) and that they are often perceived as 'difficult patients' because of this. Being aware of your own emotions (often strong feelings of anger or anxiety) and taking a nonjudgemental and empathic stance during assessment can be greatly beneficial, as well as providing insight into the diagnosis itself.

A number of self-rating questionnaires that focus on personality traits are available. These can be helpful in the diagnosis of personality disorder; however, they should not be used as a substitute for a comprehensive clinical history. Structured interviews are also available, although these tend to be used for research purposes and are seldom used clinically.

Examination and investigation

There are no specific physical signs that help in the diagnosis of personality disorders. However, the consequences of associated behaviours may be seen on examination or investigation (e.g. marks from self-inflicted lacerations or burns, musculoskeletal injuries from assaults or accidents, the sequelae of drug or alcohol misuse and sexually transmitted infections following promiscuity).

COMMUNICATION

It is difficult to confirm or to exclude the diagnosis of a personality disorder without taking a reliable collateral history to establish pervasiveness and stability of presentation. It can be difficult for patients to comment on this objectively, especially if they are in a state of distress.

DIFFERENTIAL DIAGNOSIS

A personality disorder should not be diagnosed if symptoms are better explained by a physical problem, substance misuse or a mental illness. Almost all the mental illnesses described in this book can feature some of the behaviours that characterize personality disorders. Examples include social withdrawal, suspiciousness and odd ideas in schizophrenia; self-harm, low mood and poor self-image in depression; aggression, irresponsibility and impulsivity in substance

misuse or mania (see Table 17.2). The diagnostic task is also complicated by the observation that many patients with a major mental illness or intellectual disability also have a concurrent personality disorder. A personality disorder should only be diagnosed when the clinical features begin in adolescence or early adulthood, are relatively stable over time and do not only occur during an episode of a major mental illness (e.g. depressive, manic, psychotic episode).

When an individual develops a dramatic personality change after a period of normal personality functioning, consider an organic personality disorder or a personality change that occurs secondary to experiencing a catastrophic event or developing a severe psychiatric illness.

HINTS AND TIPS

Remember that Cluster A personality disorders may present with features similar to the psychotic disorders (e.g. suspiciousness, social withdrawal and eccentric beliefs) but are differentiated by the absence of true delusions or hallucinations.

Table. 17.2 Differential diagnosis for common presenting problems in personality disorder

Presenting problem	Potential personality disorder	Differentials to consider (also consider 'no psychiatric disorder' in all cases)
Cluster A		
Suspiciousness	Paranoid	Schizophrenia
Difficulty forming relationships	Borderline (emotionally unstable), schizoid, paranoid, schizotypal	Autism spectrum disorder
Intrusive images, voices or thoughts	Borderline (emotionally unstable), schizotypal	OCD, schizophrenia, PTSD, substance abuse
Cluster B		
Chronic mood problems	Borderline (emotionally unstable)	Recurrent depressive disorder, bipolar affective disorder, dysthymia, cyclothymia, ADHD, substance use (especially alcohol dependence)
Impulsivity	Borderline (emotionally unstable), antisocial (dissocial)	ADHD, substance abuse
Frequent offending	Borderline (emotionally unstable), antisocial (dissocial)	ADHD
Suicidal tendencies	Borderline (emotionally unstable)	Depressive episode
Grandiosity	Narcissistic, histrionic	Mania
Cluster C		
Chronic anxiety	Dependent, avoidant	Generalized anxiety disorder, social anxiety, recurrent depressive disorder, substance abuse

ADHD, attention deficit hyperactivity disorder; OCD, obsessive-compulsive disorder; PTSD, posttraumatic stress disorder.

DISCUSSION OF CASE STUDY

Miss BP has a chronic condition that first presented in adolescence and has changed little over time. She has a number of maladaptive and inflexible personality traits that manifest as repeated self-harm, suicidal behaviour, impulsivity (promiscuity, binge drinking), fluctuations in mood and a marked fear of abandonment by her mother. These characteristics are consistent with a diagnosis of an emotionally unstable personality disorder, borderline type. It would be important to exclude another mental illness that may co-exist with the personality disorder, such as depression or harmful use/dependence on alcohol. Note that there is an association between emotionally unstable personality disorder and childhood trauma, including physical, emotional and sexual abuse.

Now go on to Chapter 24 which deals with personality disorders and their management.

Chapter Summary

- A personality disorder is when someone has ways of thinking, feeling or behaving that:
  - Are stable over time and context
  - Manifest in adolescence or early adulthood
  - Cause significant distress to the patient or those around them
- The classification of personality disorders is a controversial topic currently being reviewed.
- Many people have both a personality disorder and a mental disorder.
- A personality disorder should not be diagnosed if symptoms are better explained by a physical problem, substance abuse or a mental disorder.

The patient with neurodevelopmental problems

CASE SUMMARY

John, aged 9 years, was assessed by the child and adolescent mental health team after his teacher told his parents she thought John might have Attention Deficit Hyperactivity Disorder (ADHD). She had noticed that he was a bright child but made a lot of careless mistakes in his homework, which he often forgot to bring to school. He had always been very talkative, which initially endeared him to his peers, but lately he had fallen out with some friends as they said he never let them get a word in. He had also always been an active boy and had been picked for his school football team. However, the coach had dropped him after John failed to notice the ball coming in his direction on a number of occasions, seemingly staring off into space. His high activity levels were becoming increasingly noticeable as he got older and his peers became better able than him to sit through a class. John's parents were initially surprised by the suggestion but on reflection agreed that he often did things without thinking (he broke an arm last year after leaping out of a tree) and they had never considered going to the cinema as a family because they knew John would not be able to sit through a film. There were no concerns that they were not looking after John well. John told the psychiatrist that he generally felt cheerful, had no physical problems and did not have any problems seeing or hearing. In fact, he thought he had extra good hearing because he seemed to notice things other people did not, such as bird calls outside the classroom.

(For a discussion of the case study see the end of the chapter).

DEFINITIONS

Neurodevelopmental disorders are common and increasingly identified throughout a normal life span. You will encounter patients with them in all branches of psychiatry. They are disorders where abnormal development of the central nervous system leads to impairments in brain function, for example, seizures (epilepsy), abnormal movements (tics) and abnormal learning and memory (intellectual disability). The severest neurodevelopmental disorders tend to present early and are assessed and diagnosed by paediatricians. Disorders that primarily influence subtle aspects of cognition are more likely to present with behavioural difficulties in children of school age and are assessed and diagnosed by psychiatry. Because of increasing awareness of neurodevelopmental disorders in both the public and among health professionals, some people who had difficulties that were not assessed in childhood and that have persisted into adulthood are now seeking assessment for neurodevelopmental disorders as adults.

The concept of neurodevelopmental disorders is evolving. Recent classification changes have given them increasing precedence, with the Diagnostic and Statistical Manual of Mental Disorders, 5th Edition (DSM-5) and the most recent draft of the International Statistical Classification of Diseases and Related Health Problems, 11th edition (ICD-11; not yet published) including them as a diagnostic category in their own right. Some disorders not historically viewed as neurodevelopmental may be categorized as such in due course, for example, brain changes in schizophrenia and bipolar disorder probably occur from a young age, but symptoms only manifest from adolescence or early adulthood. These disorders are covered in Chapters 9 and 10 in this book. Personality disorders also overlap conceptually with neurodevelopmental disorders: both describe dysfunctional patterns of behaviour with onset in childhood causing significant impairment to the patient or others. These are covered in Chapter 17.

This chapter covers the common neurodevelopmental problems that present to psychiatry: difficulties with learning, socializing, paying attention and controlling movements. In defining disorders involving these abilities, it is crucial to recognize that performance in these areas varies normally within the healthy population (see Fig. 18.1). A disorder is only diagnosed if:

1. The person has characteristics that are significantly outwith the typical range.
2. These characteristics are associated with functional impairment (i.e. problems in social, occupational or adaptive functioning).

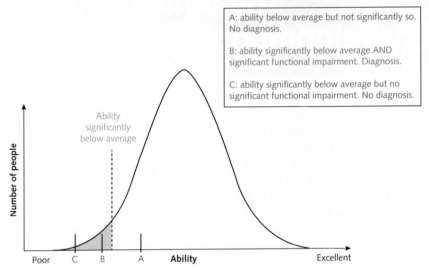

A: ability below average but not significantly so. No diagnosis.

B: ability significantly below average AND significant functional impairment. Diagnosis.

C: ability significantly below average but no significant functional impairment. No diagnosis.

Fig. 18.1 Core criteria for a diagnosis of a neurodevelopmental disorder.

CLINICAL FEATURES AND DIFFERENTIAL DIAGNOSIS

Problems with learning

Global

A generalized problem with learning new information and skills can arise through physical or mental health problems, sensory impairments or psychosocial adversity. If these are excluded, a diagnosis of intellectual disability should be considered.

Intellectual disability is an umbrella term used to describe diverse difficulties that manifest as significant intellectual impairment associated with a diminished ability to adapt to the normal demands of daily living, arising during the developmental period (normally in early childhood). These disorders are generally caused by an interruption in the normal development of the brain resulting from a variety of problems. Intellectual disability is a lifelong condition.

Adaptive functioning is a measure of how patients cope with activities of living such as communication, self-care, social skills and academic and vocational skills. This is assessed by a thorough developmental, psychiatric and medical history from the patient's parents and other care providers.

Intellectual functioning is usually defined by the intelligence quotient (IQ). This can be assessed by standardized intelligence tests (e.g. Wechsler Intelligence Scales for Children – WISC). An IQ of 70 or below, which is two standard deviations below the mean (IQ = 100), represents sub-average intellectual functioning. It is important to remember the limitations of using standardized testing instruments. Many standardized tests tend to be aimed at people of (or around) average intelligence and may be unsuitable for patients with more severe difficulties. Also, differences in native language and background, as well as

sensory, motor or communication difficulties may lead to patients obtaining falsely low IQ scores. Therefore patients obtaining IQ scores lower than 70 should not be diagnosed as having intellectual disability if there is no evidence of significant impairments in adaptive functioning.

In addition to the impairment of adaptive functioning, patients may have clinical features associated with the specific cause of their intellectual disability (e.g. Down syndrome: epicanthic folds with oblique palpebral fissures, broad hands with single transverse palmar crease, flattened occiput, cardiac septal defects). Other features associated with intellectual disabilities include aggression, self-injurious behaviour, repetitive stereotypical motor movements and poor impulse control. Up to a third of people with an intellectual disability have a comorbid psychiatric illness, most commonly schizophrenia (4%), which occurs at a higher rate in individuals with learning disabilities than in the general population.

Intellectual disabilities are classified as mild, moderate, severe and profound, according to the degree of intellectual and adaptive impairment. Table 18.1 summarizes the clinical features of the degrees of intellectual disabilities. However, this is simplified and difficulties experienced can vary from person to person.

HINTS AND TIPS

Whereas dementia describes a loss of cognitive ability already acquired, intellectual disability describes the failure to develop a normal level of cognitive functioning. However, individuals with Down syndrome are also at very high risk for developing Alzheimer disease in later life.

The terms 'intellectual disability' and 'learning difficulty' are often confused. A learning difficulty refers in general to any condition that impairs learning and is most often not associated with a global reduction in IQ. A specific learning difficulty is impairment in one particular type of learning (e.g. dyslexia, dyscalculia). An 'intellectual disability' is where learning difficulties are also associated with IQ <70 and impairments in adaptive functioning.

Specific

Some disorders are characterized by the disturbed acquisition of a *specific* cognitive or motor function during a child's development (e.g. language, reading, spelling, arithmetical ability and motor skills). If other areas of cognitive functioning are normal, a child may have a specific reading disorder (developmental dyslexia) but be of normal intelligence and have no problem with writing or mathematics. In some children, the consequences of the difficulty (e.g. school problems, bullying) might lead to secondary emotional or behavioural problems.

Problems with social interaction and communication

Social interaction is one of the most complex tasks the brain has to negotiate and many factors can influence social ability.

Children

Parents, health visitors or teachers may raise concerns about a child's ability to communicate and interact socially. It is important to exclude an influence of physical or mental health problems, sensory impairments or psychosocial adversity. Intellectual disability reduces social abilities, but if the social impairments are more marked than would be expected for the degree of intellectual disability, they can be diagnosed separately. Differentials are shown in Box 18.1 and clinical features of the neurodevelopmental causes of social difficulty are described below. Selective mutism and reactive attachment disorder are described in Chapter 30.

Autism spectrum disorder

The three characteristic features of autism manifest within the first 3 years of life and include:

1. *Impairment in social interaction* as evidenced by the poor use of nonverbal behaviour (e.g. eye contact, facial expression, gestures) and a failure to develop and to share in the enjoyment of peer relationships

Table 18.1 Degrees of intellectual disability

Degree of intellectual disability	Intelligence quotient (IQ) range	Adaptive functioning
Mild (85% of cases)	50–69	Difficulties may be subtle and difficult to identify. Often only identified at a later age. Difficulties in academic work (reading and writing) but greatly helped by educational programmes. Usually capable of unskilled or semi-skilled manual labour. May be able to live independently or with minimal support.
Moderate (10% of cases)	35–49	Language and comprehension limited. Self-care and motor skills impaired, may need supervision. May be able to do simple practical work with supervision. Rarely able to live completely independently.
Severe (3%–4% of cases)	20–34	Marked degree of motor impairment. Little or no speech during early childhood; may learn to talk in school-age period. Capable of only elementary self-care skills. May be able to perform simple tasks under close supervision.
Profound (1%–2% of cases)	<20	Severely limited in ability to communicate their needs. Often severe motor impairment with restricted mobility and incontinence. Little or no self-care. Often require residential care.

BOX 18.1 DIFFERENTIAL DIAGNOSIS FOR SOCIAL AND COMMUNICATION DIFFICULTIES IN CHILDREN

Normal for age

Secondary to sensory impairment (e.g. deafness)

Secondary to mental or physical health problem (e.g. depression, childhood schizophrenia, uncontrolled epilepsy)

Secondary to psychosocial adversity (e.g. emotional abuse)

Intellectual disability

Autism spectrum disorder

Rett syndrome

Childhood disintegrative disorder

Attention deficit hyperactivity disorder

Reactive attachment disorder

Conduct disorder

Selective mutism

Specific language impairment

Specific movement disorder

2. *Impairment in communication* as evidenced by poor development of spoken language; extreme difficulty in initiating or sustaining conversation; repetitive use of idiosyncratic language and lack of imitative or make-believe play

3. *Restricted, stereotyped interests and behaviours* as evidenced by intense preoccupations with interests such as dates, phone numbers and timetables; inflexible adherence to routines and rituals; repetitive, stereotyped motor movements such as clapping, rocking or twisting and an unusual interest in parts of hard or moving objects

In addition to these diagnostic features, patients may also exhibit behavioural problems such as aggressiveness, impulsivity and self-injurious behaviour. Although children with autism can be of normal intelligence, 50% have significant intellectual disabilities. Epilepsy develops in about 25%–30% of cases.

Asperger syndrome (or 'high functioning autism') is a subtype of autism where there are no significant abnormalities in language acquisition and ability or in cognitive development and intelligence. Although Asperger syndrome is a diagnosis in ICD-10, it is not included as a separate diagnostic category in DSM-5 or in the latest draft of ICD-11 (to be published). The term 'pervasive developmental disorder' is now used synonymously with autism spectrum disorder.

Rett syndrome

Rett syndrome, which has almost only been seen in girls, is caused by mutations in the gene MECP2 located on the X chromosome and can arise sporadically or from germline mutations. It is initially characterized by an apparently normal antenatal development with a normal head circumference at birth, followed by an apparently normal psychomotor development in the first 5 months after birth. From 6 months to 2 years of age, a progressive and destructive encephalopathy results in a deceleration of head growth; loss or lack of development of language and loss of purposeful hand movements and fine motor skills, with subsequent development of stereotyped hand movements (e.g. midline hand-wringing). After a decade, most girls are bound to a wheelchair with incontinence, muscle wasting and rigidity and almost no language ability.

Childhood disintegrative disorder (Heller syndrome)

This disorder, which is more common in boys, is characterized by about 2 years of normal development, followed by a loss of previously acquired skills (language, social and adaptive skills, play, bowel and bladder control and motor skills) before age 10 years. It is also associated with an autism-like impairment of social interaction as well as repetitive, stereotyped interests and mannerisms. Thus, after the deterioration, these children may resemble autistic children.

Adults

In adults presenting with social difficulties, the main differentials are shown in Box 18.2. It is paramount to take a history of the time course of difficulties: have they been present from a young age or only since adulthood? Patients

BOX 18.2 DIFFERENTIAL DIAGNOSIS FOR SOCIAL AND COMMUNICATION DIFFICULTIES IN ADULTS

Within normal range

Intellectual disability

Autism spectrum disorder

Personality disorder
- Schizoid
- Schizotypal
- Anankastic (obsessive-compulsive)
- Emotionally unstable
- Dissocial

Secondary to other psychiatric disorder
- Social phobia
- Generalized anxiety disorder
- Depression
- Negative symptoms of schizophrenia

Brain injury (e.g. traumatic, cerebrovascular accident, infection, inflammation)

Neurodegeneration (e.g. dementia)

themselves usually struggle to provide an objective account of this, so it is essential to obtain a collateral developmental history from someone who knew the patient well as a child. This can be a parent, a teacher, an older sibling or in written form, for example, school reports. The validity of any diagnosis of this sort in adulthood increases with the number of sources of collateral information available.

If impairments in communication and social abilities have had onset or significantly worsened in adulthood, then it is important to exclude other conditions that could have caused this, for example, a traumatic brain injury, frontotemporal dementia, a depressive episode or schizophrenia.

Anxiety and depression are often comorbid with autism in adults. A primary diagnosis of social anxiety can be distinguished from an autism spectrum disorder in that there should be no associated problems in communication or restricted interests and social abilities should be intact (e.g. able to make normal eye contact). In generalized anxiety disorder, anxiety covers many areas, not just social situations.

Personality disorders can be distinguished from autism by the associated features (see Chapter 17), for example, finding little pleasure in anything in schizoid personality disorder, magical thinking in schizotypal personality disorder, a desire for perfection in anankastic personality disorder, feelings of emptiness and frequent self-harm in emotionally unstable personality disorder and the ability to read social situations, but to disregard social obligations, in dissocial personality disorder.

Clinical features of autism spectrum disorders in adults vs. children are shown in Table 18.2. In adults presenting for the first time with a possible diagnosis of autism, intellectual disability is rare, and impairments tend to be milder than in those diagnosed in childhood. Because difficulties are likely to be at the milder end of the spectrum, it is very important to clarify the severity of the person's difficulties and the degree to which they impact their life (e.g. problems in initiating or sustaining employment, education and/or relationships). Your own mental state examination

(see Table 18.4) and a collateral history are crucial. Not everyone who has difficulty in interacting has autism or any other psychiatric diagnosis!

Problems with attention

Children

In a child described as paying poor attention, it is important to exclude an influence of physical or mental health problems, sensory impairments or psychosocial adversity. Intellectual disability reduces the ability to pay attention, but if this is more marked than would be expected for the degree of intellectual disability, it can be diagnosed separately. Differentials are shown in Box 18.3 and clinical features of the key neurodevelopmental cause of inattention (attention deficit hyperactivity disorder; ADHD) is described below.

Conduct disorder and reactive attachment disorder are described in Chapter 30. They can be distinguished from ADHD in that in conduct disorder the child breaks rules deliberately rather than impulsively and resists completing tasks because they do not wish to conform, rather than being unable to sustain attention. In reactive attachment disorder, a child may appear socially disinhibited, as with ADHD, but will struggle to form any sustained relationships, which is not the case for ADHD.

HINTS AND TIPS

Sensory processing abnormalities such as hypersensitivity to sound or touch are common in autism spectrum disorders and attention deficit hyperactivity disorder. The presence of such abnormalities increases the likelihood of a neurodevelopmental diagnosis but is not required for a diagnosis.

Table 18.2 Clinical features of autism spectrum disorder presenting at different ages

	Examples	
	Presenting in childhood	Presenting in adulthood
Domain		
Impaired social interaction	Not interested in peers. Little eye contact.	Not able to make small talk. Doesn't pick up social cues.
Impaired communication	Delayed speech.	Pedantic, overly formal use of language.
Restricted, stereotyped interests and behaviours	Intense interest in physical aspects of objects or numbers (e.g. lining up milk bottle tops). Inflexible adherence to routine. Repetitive movements (e.g. clapping, rocking).	Intense interest in objects or numbers, often enjoyment gained from categorizing or collecting (e.g. listing train timetables). Inflexible adherence to routine. Repetitive movements less common.

BOX 18.3   DIFFERENTIAL DIAGNOSIS FOR ATTENTION DIFFICULTIES IN CHILDREN

Normal for age
Secondary to sensory impairment (e.g. myopia)
Secondary to mental or physical health problem (e.g. anxiety, restlessness due to pain)
Secondary to psychosocial adversity (e.g. hunger)
Intellectual disability
Attention deficit hyperactivity disorder
Conduct disorder
Reactive attachment disorder
Tourette syndrome or dyskinesia
Specific learning difficulty

Attention deficit hyperactivity disorder

Problems in the three domains below should be present, causing significant functional impairment in at least two settings (e.g. school and home) for at least 6 months:

1. *Impaired attention*: Rather than failing to pay attention children pay more attention to more cues and are unable to eliminate unnecessary cues. This may manifest as difficulty completing work or play tasks; not listening when being spoken to; being highly distractible – moving from one activity to another; reluctance to engage in activities that require a sustained mental effort (e.g. schoolwork) unless very interested in the task (e.g. video games); being forgetful or regularly losing things.
2. *Impulsivity*: Children with ADHD are unable to suppress impulses and therefore respond to all impulses. This may manifest as difficulty awaiting turn, interrupting others' conversations or games or prematurely blurting out answers to questions.
3. *Hyperactivity*: Children with ADHD fail to pause and to consider options and consequences prior to acting. This may manifest as restlessness, incessant fidgeting, running and jumping around in inappropriate situations, excessive talkativeness or noisiness or difficulty engaging in quiet activities.

HINTS AND TIPS

When assessing a person's ability to concentrate, remember to take their developmental stage into account. A rule of thumb is that a preschool child would be expected to be able to concentrate for at least 3 minutes, a child at primary school for at least 10 minutes and an adolescent for at least 30 minutes.

Adults

In adults presenting with attentional difficulties, the main differentials are shown in Box 18.4. As with social impairment, it is paramount to take a history of the time course of difficulties with a collateral developmental history from someone who knew the patient well as a child or contemporaneous documentation such as school reports.

If impairments in attention have had onset or significantly worsened in adulthood, then it is important to exclude other conditions that could have caused this, for example, a traumatic brain injury, dementia, a depressive episode or anxiety. Bipolar affective disorder can present with mood instability similar (but more severe) than that seen in ADHD. The use of substances, particularly amphetamines, must be excluded.

Emotionally unstable personality disorder overlaps with ADHD in terms of impulsivity and rapid emotional variation. However, ADHD is not associated with feelings of emptiness or self-harm. Dissocial personality disorder overlaps with ADHD in that both are associated with law breaking and often found in prison populations. However, in ADHD the offences tend to be committed impulsively whereas in dissocial personality disorder there is more likely to be premeditation.

HINTS AND TIPS

The symptoms of neurodevelopmental disorders overlap with the symptoms of many other psychiatric disorders and it is important to be aware of the possibility of a missed neurodevelopmental diagnosis. This applies particularly to patients with atypical patterns of symptoms or response (e.g. rapid cycling bipolar, treatment-resistant depression) and to patients with several diagnoses, none of which quite seem to fit.

Clinical features of ADHD in adults vs. children are shown in Table 18.3. In adults presenting for the first time with a possible diagnosis of ADHD, impairments tend to be milder than in those diagnosed in childhood. Because difficulties are likely to be at the milder end of the spectrum, it is very important to clarify the severity of the person's difficulties and the degree to which they impact their life. Your own mental state examination (see Table 18.4) and a collateral history are crucial. Not everyone who gets bored easily has ADHD or any other psychiatric diagnosis.

BOX 18.4 DIFFERENTIAL DIAGNOSIS FOR ATTENTION DIFFICULTIES IN ADULTS

Within normal range
Secondary to substance abuse
Intellectual disability
Attention deficit hyperactivity disorder
Personality disorder
- Emotionally unstable
- Dissocial

Secondary to other psychiatric disorder
- Bipolar affective disorder
- Generalized anxiety disorder
- Depression

Brain injury (e.g. traumatic, cerebrovascular accident, infection, inflammation)
Neurodegeneration (e.g. dementia)

Table 18.3 Clinical features of attention deficit hyperactivity disorder presenting at different ages

Domain	Examples	
	Presenting in childhood	**Presenting in adulthood**
Inattention	Poor self-organization (e.g. loses school jumper). Needs instructions repeated. Careless mistakes in schoolwork.	Frequently loses important items (e.g. keys, wallet, phone). Struggles to complete administrative tasks.
Impulsivity	Shouts out answers to questions. Difficulty waiting turn. Easily led. Risk taker.	Makes reckless decisions. Completes others' sentences. Avoids queuing.
Hyperactivity	Moves around inappropriately. Excessively talkative, goes off on tangents.	Movement less of a problem in adulthood. May avoid situations where sitting still is expected (e.g. cinema, theatre). Over-talkative with tangential conversation.

Table 18.4 Mental state abnormalities in people with neurodevelopmental disorders

Disorder	Typical findings on mental state examination
Intellectual disability	*Very dependent on severity of disability.* Struggles to understand your questions. Gives short answers with limited vocabulary. Dysarthric.
Autism spectrum disorder (ASD)	Reduced eye contact. Does not pick up on social cues (e.g. when it is the end of the appointment). Speech may have limited intonation, be oddly accented or be unusually formal or pedantic. Talks excessively about topics of particular interest to them, does not take turns as in a normal conversation. Affect unreactive or odd, not able to use facial expression to communicate naturally.
Attention deficit hyperactivity disorder (ADHD)	Adults may be fidgety. Children may get up from chair, play noisily with toys, run around waiting room, shout. Person may talk at length in a tangential fashion. They may speak over you or finish your sentences. Information may need to be repeated. Easily distracted by external noises (e.g. traffic or a distant telephone).
Tourette syndrome	Tics. Features of comorbid attention deficit hyperactivity disorder.

Problems with controlling movements

Abnormal movements can result from a diverse range of problems, for example, orthopaedic, rheumatological, neurological or nutritional problems. Those covered here are those that are thought to be due to a problem with cortical processing of the coordination of movement (see Table 18.5), rather than a problem with the mechanics of a movement.

Developmental motor coordination disorder/ specific developmental disorder of motor function

This disorder is characterized by significantly impaired gross and fine motor skills in the absence of intellectual disability, sufficient to cause marked functional impairment. For example, very slow or inaccurate when catching a ball, walking or riding a bike (gross), or using scissors, cutlery zippers or pens (fine). This generally improves with age.

Table 18.5 Types of motor abnormality

Abnormality	Description	Examples
Tic	Quick, sudden, movement arising unpredictably, generally occurring for a brief time. Often stereotyped (i.e. the same movement) and recurrent, but not rhythmic. Suppressible and suggestible. Usually occurs at age 5–7 years.	Eye-blinking, mouth twitching, grunting (simple) or shouting out words, squatting, twirling while walking, making obscene gestures (complex).
Stereotypy	Identical, nonfunctional movement repeated many times. Arises in a fixed, predictable manner. Person can be distracted from movement but cannot voluntarily suppress. Usually occurs by age 2 years.	Hand flapping, twisting, rocking, head banging, grimacing, humming, grunting.
Mannerism	Goal-directed movement that individual performs frequently in a way unique to them. Under voluntary control. May be bizarre if in response to delusional idea.	Twirling hair, rolling eyes, clearing throat (common, part of personality). Jerking head, twiddling finger movements (rarer, bizarre).

Tourette syndrome

Tics are sudden, repetitive, nonrhythmic motor movements or vocalizations (see Table 18.5). They are usually preceded by a premonitory feeling of discomfort. They are involuntary; however, they can be voluntarily suppressed (although this can be very difficult, like trying to suppress the urge to sneeze). They are also often suggestible (i.e. can be provoked by discussing them or by observing others' tics) and become more prominent during times of stress. Tics are divided into:

- Simple motor tics (e.g. eye-blinking, neck-jerking, facial grimacing)
- Simple vocal tics (e.g. grunting, coughing, barking, sniffing)
- Complex motor tics (e.g. jumping, touching self, copropraxia (use of obscene gestures))
- Complex vocal tics (senseless repetition of words, coprolalia (use of obscene words or phrases))

Tourette syndrome is characterized by the presence of both multiple motor tics and one or more vocal tics for more than 1 year. The motor tics usually present by age 7 years, although tics can present as early as 2 years of age. Obsessive compulsive disorder and ADHD are common comorbidities.

ASSESSMENT

See Figure 18.2 for an overall approach to assessing neurodevelopmental conditions.

History

The following questions may be helpful in screening for the disorders below:

Learning difficulty (see Box 18.5 for communication tips)
- Do you have problems looking after yourself?
- Do you have problems with reading? Or writing? Or maths?
- Is it difficult to understand what people are saying?

Autism spectrum disorder
- What is a friend?
- What are your hobbies?
- How would you know if someone was sad?
- What would you do if someone was sad?
- Can you make small talk?

ADHD
- When did you last lose your bank card/phone/keys?
- Do you often make careless mistakes?
- Have you been told you don't listen?
- Are you distracted easily by background noises?
- Are you fidgety?
- What's it like inside your head?

(people with ADHD will often answer that it is busy and chaotic)

Tourette syndrome
- Do you find yourself making pointless movements or sounds?
- Do you get an urge beforehand?
- Can you suppress the urge? (Like with a sneeze or an itch?)
- What happens if you suppress it?

(People with Tourette syndrome report discomfort)

Examination

- Assess for physical signs suggestive of a syndromic intellectual disability, for example, large ears in Fragile X.
- Assess for physical disorders that could cause the presenting complaint.

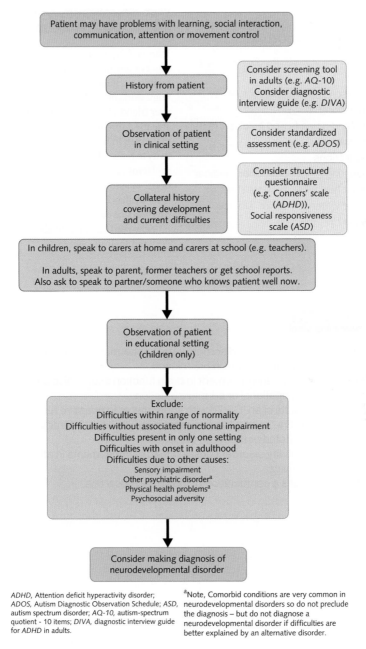

Patient may have problems with learning, social interaction, communication, attention or movement control

History from patient

Consider screening tool in adults (e.g. AQ-10)
Consider diagnostic interview guide (e.g. *DIVA*)

Observation of patient in clinical setting

Consider standardized assessment (e.g. *ADOS*)

Collateral history covering development and current difficulties

Consider structured questionnaire (e.g. Conners' scale (*ADHD*)), Social responsiveness scale (*ASD*)

In children, speak to carers at home and carers at school (e.g. teachers).

In adults, speak to parent, former teachers or get school reports. Also ask to speak to partner/someone who knows patient well now.

Observation of patient in educational setting (children only)

Exclude:
Difficulties within range of normality
Difficulties without associated functional impairment
Difficulties present in only one setting
Difficulties with onset in adulthood
Difficulties due to other causes:
Sensory impairment
Other psychiatric disorder[a]
Physical health problems[a]
Psychosocial adversity

Consider making diagnosis of neurodevelopmental disorder

ADHD, Attention deficit hyperactivity disorder; *ADOS*, Autism Diagnostic Observation Schedule; *ASD*, autism spectrum disorder; *AQ-10*, autism-spectrum quotient - 10 items; *DIVA*, diagnostic interview guide for *ADHD* in adults.

[a]Note, Comorbid conditions are very common in neurodevelopmental disorders so do not preclude the diagnosis – but do not diagnose a neurodevelopmental disorder if difficulties are better explained by an alternative disorder.

Fig. 18.2 Approach to neurodevelopmental disorder assessment.

- Complete a mental state examination focusing on behaviours suggestive of the neurodevelopmental disorder you are assessing for (see Table 18.4).

Investigations

No specific investigations are required to make a diagnosis of a neurodevelopmental disorder. Genetic testing is increasingly used in identifying the cause of intellectual disability, but it is not required for the diagnosis. Some investigations may be useful in excluding differentials or in identifying suspected comorbidities, for example, an EEG in someone with repetitive movements to exclude epilepsy, thyroid function in someone who has become restless and lost weight to exclude hyperthyroidism.

BOX 18.5 COMMUNICATION CONSIDERATIONS IN INTELLECTUAL DISABILITY

Allow extra time

Speak first to the person with the intellectual disability, not their carer

Assess their understanding early and involve them as much as possible

Ask short, simple questions

Use literal, direct language, not abstract or medical terms (e.g. 'Does it hurt when you pee?' rather than 'How are your waterworks?' or 'Do you experience dysuria?')

DISCUSSION OF CASE STUDY

John is likely to meet criteria for ADHD, although a school observation needs to be arranged. He has problems maintaining attention (e.g. completing schoolwork, remembering homework, on the football pitch), impulse control (e.g. talking over friends, jumping out of trees) and hyperactivity (e.g. not able to sit through a class or a film) that are more severe than those seen in his peers. He may also have sensory hypersensitivity to noise. His difficulties occur in multiple settings. These problems are causing him functional impairment in educational attainment, socializing and risks to his person. There is no evidence of intellectual disability, sensory impairment, psychosocial adversity or physical or mental health problems.

Now read Chapter 29 about neurodevelopmental disorders and their management.

● Chapter Summary

- Neurodevelopmental disorders are disorders where abnormal development of the central nervous system leads to impairments in brain function.
- To be classed as a disorder, an impairment in brain function should also cause an impairment in social, occupational or adaptive function.
- Intellectual disability results in an IQ <70 with impairments in adaptive functioning.
- Autism spectrum disorders cause a triad of impairments in social interaction, communication and restricted or repetitive behaviours.
- Attention deficit hyperactivity disorder causes a triad of impairments in attention, impulsivity and hyperactivity.
- Tourette syndrome causes a combination of motor and vocal tics.

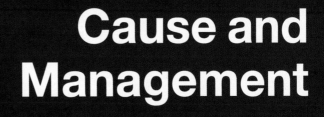

Cause and Management

Dementia and delirium

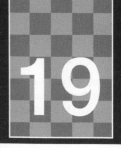

This chapter discusses the most common disorders associated with the complaints described in Chapter 7, which you might find helpful to read first.

DEMENTIA

Epidemiology

The overall prevalence of dementia is approximately 1% of the total UK population, rising sharply with increasing age. Fig. 19.1 illustrates the increasing prevalence of dementia with age. The prevalence in persons aged 65 years or over is approximately 7%, in those over 80 years about 20% and in those over 90 years of age around 30%. Dementia that manifests before the age of 65 years is referred to as early-onset. This arbitrary age cut-off is sometimes important when determining which service will treat a patient (see Chapter 31). Alzheimer dementia is more common in women and vascular dementia more common in men.

Dementia is a syndrome due to various diseases, most commonly neurodegeneration or vascular damage as below:

- Alzheimer dementia, 62% of cases
- Vascular dementia, approximately 17%
- Combined Alzheimer and vascular ('mixed') dementia, approximately 10%

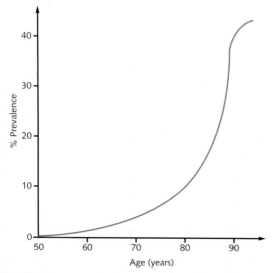

Fig. 19.1 Graph showing increasing prevalence of dementia with age.

- Dementia with Lewy bodies (DLB), 4%
- Frontotemporal dementia, approximately 2% (20% of early onset dementia)
- Parkinson dementia 2%
- Other causes of dementia 3%

Aetiopathology

Each type of dementia will be discussed separately.

Alzheimer dementia

Alzheimer dementia (AD) is classified as:

- Early onset (onset before age 65 years, usually familial, with relatives also affected before age 65 years)
- Late onset/sporadic (onset after age 65 years, either no family history or relatives affected after age 65 years)

At present, the cause of most cases of AD is unknown. It appears to be a combination of multifactorial genetic risk factors, vascular risk factors and other uncertain environmental factors. The characteristic pathological changes are:

1. Beta-amyloid **plaques** between neurones
2. Neurofibrillary **tangles** of hyperphosphorylated tau inside neurones

It is unclear whether either of these changes are a cause or a consequence of neuronal damage and death. The abnormalities generally begin in the medial temporal lobe (where key structures relating to memory are located) before becoming more diffuse, resulting in generalized cortical atrophy and compensatory ventricular enlargement. Degeneration of cholinergic neurons in the nucleus basalis of Meynert leads to a deficiency of acetylcholine, which can be partially reversed by some anti-dementia medications (cholinesterase inhibitors). These drugs can temporarily slow the loss of cognitive function but not reverse or ultimately prevent it.

Genetic factors

Late-onset AD. First-degree relatives of people with AD have a threefold increased risk for developing AD themselves. The most important gene associated with late-onset AD is the gene that codes a protein involved in cholesterol metabolism called apolipoprotein E (ApoE), which is encoded by three different common alleles (ε2, ε3 and ε4). Individuals who inherit one copy of the ApoE ε4 allele are at a roughly threefold increased risk for developing AD and those with two copies are at a roughly 10-fold increased risk. However, other environmental and genetic factors must be involved because having two ApoE ε4 alleles does not guarantee the development of AD and many patients with AD have no copies of the allele. Genome-wide association studies have identified approximately 20 genes in which polymorphisms contribute a small increase in risk for AD. These genes are involved in amyloid processing, lipid transport and metabolism, endocytosis and immune response.

Early-onset AD. Some forms of early-onset familial AD are inherited in an autosomal dominant fashion. Three genes have been isolated so far:

- Amyloid precursor protein – chromosome 21
- Presenilin-1 – chromosome 14
- Presenilin-2 – chromosome 1

These genes are all involved in metabolism of the amyloid protein. These autosomal dominant dementias present between the ages of 30 and 60 years, sometimes as early as 28 years of age when there is a mutation at presenilin 1.

Adults with trisomy 21 (Down syndrome) invariably develop neuropathological changes similar to AD by middle age and many will develop dementia. This has been attributed to triplication and over-expression of the gene for amyloid precursor protein (APP).

HINTS AND TIPS

You should be aware of four genes in Alzheimer dementia (AD) – one in late-onset AD, and three in early-onset autosomal dominant AD:

- In late-onset AD, the ApoE ε4 allele increases an individual's susceptibility to develop AD.
- In early-onset AD, the possession of a mutated version of one of three genes, amyloid precursor protein, presenilin-1 and presenilin-2, is strongly associated with development of AD.

Late-onset sporadic AD accounts for the overwhelming majority of all AD cases.

Nongenetic factors

The main environmental risk factors for AD are vascular (see Box 19.1). It is unclear whether vascular insufficiency in part causes the plaques and tangles seen in AD or whether vascular damage reduces the brain's reserve, making a given amount of neurodegeneration more likely to manifest clinically. Head injury and low educational attainment are also risk factors.

HINTS AND TIPS

Neurodegeneration seems to be associated with misplaced proteins: Alzheimer disease, dementia with Lewy bodies and frontotemporal dementia all involve the accumulation of degradation-resistant protein aggregates (see Table 19.1 for more detail).

BOX 19.1 NONGENETIC RISK FACTORS FOR ALZHEIMER AND VASCULAR DEMENTIA

Vascular	Both	Alzheimer
Previous stroke	Smoking	Head injury
Atrial fibrillation	Hypertension	Low educational attainment
	Diabetes	
	Hypercholesterolaemia	
	Previous myocardial infarct	
	Obesity	
	Late onset depression	

HINTS AND TIPS

The National Institute for Health and Care Excellence (2015) recommends that individuals reduce their risk for dementia in later life by quitting smoking, being more active, reducing alcohol, eating healthily and maintaining a healthy weight.

Vascular dementia

The cause of vascular dementia is presumed to be multiple cortical infarctions or many small subcortical infarctions in white matter (Binswanger disease) resulting from widespread cerebrovascular disease. On occasions, vascular dementia can arise from a single infarct in a strategic area. As with both Alzheimer dementia and cerebrovascular disease, vascular dementia is closely associated with increasing age. In rare cases, the disease is linked to *NOTCH3*, a gene on chromosome 19 involved in vascular smooth muscle cells response to injury (cerebral autosomal dominant arteriopathy with subcortical infarcts and leukoencephalopathy; CADASIL). The risk factors for developing vascular dementia are the same as for cerebrovascular disease in general (Box 19.1).

Lewy body dementias

Dementia with Lewy bodies and Parkinson disease dementia are now viewed as part of a continuum with the umbrella term Lewy body dementias (LBD). They have the same pathogenesis and as both diseases progress they become increasingly similar. Both are associated with the deposition of Lewy bodies: neuronal inclusions composed of abnormally phosphorylated neurofilament proteins aggregated with ubiquitin and α-synuclein. The initial distribution of Lewy bodies probably determines which symptoms occur first and hence which diagnosis is given

Table 19.1 Neuropathology of dementia

Dementia type	Abnormal protein(s)	Macroscopic findings	Microscopic findings
Alzheimer dementia	Beta amyloid Tau	Generalized cerebral atrophy, beginning in medial temporal lobes	Extracellular amyloid plaques Intracellular neurofibrillary tangles containing hyperphosphorylated tau and ubiquitin
Frontotemporal dementia (a heterogeneous collection of dementias including Pick disease and progressive supranuclear palsy)	Tau TDP FUS	Atrophy of frontal and temporal lobes, particularly anteriorly	Intracellular aggregates of tau, TDP or FUS.
Dementia with Lewy bodies	α-synuclein	Mild atrophy frontal, parietal, occipital lobes	Lewy bodies (intracellular aggregates of α-synuclein and ubiquitin) in cortex
Parkinson disease (dementia point prevalence of 25%, increasing with duration)	α-synuclein	Atrophy of substantia nigra and locus coeruleus	Lewy bodies in brainstem nuclei
Huntington disease	Huntingtin	Marked atrophy of basal ganglia and often frontal lobes	Intracellular aggregates of huntingtin and ubiquitin
Creutzfeldt–Jakob disease	Prion protein	Spongiform changes throughout cortex and subcortical nuclei	Extracellular prion protein plaques, particularly in cerebellum
Vascular dementia	None identified (in most cases)	Infarction – multiple small infarcts, or single large or strategic infarct	Infarcted grey and or white matter

FUS, Fused-in-sarcoma protein; TDP, TAR DNA-binding protein with molecular weight 43 kDa.

initially. Early deposition in the brain stem is thought to underlie the rapid eye movement (REM) sleep behaviour disorder that often precedes the onset of LBD by several years (see Chapter 25). Deposition in the substantia nigra, with associated neuronal death, results in parkinsonism. Deposition in the cortex results in cognitive impairment and hallucinations.

Familial cases of dementia with Lewy bodies are rare but can be caused by mutations in the genes coding for α-synuclein (*SNCA*), an intracellular signalling protein (LRRK2) and lysosomal processing. Fifteen percent of people with Parkinson disease have a family history of the disorder, associated with mutations in the same genes as dementia with Lewy body and with mutations in genes coding for proteins involved in the ubiquitin-proteasome system (e.g. parkin).

The syndrome of parkinsonism (as opposed to the specific disorder of idiopathic Parkinson disease) can be due to any injury to the basal ganglia: cerebrovascular disease, head injury, carbon monoxide poisoning, dopamine antagonists (including antipsychotic medication) or other neurodegenerative disorders (e.g. Parkinson-plus syndromes such as progressive supranuclear palsy).

HINTS AND TIPS

If dementia occurs at the same time or within a year of onset of parkinsonism, dementia with Lewy bodies is diagnosed. If dementia occurs more than a year after well-established Parkinson disease, Parkinson disease with dementia is diagnosed. The umbrella term Lewy body dementia describes both disorders.

RED FLAG

It is important to recognize Lewy body dementias as they require a specific management approach. Key features supporting Lewy body dementia rather than Alzheimer dementia are visual hallucinations and parkinsonism early in dementia, and a history of rapid eye movement sleep behaviour disorder.

Frontotemporal dementia

Frontotemporal dementias are a heterogeneous group of neurodegenerative disorders associated with degeneration of the anterior part of the brain. Their pathology and presentation overlap with motor neurone disease. There are three main variants: behavioural and primary progressive aphasia, which is subdivided into nonfluent and semantic variants (see Table 7.4). Macroscopically, they are associated with bilateral atrophy of the frontal and anterior temporal lobes (atrophied paper-thin gyri known as 'knife-blade atrophy') and degeneration of the striatum. Microscopically, three main types of intracellular inclusion body have been identified, containing mainly tau (e.g. Pick bodies; 30%–50% cases) the TAR DNA-binding protein (50% of cases) or the fused-in-sarcoma protein (10% of cases). Mutations in genes encoding three proteins account for around 60% of familial frontotemporal dementia: tau (microtubule stabilization), C9orf72 (endosomal trafficking) and progranulin (a protein involved in neuronal repair and lysosomal degradation).

COMMUNICATION

Pick disease is strictly a neuropathological diagnosis requiring the presence of Pick bodies at post-mortem, but previously it was used to mean the clinical diagnosis of any type of frontotemporal dementia.

Huntington disease

Huntington disease has autosomal dominant inheritance with complete penetrance. It is caused by an excessive number of trinucleotide (CAG) repeat sequences, usually more than 40, in the gene encoding the protein 'huntingtin'. The length of the abnormal trinucleotide repeat sequence is inversely correlated to the age of onset of the disease. This abnormal protein is associated with neuronal death, particularly in the basal ganglia, giving rise to the distressing motor signs of the disease.

Creutzfeldt–Jakob disease and other prion-related diseases

A prion is an infectious protein. All the prion-related dementias result in a spongiform degeneration of the brain in the absence of an inflammatory immune response, associated with the deposition of the prion protein (PrP) in the form of beta pleated sheets.

A number of prion diseases exist: kuru (prion transmitted by cannibalism of neural tissue, described in the highland tribes of New Guinea), Gerstmann–Sträussler syndrome (autosomal dominant condition caused by mutation of PrP gene on chromosome 20), scrapie in sheep and BSE (bovine spongiform encephalopathy) in cattle.

Most cases of Creutzfeldt–Jakob disease (CJD) appear to be sporadic, affecting people aged in their 50s, although it can be transmitted iatrogenically (e.g. via infected corneal transplants and surgical instruments). It presents with a rapidly progressing dementia with cerebellar ataxia and myoclonic jerks over 6–8 months. The electroencephalogram (EEG) characteristically shows stereotyped sharp wave complexes.

New variant CJD (nvCJD) is thought to be secondary to the ingestion of BSE-infected beef products. It typically presents in young adults with mild psychiatric symptoms such as depression and anxiety preceding the development of ataxia, dementia and finally death over a period of 18 months. There are no characteristic EEG changes, although nvCJD may have a characteristic MRI picture: a bilaterally evident high signal in the pulvinar (post-thalamic) region. As a result of public health measures, the incidence of this rare disorder has declined further, only affecting one or two people per year in the UK since 2012.

HIV-related dementia

Infection with the human immunodeficiency virus (HIV) is thought to cause direct damage to the brain in addition to the complications of HIV infection, such as opportunistic infections (cerebral cytomegalovirus infection, cryptococcosis, toxoplasmosis, tuberculosis, syphilis) and cerebral lymphoma. HIV encephalopathy presents clinically as a subcortical dementia and neuropathological examination shows diffuse multifocal destruction of the white matter and subcortical structures.

Assessment, clinical features, investigations and differential diagnosis

Discussed in Chapter 7.

Management

There is no cure for any of the neurodegenerative forms of dementia. Although the prognosis is invariably continued deterioration, considerable improvements in the quality of patients' lives are possible through a variety of psychosocial and pharmaceutical approaches. The principles of management are:

- Treating the underlying cause if possible (e.g. hypothyroidism, modifying vascular risk factors)
- Slowing down the rate of cognitive decline using anti-dementia drugs if indicated
- Managing associated disorders or complications (e.g. aggression, depression, psychotic symptoms)
- Addressing resulting functional problems (e.g. kitchen skills, financial management, social isolation)
- Providing advice and support for carers
- Advising on legal measures to prepare for loss of capacity (e.g. Power of Attorney, Advance Statements)

Specific management strategies

Maintaining cognitive functioning

Alzheimer dementia:

- The cholinesterase inhibitors, donepezil, rivastigmine and galantamine, are recommended by National Institute for Health and Care Excellence (NICE; 2011) for patients with mild-moderate Alzheimer dementia. Up to half the patients given these drugs will show a slower rate of cognitive decline and possible improvement in behavioural and psychological symptoms.
- Memantine, is recommended by NICE (2006) for those with moderate to severe Alzheimer dementia or for those who cannot tolerate cholinesterase inhibitors. It is an N-methyl-D-aspartate (NMDA) receptor antagonist, thought to reduce excitotoxic damage by blocking NMDA receptors and preventing the influx of calcium.

Vascular dementia: Cholinesterase inhibitors are not recommended (NICE 2006). The cornerstone of treatment is preventing further strokes by ensuring vascular risk factors are optimally managed. In mixed Alzheimer/vascular dementia, cholinesterase inhibitors can be prescribed.

Lewy body dementias: Cholinesterase inhibitors are recommended. Rivastigmine has the most evidence of benefit in both Lewy body dementia and dementia associated with Parkinson disease.

Frontotemporal dementias: Cholinesterase inhibitors can worsen behavioural abnormalities and are not usually recommended.

Structured group cognitive stimulation programmes can be of benefit in mild to moderate dementia of all types.

Reducing behavioural and psychological symptoms of dementia

- Behavioural and psychological symptoms of dementia (BPSD) are the noncognitive symptoms of dementia, including anxiety, agitation, delusions, hallucinations, aggression, wandering and sexual disinhibition (see Chapter 7).
- If a patient develops BPSD, carefully assess for a change in their physical health, including pain. People with dementia may find it very difficult to communicate discomfort. Consider medication side-effects including constipation. Assess for depression. Consider also a change in the person's environment – are they troubled by noise, extremes of temperature, other people's behaviour?
- NICE (2006) recommends aromatherapy, massage, animal-assisted therapy, multisensory stimulation or therapeutic use of music or dancing for agitation.
- Pharmacological treatment can be considered for disturbed behaviour such as aggression or agitation that does not respond to nonpharmacological strategies and is causing significant distress or risk. Anxiolytic medication such as trazodone can be useful because of its relatively benign side-effect profile. Benzodiazepines should be avoided if at all possible because they worsen cognition, predispose to delirium, increase fall risk and may paradoxically disinhibit (and make more aggressive) those with dementia.

- Psychotic symptoms do not require treatment if they are not distressing to the patient nor causing risk to others. If there is felt to be significant distress, a trial of an antipsychotic can be considered. Consider and document the increased risk for cerebrovascular events. Discontinue if there is no benefit within 12 weeks.
- Depression in dementia is managed similarly to depression in older adults but with even more care taken to avoid anticholinergic drugs, which can worsen cognition.

HINTS AND TIPS

Most medications should be prescribed at lower doses in older adults. In general, prescribe according to the rule 'start low and go slow'. This is particularly true when prescribing psychotropic medications for those with vulnerable brains (e.g. dementia) where doses a tenth of what would be used in a younger adult can be sufficient.

Legal issues

- People with dementia are likely in due course to lose the capacity to be able to make decisions about their welfare and financial affairs. It is advisable to arrange Power of Attorney as early as possible, before the person loses capacity to authorize this. They may also wish to consider an Advance Statement.
- People with dementia may lose the ability to drive safely and they and their carers should be advised to notify the Driver and Vehicle Licensing Agency (DVLA) and their insurer of their diagnosis.

RED FLAG

- Benzodiazepines should be avoided if at all possible in most patients with dementia, as they are particularly vulnerable to their adverse effects such as sedation, falls and delirium.
- Remember that 50% of patients with dementia with Lewy bodies will have a catastrophic reaction to antipsychotics (even atypicals), precipitating potentially irreversible parkinsonism, impaired consciousness, severe autonomic symptoms and a two- to threefold

increase in mortality. Benzodiazepines and cholinesterase inhibitors are safer in this group of patients. This exemplifies the need to exercise caution when prescribing antipsychotics and the importance of differentiating the various types of dementia.

Course and prognosis

The course of dementia is invariably progressive. Around a third of people with dementia live in residential care. Dementia is a life-shortening illness directly and indirectly, because it reduces the ability to communicate and tolerate management of physical problems. A diagnosis of dementia roughly halves a person's remaining life expectancy. The average duration of survival from the time of diagnosis of a late-onset dementia is 4 years, although there is a wide range.

DELIRIUM

Epidemiology

Most research into the epidemiology of delirium concentrates on older adults, who, along with infants and young children, are more vulnerable to this disorder. The prevalence in hospitalized, medically ill patients ranges from 10% to 30%. Between 10% and 35% of patients over the age of 65 years are delirious on admission and a further 10%–40% develop a delirium during hospitalization, with incidence increasing up to 87% in those admitted to intensive care. Patients with dementia are at an increased risk for developing a delirium; up to two-thirds of cases of delirium occur in patients with dementia.

Aetiology

Delirium is a final common pathway of disrupted homeostasis. It is nearly always multifactorial. In healthy individuals, multiple severe insults are required to cause it (e.g. head injury followed by sedative medication followed by surgery). In those with vulnerable brains (e.g. dementia), a minor insult is sufficient (e.g. constipation or a urinary tract infection). The commonest causes are medication (most commonly anticholinergics, opiates or benzodiazepines) or systemic illness, particularly infection. See Box 7.1 for a fuller list. Sometimes no cause is found – this does not preclude the diagnosis. Around a third of cases are viewed as preventable.

The pathophysiological mechanism remains unclear and may vary with cause. Suggested mechanisms include: aberrant stress response (neurotoxic effects of excess glucocorticoids), disrupted blood–brain barrier (allowing entry of toxins and cytokines to the brain) and impaired cholinergic neurotransmission.

HINTS AND TIPS

The cause of delirium is almost always multifactorial. This means prevention and management should address multiple factors too.

Assessment, clinical features, investigations and differential diagnosis

Discussed in Chapter 7.

Management

Delirium can be highly distressing for patients and anxiety-provoking for medical ward staff who are not experienced in dealing with agitated patients. It can also be very distressing for the families and friends of the patient. Fortunately, it is treatable if managed appropriately and urgently. See Fig. 19.2 for a management algorithm incorporating recommendations by NICE (2010). General principles of management are as follows:

- Hospitalization is essential: delirium is a medical emergency (unless prior ceiling of care discussions have concluded that this is not appropriate).
- Vigorously investigate and treat any underlying medical condition.
- Always assess medication use, including over-the-counter treatments: this is a high yield intervention.
- To limit confusion and foster trust, try to ensure that the patient is nursed by the same staff consistently.
- Merely the physical presence of a reassuring person is often enough to calm a distressed patient.
- Maximize visual acuity (e.g. glasses, appropriately lit environment) and hearing ability (e.g. hearing aid, quiet environment) to avoid misinterpretation of stimuli.
- Encourage a friend or family member to remain with the patient to help comfort and orientate them.
- Clocks, calendars and familiar objects may be helpful with orientation.
- Avoid medication unless the patient's agitation is causing them extreme distress, a significant risk to themselves or others or preventing them from receiving essential medical investigations or treatment.
- Antipsychotics, especially low-dose haloperidol, are generally effective in treating delirious symptoms, in part due to their sedative qualities, but perhaps also due to their effects on the dopamine–acetylcholine balance.

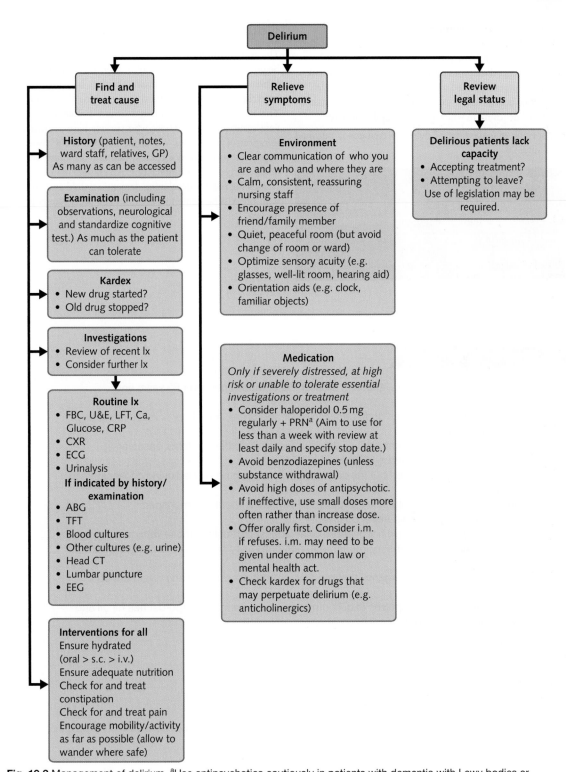

Delirium

Find and treat cause

History (patient, notes, ward staff, relatives, GP) As many as can be accessed

Examination (including observations, neurological and standardize cognitive test.) As much as the patient can tolerate

Kardex
- New drug started?
- Old drug stopped?

Investigations
- Review of recent Ix
- Consider further Ix

Routine Ix
- FBC, U&E, LFT, Ca, Glucose, CRP
- CXR
- ECG
- Urinalysis
If indicated by history/ examination
- ABG
- TFT
- Blood cultures
- Other cultures (e.g. urine)
- Head CT
- Lumbar puncture
- EEG

Interventions for all
Ensure hydrated
(oral > s.c. > i.v.)
Ensure adequate nutrition
Check for and treat constipation
Check for and treat pain
Encourage mobility/activity as far as possible (allow to wander where safe)

Relieve symptoms

Environment
- Clear communication of who you are and who and where they are
- Calm, consistent, reassuring nursing staff
- Encourage presence of friend/family member
- Quiet, peaceful room (but avoid change of room or ward)
- Optimize sensory acuity (e.g. glasses, well-lit room, hearing aid)
- Orientation aids (e.g. clock, familiar objects)

Medication
Only if severely distressed, at high risk or unable to tolerate essential investigations or treatment
- Consider haloperidol 0.5 mg regularly + PRN[a] (Aim to use for less than a week with review at least daily and specify stop date.)
- Avoid benzodiazepines (unless substance withdrawal)
- Avoid high doses of antipsychotic. If ineffective, use small doses more often rather than increase dose.
- Offer orally first. Consider i.m. if refuses. i.m. may need to be given under common law or mental health act.
- Check kardex for drugs that may perpetuate delirium (e.g. anticholinergics)

Review legal status

Delirious patients lack capacity
- Accepting treatment?
- Attempting to leave?
Use of legislation may be required.

Fig. 19.2 Management of delirium. [a]Use antipsychotics cautiously in patients with dementia with Lewy bodies or parkinson disease (see earlier) or with a prolonged QTc. Use benzodiazepines instead. *ABG*, arterial blood gas; *Ca*, calcium; *CRP*, C-reactive protein; *CT*, computed tomography; *CXR*, chest X-ray; *ECG*, electrocardiogram; *EEG*, electroencephalogram; *FBC*, full blood count; *GP*, general practitioner; *i.m.*, intramuscular; *i.v.*, intravenously; *LFT*, liver function test; *PRN*, when necessary; *s.c.*, subcutaneous; *TFT*, thyroid function test; *U&E*, urea and electrolytes.

- Olanzapine can be given if haloperidol is ineffective or contraindicated (e.g. history of dystonia, long QTc). Low doses should be given initially (e.g. 2.5 mg).
- Avoid benzodiazepines unless the patient is at high risk and has not responded to haloperidol, as they tend to prolong delirium. The exception is alcohol- or substance-related delirium, in which they are highly effective.

The specific management of delirium tremens is outlined in Chapter 20.

RED FLAG

Remember that delirium indicates the presence of a medical condition that should be managed on a medical, not a psychiatric, ward. Remember this when making referrals.

Course and prognosis

The average duration of a delirium is 7 days, but delirium can be prolonged for weeks or months, even after the initial insult is treated. Inpatients who develop delirium have an increased mortality, with around a third dying during that admission. This is unsurprising given that delirium is often a sign of severe systemic illness. Those who survive have an increased duration of admission, are at increased risk for complications such as pressure sores and falls and are more likely to be discharged to institutional care. An episode of delirium increases the risk for developing dementia sixfold and, in those with preexisting dementia, delirium can accelerate cognitive decline.

Chapter Summary

- Dementia is very common, affecting around 7% of those aged over 65 years and increasing with age.
- The four commonest types of dementia in older adults are: Alzheimer > vascular > Lewy body > frontotemporal.
- Neurodegenerative dementia arises due to abnormally folded proteins, vascular dementia due to one or many infarcts.
- Dementia cannot be cured but the commonest forms can be slowed using cholinesterase inhibitors.
- Behavioural and psychological symptoms of dementia should be managed nonpharmacologically wherever possible.
- Delirium is very common in hospitalized older adults, particularly those with preexisting cognitive impairment, sensory impairment, polypharmacy or who are severely unwell. Think delirium!
- Delirium is a medical emergency that requires prompt assessment and treatment of causes.
- Management of the symptoms of delirium requires environmental approaches for all and medication for a minority.

Alcohol and substance-related disorders

This chapter discusses the disorders associated with the complaints described in Chapter 8, which you might find helpful to read first. Alcohol-related disorders will be presented first, followed by other psychoactive substances.

ALCOHOL DISORDERS

Epidemiology

Alcohol use is declining in the UK but is still associated with high morbidity and mortality and overall is the most harmful psychoactive substance in common use (see Fig. 20.1). Middle-aged people are the most likely to drink dependently and to die of complications from alcohol abuse. Men are more likely to drink excessively than women. See Table 20.1.

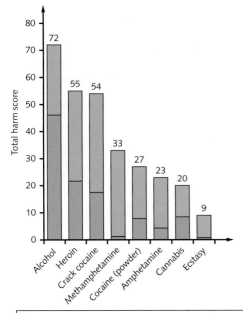

Harm to others (e.g. crime, RTA, violence, child neglect, economic cost)

Harm to user (e.g. mental health problem, physical health problem, death, loss of income, loss of relationships)

Fig. 20.1 Relative harmfulness of commonly used psychoactive substances. *Alcohol causes the most harm to others with heroin and crack cocaine causing the most harm to users. When scores are combined, alcohol is the most harmful substance. RTA, Road traffic accidents. (Modified from Nutt, DJ et al., (2010), Drug harms in the UK: a multicriteria decision analysis. Lancet, 376 (9752); 1558–1565.)*

Table 20.1 Epidemiology of alcohol use[a]

	Prevalence within adults in England in 2014, 2015 or 2016	Association with gender and age
Alcohol use	57% drank any alcohol within the last week (*this proportion is gradually reducing*)	63% men, 51% women Age 16–24 years least likely to drink
Hazardous use of alcohol (>8 (male) or 6 (female) units/ alcohol in 1 day)	15% binge drank within previous week	Male to female ratio 1:1 Age 16–24 years most likely to binge
Alcohol dependence	1.4%	Male to female ratio 3:1 Highest dependency rates in 25–64-year-olds
Hospital admissions related to alcohol	7% of **all** hospital admissions (1.1 million)	Male to female ratio 2:1 Most admissions in 55–74-year-olds
Deaths related to alcohol	1.4% of all deaths (7000)	Male to female ratio 2:1 Highest death rate in 55–64-year-olds

[a] *These are self-report values; alcohol sales figures show actual consumption is higher.*

Aetiology

The causes of alcohol dependence are multifactorial and are determined by biological, psychological and sociocultural factors.

Genetic and biochemical factors

Strong evidence shows a genetic component to alcohol dependence. Family studies show an increased risk for dependence among relatives of dependent individuals. Twin studies indicate that monozygotic twins have a higher concordance rate than dizygotic twins and adoption studies indicate a heritable component. The nature of this influence is unclear. It may operate at the level of heritable personality characteristics or it might relate to the body's inherited biochemical susceptibility to alcohol and its consequences. For example, 50% of East Asians have a deficiency in mitochondrial aldehyde dehydrogenase, leading to flushing and palpitations after small quantities of alcohol; this may explain reduced rates of consumption and dependence in these cultures.

From a biochemical perspective, chronic alcohol consumption influences a range of receptors and intracellular signalling proteins to cause long-term changes in plasticity in reward pathways, and to cause epigenetic changes. Some of the systems implicated are decreasing activity (down-regulation) of γ-aminobutyric acid (GABA) systems and increasing activity (up-regulation) of glutamate (mainly N-methyl-D-aspartate, or NMDA) systems.

Psychological factors

Behavioural models explain dependence in terms of operant conditioning where:

- Positive reinforcement occurs when the pleasant effects of alcohol consumption reinforce drinking behaviour (despite adverse social and medical consequences).
- Negative reinforcement occurs when continued drinking behaviour is reinforced by the desire to avoid the negative effects of alcohol withdrawal symptoms.

An alternative behavioural explanation is the observational learning theory (modelling), which suggests that patterns of drinking are modelled on the drinking behaviour of relatives or peers. Family studies support the idea that drinking habits follow those of older relatives.

The presence of psychiatric (anxiety, bipolar affective disorder, depression, schizophrenia) or physical illness appears to increase the risk for alcohol abuse and dependence, although differentiating cause and effect can be difficult (see Chapter 8). There is also evidence linking alcohol dependence with antisocial and borderline personality traits. Possible explanations for this could include any of the following: attempts to self-medicate to relieve symptoms, the use of alcohol as a (maladaptive) coping mechanism, the lack of a supportive environment, impulsivity, or the lack of insight into the risks associated with excessive alcohol.

Social and environmental factors

The cultural attitude towards alcohol affects the prevalence of alcohol-related problems (e.g. lower rates in Jewish societies as opposed to Mediterranean countries). Enormous cross-cultural variation in the way that people behave when drinking alcohol has been noted (e.g. alcohol consumption in the UK, US and Australia is associated with antisocial behaviour and violence, while in Mediterranean countries it is generally more peaceful), suggesting that the effect that alcohol has on behaviour is linked to social and cultural factors rather than solely to the chemical effects of ethanol. Alcohol consumption is greatly affected by price; strong evidence exists to suggest that the more affordable alcohol is, the more is consumed and the more harm results (see Fig. 20.2).

There is an association between certain occupations and deaths from alcoholic liver disease. The highest risk professions are members of leisure and catering trades (publicans especially), doctors, journalists and those involved with shipping and travel. Furthermore, higher rates of dependence are noted in unskilled workers and the unemployed compared with those with higher incomes. This may be partly explained by the 'social drift' caused by alcohol dependence (see Box 8.2).

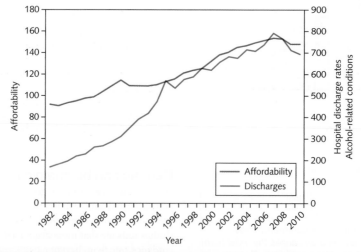

Fig. 20.2 Increasing alcohol affordability is associated with increasing alcohol-related harm. *Alcohol has become around 45% more affordable in the UK since 1980, and alcohol-related hospital admissions have quadrupled. As the affordability of alcohol has increased, so has the number of hospital discharges for alcohol-related conditions (rates shown here are per 100,000 people in the population of Scotland). This is the rationale for minimum unit pricing. Modified from Scottish Government (2012). Framework for Action: Changing Scotland's Relationship with Alcohol. Available at: https://www.gov.scot/Publications/2009/03/04144703/14.)*

The frequency of significant life events increases the risk for harmful drinking. Although the anxiolytic properties of alcohol are often used as a means of coping with stress, the social and physical complications of heavy drinking often lead to further stress.

Assessment, clinical features, investigations and differential diagnosis

Discussed in Chapter 8.

Management

The management of alcohol-related problems varies markedly depending on the pattern of use. Advice about reducing intake may be sufficient for hazardous drinkers and can be delivered by general practitioners (GPs) or any health care professional. See the box below for guidance on how to deliver a brief alcohol intervention. Up to a third of people with alcohol problems manage to abstain from alcohol without any formal treatment or self-help programme. Dependent drinkers may require a more intensive intervention, delivered by a specialist alcohol advisory service. Management of the latter group can be considered as having two overlapping objectives: the treatment of alcohol withdrawal and the longer-term maintenance of abstinence.

HINTS AND TIPS

Components of a brief alcohol intervention (FRAMES)

Research has shown that the features below contribute to the effectiveness of a brief alcohol intervention. Remember the acronym FRAMES:

F - Feedback – after taking a history or using a screening tool, point out the patient's alcohol problem and/or how alcohol may have contributed to their presenting complaint.

R - Responsibility – the decision whether or not to change is the patient's responsibility. Emphasizing this is less likely to trigger resistance.

A - Advice – clearly state that cutting down or stopping alcohol will reduce the patient's risk for future health problems.

M - Menu – provide a range of options the patient can use for change (e.g. a substance diary, alternative activities to drinking, identifying and

avoiding high-risk situations, attending mutual aid groups). Encourage the patient to select one or two to begin with.

E - Empathy - be warm, reflective and understanding

S - Self-efficacy – help the patient to feel confident they can make the proposed changes. Encourage the patient to describe their ability to make the change in their own words, for example: 'Do you think this is a change you'll be able to make?'.

Treatment of alcohol withdrawal

All clinicians need to be able to recognize alcohol withdrawal because of its high mortality and morbidity. The treatment of the alcohol withdrawal syndrome is commonly termed 'detoxification'. The following points are important:

- For the majority of patients, an outpatient or community-based detoxification will be safe and effective.
- Contraindications to detoxification in the community include severe dependence, a history of withdrawal seizures or delirium tremens, an unsupportive home environment, significant physical or psychiatric comorbidity, advanced age, pregnancy, or a previous failed community detoxification. In these cases, inpatient detoxification is advised.
- Unplanned, short notice detoxification should only be undertaken if absolutely necessary (e.g. if a patient has to be an inpatient for another reason). In general, detoxification works best when it is planned in advance to allow the perpetuating factors for dependence to be addressed alongside detoxification.
- In order to relieve severe symptoms and reduce the risk for developing seizures or delirium tremens, a drug with similar neurochemical effects to alcohol is prescribed, usually a benzodiazepine (such as chlordiazepoxide, diazepam or lorazepam). Initially, high doses are given, which are gradually reduced over 5–7 days.
- Medication may not be necessary if the patient has been drinking less than 15 units/day (men) or 10 units/day (women) and has no current or previous withdrawal symptoms.
- Alcohol withdrawal is a high-risk time for precipitating Wernicke encephalopathy (brain damage due to thiamine deficiency). Thiamine is therefore given prophylactically to those undergoing alcohol withdrawal. If a patient is well nourished and otherwise physically well, oral supplements are recommended. However, parenteral thiamine (Pabrinex) is needed if there is any suspicion of the onset of Wernicke, if someone is acutely physically unwell for any reason, if

they are admitted to hospital, if they are malnourished or if they have decompensated liver disease.

- Every time the brain withdraws from alcohol it is at risk for delirium with persistent cognitive impairment. However, continuing alcohol also places the individual at risk for brain damage. If a person relapses after detox, it is usually recommended to wait for at least 6 months before initiating a further detox, to balance the risk for brain damage due to withdrawal vs, ongoing use.
- Acamprosate is given in some centres because of its potential neuroprotective effect during alcohol withdrawal.

The box below summarizes the management of delirium tremens and Wernicke encephalopathy.

MANAGEMENT OF DELIRIUM TREMENS

Emergency hospitalization essential

Physical examination and investigations:

Thorough search for alternative cause of delirium associated with alcohol use, for example

- Infection
- Head injury
- Liver failure
- Gastrointestinal haemorrhage

Assess for signs of:

- Wernicke encephalopathy

Medication:

Control withdrawal symptoms and reduce risk for seizures

- Large doses of a drug with similar neurochemical actions to alcohol (e.g. benzodiazepines. Intravenous therapy seldom needed). Also prevents and controls seizures.
- Follow local guidelines regarding dosage and choice of benzodiazepine: in general, dosage is symptom driven (e.g. using CIWA) or follows a reducing regime.
- Only use antipsychotics (e.g. haloperidol) for severe psychotic symptoms (risk for lowering seizure threshold).

Prophylaxis against or treatment of Wernicke Encephalopathy

- Large dosages of parenteral (intramuscular or slow intravenous) thiamine – two Pabrinex ampoules twice daily for 5 days. Oral thiamine is not adequate in delirium tremens.

Monitoring of temperature, fluid, electrolytes and glucose:

- Risk for hyperthermia, dehydration, hypoglycaemia, hypokalaemia, hypomagnesaemia

General principles for managing delirium (see Chapter 19)

COMMUNICATION

Some patients think that 'detoxification' refers to the treatment of alcohol dependence. However, it only refers to the management of physical and psychiatric symptoms of withdrawal. Treating alcohol dependence involves addressing biological, psychological and social factors that may have precipitated and perpetuated its development.

RED FLAG

Delirium tremens is a medical emergency that is common on medical and surgical wards. Despite appropriate care and treatment, it is associated with a mortality of 5%–15% (estimated to be as high as 35% if untreated), emphasizing the need for prompt recognition and appropriate treatment. Make sure that you know the symptoms (Chapter 8) and management well.

Maintenance after detoxification

Remaining abstinent from alcohol is not as simple as a successful detoxification. Often the period post-detoxification highlights psychosocial issues to the patient that intoxication had previously allowed them to ignore. This may include the reasons they started to drink to excess in the first place and the damage they have done to themselves and others subsequent to becoming dependent. For this reason, psychosocial interventions are crucial in allowing the patient to process emotional distress and to develop a new network of friends with similar experiences who are now sober. Recovery can be a transformational process, with changes far wider reaching than simply achieving abstinence.

Psychosocial interventions

Not all interventions are suited to all patients, but the huge range available means there will be something that meets the needs of everyone. Many interventions include assessing where a patient's motivation for change is using Prochaska and DiClemente's stages of change model (Fig. 20.3). The

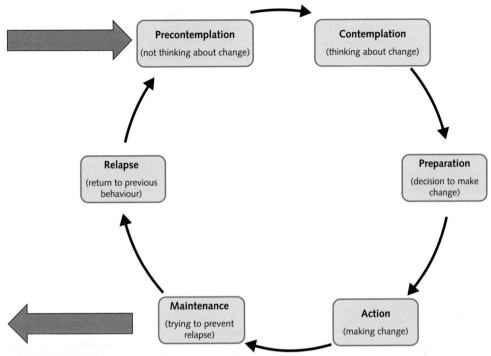

Fig. 20.3 Prochaska and DiClemente stages of change. (Adapted with permission from Prochaska JO, et al. *In search of how people change; applications to addictive behaviours*. Am Psychol. 1992;47:1102–14)

various forms of psychosocial intervention that have been shown to be effective in managing alcohol problems include:

- Motivational interviewing (see Chapter 3)
- Cognitive behavioural therapy (CBT): focusing on cue exposure, relapse prevention work, behavioural contracting, dealing with trauma symptoms
- Mutual aid organizations
  - 12-step fellowship organizations (e.g. Alcoholics Anonymous): based around a 12-step programme of spiritual and personal development
  - SMART recovery uses CBT to facilitate group self-help
- Social support: social workers, probation officers and citizens' advice agencies may be able to help with homelessness, criminal charges and debt

HINTS AND TIPS

For every person who drinks to excess, multiple others are adversely affected. The families of people who misuse alcohol or other substances can also benefit from mutual aid through organizations such as Al-Anon. Support for families can also indirectly help the user.

- Residential rehabilitation communities: these can provide intensive periods of structured holistic support (e.g. 12 weeks or longer) in the difficult period immediately following detoxification.
- Peer support

Pharmacological therapy

Various pharmacological strategies have been shown to be useful in the maintenance of abstinence from alcohol. They should be offered as an adjunct to appropriate psychosocial measures:

- Disulfiram (Antabuse): blocks the aldehyde dehydrogenase enzyme, causing an accumulation of acetaldehyde if alcohol is consumed. This causes unpleasant symptoms of anxiety, flushing, palpitations, headache and nausea very soon after alcohol consumption. It is contraindicated in patients with heart failure, stroke or coronary heart disease and caution is advised in people with hypertension, severe liver disease, cognitive impairment, psychosis and personality disorder.
- Acamprosate (Campral): enhances GABA transmission and inhibits glutamate transmission via NMDA receptors and appears to reduce the likelihood of relapse after detoxification by reducing craving. It is safe to use while drinking.

- Naltrexone (Nalorex) and nalmefene (Selincro): block opioid receptors, and appear to both reduce cravings for alcohol, and – when taken in conjunction with normal drinking – reduce the pleasant effect of alcohol, therefore decreasing the desire to drink and the amount consumed.
- The use of antidepressants and benzodiazepines is not recommended as pharmacological means for the maintenance treatment of abstinence from alcohol.

Course and prognosis

Alcohol dependence has a variable course and is often associated with numerous relapses. However, the prognosis is not as poor as is often thought, with around 50%–60% of people with alcohol dependence showing abstinence or significant functional improvement 1 year after treatment. Good prognostic indicators include being in a stable relationship, employment, having stable living conditions with good social supports, lack of cognitive impairment and having good insight

and motivation. People with any alcohol use disorder have an increased risk for death compared to age-matched controls (threefold in men, fivefold in women). Alcohol dependence is associated with a 12-fold increase in the risk for completed suicide, with deaths through accidents, cancer and cardiovascular disease also common.

OTHER PSYCHOACTIVE SUBSTANCES

Epidemiology

In 2014, 29% of adults in England and Wales had tried a recreational substance (35% of men and 23% of women). In 2016, 1 in 12 young or middle-aged adults (aged 16–59 years) in England and Wales had used a recreational substance within the last year. Cannabis, cocaine and ecstasy are the most commonly used recreational drugs in the UK. Use is most

Table 20.2 Epidemiology of substance use

	Prevalence within adults in England in 2014, 2015 or 2016	Association with gender and age
Within the last year, in 18–59-year-olds:		
Recreational drug use	8% (this proportion is gradually reducing)	Male to female 2:1 (12% vs 5%) Younger people more likely to have used (18% aged 16–24 years)
Cannabis use	6.5% (this proportion is gradually reducing) 37% of users are frequent users (more than once a month)	Male to female 2:1 (9% vs 4%)
Cannabis dependence	2.3% of general adult population show signs of dependence	Male to female 2:1 (3.7% vs 1.6%)
Cocaine use (powder)[a]	2.2% (majority once or twice a year)	Male to female 3:1 (3.3% vs 1.2%)
Ecstasy (MDMA) use	1.5% (majority once or twice a year)	Male to female 3:1 (2.2% vs 0.8%)
New psychoactive substance use	0.7%	Male to female 3:1 (1.1% vs 0.4%) Younger people more likely to have used (2.6% aged 16–24 years)
Opioid dependence	0.3%	Male to female 4:1 (0.4% vs 0.1%) Commonest in 25–44-year-olds
Hospital admissions related to recreational drugs (mental and behavioural problems, poisoning)	Approximately 0.7% of all hospital admissions (100,000)	Male to female 3:1 Over half of admissions in 25–44-year-olds
Deaths related to recreational drugs	0.5% of all deaths (2500) (drug-related deaths are increasing)	Male to female 3:1 Over half of deaths occurred in 30–49-year-olds 80% died via unintentional overdoses

[a] *Crack cocaine is smoked. Powder cocaine is snorted or injected. Crack cocaine's effects have faster onset and it is more likely to be associated with addiction. In the UK crack cocaine is much less commonly used than powder cocaine.*

common among men and among young people. Fewer than 1 in 100 people have used a novel psychoactive substance within the last year. Opioid use is rare by comparison with other drug use but has the highest morbidity and mortality. See Fig. 20.1 and Table 20.2.

Aetiology

Occasional or experimental use of recreational substances is not the same as drug dependence. However, ongoing use of recreational substances over a period of time can lead to development of a dependence syndrome, particularly drugs with a strong potential for the development of dependence (namely opioids and benzodiazepines). Using opioids for as little as 7 consecutive days can result in dependence. Dependence on any drug is associated with stimulation of the brain's 'reward system' (by increasing dopamine release in the mesolimbic pathway). Aetiological factors for recreational drug dependence are not well understood, although they appear to be related to a mixture of biopsychosocial factors. The operant conditioning model described in the alcohol section also applies to other psychoactive substances. Similarly, price, availability and cultural attitudes appear to be key factors influencing the use of recreational substances. In addition, social deprivation, childhood adversity, a family environment of substance abuse, conduct disorder in childhood, antisocial personality disorder and severe mental illness all increase the likelihood of substance misuse problems.

Assessment, clinical features, drug classification and differential diagnosis

Discussed in Chapter 8.

Management

Management of recreational drug dependence involves

- Harm-reduction of continued use
- Physical detoxification (if a withdrawal syndrome exists)
- Maintenance of abstinence if patient wishes to stop using

A detailed description of management strategies regarding the use of all recreational substances is beyond the scope of this book. Patients should be directed to local substance use services (run by National Health Service or third sector staff) who will be able to direct patients towards appropriate resources. There is a great deal of information on harm reduction techniques online (e.g. Know the Score, CREW). Patients who are dependent on opioids tend to be seen by National Health Service resources because prescriptions are often involved in management. However, for many drugs there is no medication-based treatment (cannabis, cocaine, amphetamines, novel psychoactive substances). People who wish to receive help in reducing use of such substances are likely to be able to find suitable support via third sector organizations and mutual aid (e.g. fellowship organizations such as Narcotics Anonymous or Cocaine Anonymous). Key points on the treatment of opioids and benzodiazepines are described later.

Table 20.3 Opioid substitute prescribing: comparison of methadone and buprenorphine

	Methadone	Buprenorphine
Mechanism	Long acting mu opioid receptor agonist	Long acting mu opioid receptor partial agonist
Side-effects	As all opioids: constipation, sedation, euphoria, nausea. At doses above 100 mg/day, electrocardiogram to check for QTc prolongation recommended.	Less sedating, less euphoric than methadone
Overdose risk	Prolonged action increases risk for overdose if other depressants used on top	Lower risk as partial agonist
Withdrawal symptoms	A few days to weeks	A few days
Precipitated withdrawal	Does not occur	Can occur if taken by a person with opioid dependency and circulating opioids
Methods to prevent diversion	Supervised consumption	Supervised consumption or combination with naloxone (opioid antagonist which is inactive if taken orally but blocks receptors if injected (Suboxone))
Ceiling effects	None	Cannot satisfy very strong cravings as partial agonist (less suitable for people using large amounts of heroin)
Starting daily dose	10–40 mg	4–8 mg
Maintenance daily dose	Typically 60–120 mL	Typically 12–16 mg

Opioids

Opioid use is associated with high rates of drug-related death, and other health complications such as blood-borne viruses, infective endocarditis and abscesses. It is also associated with a high cost to society through unemployment, crime and child neglect. One of the primary aims when someone is opioid-dependent is to minimize the harms associated with chaotic drug use. This can be achieved through a period of stabilization with long-acting opioid substitution therapy, removing the patient's need to purchase illicit opioids to manage cravings and withdrawal. Table 20.3 compares the two forms of opioid substitution therapy recommended by NICE: methadone and buprenorphine. If they are felt equally suitable, methadone should be prescribed. However, management of opioid dependence is more than just a prescription (see Table 20.4 for the key areas to address). Establishing a therapeutic reliance with the patient where they feel in control of their management is important.

Table 20.4 Biopsychosocial management of different stages of opioid dependence

Domain	Key actions
Harm reduction	Psychoeducation Offer substitute prescribing Consider child protection and give advice on minimizing harm to children from drug use Offer • take-home naloxone kit • needle exchange • contraception advice/condoms • blood-borne virus screening (Hepatitis B and C, HIV)
Psychosocial intervention	Encourage attendance at mutual aid groups (fellowships or SMART Recovery) Signpost to extra support if needed with housing, benefits, food, debts Signpost to training and vocational opportunities Consider: • Motivational interviewing • Trauma-specific psychoeducation or CBT • Behavioural couples therapy • Family interventions • Contingency management • Residential rehabilitation
Substitute prescribing	Before initiation, confirm dependent use via toxicology screens and attendance in withdrawal (see Table 8.1) Consider methadone or buprenorphine (see Table 20.3) Initiate under supervised consumption Regular review for dose titration to be sufficient to remove cravings but not to cause intoxication Long-term aim can be stability on maintenance prescription or abstinence
Detoxification	Minimize withdrawal symptoms by providing gradual reduction in opioid substitution therapy (e.g. 5mg methadone/fortnight). Opioid withdrawal is uncomfortable and distressing, although it is not life-threatening. If required, offer symptomatic relief: • A range of symptoms: lofexidine (alpha2-adrenoreceptor agonist) • Diarrhoea: loperamide • Nausea: metoclopramide or prochlorperazine • Stomach cramps: mebeverine or hyoscine butylbromide • Pain: paracetamol or ibuprofen • Anxiety/agitation/insomnia: propranolol or diazepam (short-term only))
Abstinence	Encourage ongoing attendance at mutual aid meetings. Encourage participation in recovery community activities (e.g. cafes, sports groups). Naltrexone (an opioid antagonist) can be used to block the euphoriant effects of future opioid use. It induces withdrawal if the patient has circulating opioids. Develop a crisis plan. Ensure patient is aware how to regain rapid access to services should relapse occur.

CBT, Cognitive-behavioural therapy.

Caution must be exercised when attempting withdrawal from benzodiazepines as it can very rarely be fatal. The benzodiazepine withdrawal syndrome may include hallucinations, convulsions and delirium. Symptoms can emerge within hours to days, depending on the half-life of the benzodiazepine. Management of benzodiazepine withdrawal involves initially converting drugs with a shorter half-life (e.g. lorazepam) to drugs with a longer half-life (usually diazepam). Doses are then reduced very slowly by around an eighth every fortnight, depending on patient response. If withdrawal symptoms emerge, the rate of reduction can be slowed, but increasing the dose should be avoided if at all possible.

HINTS AND TIPS

Sudden discontinuation of a patient's long-term sleeping tablet when they are admitted to hospital can lead to a withdrawal syndrome: only consider this if the patient's condition means benzodiazepines must be avoided and ideally reduce the dose gradually.

Benzodiazepines

Benzodiazepine-dependence often arises iatrogenically when patients are prescribed benzodiazepines every day for longer than 2–4 weeks. It can also arise when patients purchase benzodiazepines illicitly. If someone is dependent on illicit benzodiazepines, they can be offered a detoxification prescription if they are truly committed to abstinence, but they should not be offered a maintenance prescription (unlike with opioids, there is no evidence that this reduces harm).

Course and prognosis

Mortality in heroin users is 12-fold that of the general population. A longitudinal study in the USA found that after two decades 28% of male heroin users had died, 18% were in prison, 23% were still using and 29% were abstinent. The median duration of opioid use is 10 years. As with alcohol, relapse rates following detoxification are high and are most likely to succeed with psychosocial support in place. A quarter to a third of people entering treatment achieve and maintain long-term abstinence.

● Chapter Summary

- Alcohol is the most harmful psychoactive substance in common use.
- Alcohol and substance problems are more common in men.
- Alcohol withdrawal is a potentially fatal condition that requires treatment with benzodiazepines and thiamine.
- Management of all alcohol and substance use disorders requires psychosocial interventions.
- Mutual aid is a key component of maintaining abstinence for many people dependent on substances.
- Harm from opioids is reduced by opioid substitute therapy.

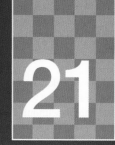
The main types of psychotic disorder are schizophrenia, schizoaffective disorder, delusional disorder and acute and transient psychoses. This chapter will concentrate on schizophrenia, the most prevalent and widely researched disorder in this group.

SCHIZOPHRENIA

History

Ideas about the disorder we now term 'schizophrenia' crystallized towards the end of the 19th century. The concept of this disorder has evolved during the 20th century. Important landmarks in the definition of this disorder are:

- 1893: Emil Kraepelin separated affective psychoses (e.g. mania) from nonaffective psychoses; he gave the term 'dementia praecox' to clinical conditions resembling the main forms of schizophrenia.
- 1911: Eugen Bleuler coined the term 'schizophrenia' (splitting of the mind); his description placed more emphasis on thought disorder and negative symptoms than on positive symptoms.
- 1959: Kurt Schneider defined first-rank symptoms, which are now the basis of criteria (a)–(d) of the International Statistical Classification of Diseases and Related Health Problems 10 (ICD-10) classification (see Boxes 9.2 and 9.3).
- 1970 to the present: The main international classification systems, ICD-10 and the Diagnostic and Statistical Manual for Mental Disorders 5 (DSM-5), have further clarified the diagnostic criteria. The main distinction between ICD-10 and DSM-5 is that the latter specifies a 6-month duration of symptoms and places a large emphasis on social or occupational dysfunction.

Epidemiology

- The incidence is approximately 15/100,000 individuals per year.
- The prevalence varies geographically but is approximately 1% in most settings.
- The lifetime risk is approximately 1% (see also Fig. 21.1).
- The age of onset is typically between late teens and mid-30s. Women have a later age of onset. Men: 18–25 years; women: 25–35 years.

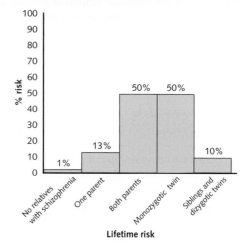

Fig. 21.1 Lifetime risk for developing schizophrenia if relatives have schizophrenia.

- Men have a higher incidence than women (ratio of 1.4:1) but equal prevalence (possibly due to a higher rate of mortality among male sufferers).
- There is an increased prevalence in lower socioeconomic classes (classes IV and V). This is more likely to be due to social drift (impairment of functioning caused by schizophrenia results in a 'drift' down the social scale) rather than social causation (poor socioeconomic conditions contribute to the development of schizophrenia).
- There is an increased incidence in urban (inner city) compared with rural areas.
- The incidence and prevalence are higher in migrants, with a relative risk of 4.6.

Aetiology

The aetiology of schizophrenia involves a complex interaction of biological and environmental factors.

Genetic

There is a strong tendency for schizophrenia to run in families. Fig. 21.1 shows the lifetime risk for developing schizophrenia if relatives have schizophrenia. Twin studies show a higher concordance rate for monozygotic twins (50%) than for dizygotic twins (10%), although this also shows that environmental factors are important, as monozygotic concordance is not 100%. Adoption studies provide further evidence for a genetic factor: babies adopted away from parents with schizophrenia to parents without retain their increased risk, whereas the risk is not increased when babies are adopted to parents with schizophrenia from biological parents without. Over 100 genetic variations associated with a small increase in risk have been identified, mainly in genes implicated in neurodevelopment, immune function, glutamatergic and dopaminergic neurotransmission and calcium signalling. Rare high penetrance genetic variations also exist, for example, deletion of a region of chromosome 22 is associated with a 30% risk for schizophrenia. The overall risk is likely to result from a complex interaction of a large number of genes, and their interaction with environmental factors.

COMMUNICATION

Schizophrenia is not purely genetic in aetiology – environment is also important. You may want to bear this in mind when discussing the diagnosis with patients and their families: parents may find a genetic description accusational, while for the patient it will have ramifications about having children themselves.

Developmental factors

Schizophrenia is associated with complications during pregnancy and birth. In addition, the observation that more people with schizophrenia are born in late winter or spring has led to the theory that schizophrenia is linked to second-trimester influenza infection. Prenatal malnutrition may also increase risk: maternal starvation early in gestation doubles the risk for schizophrenia in offspring.

Brain abnormalities

Structural and functional brain abnormalities are associated with schizophrenia, even in those with first-episode psychosis who have never received treatment. Structural imaging is not yet diagnostic, but frequently identified abnormalities include:

- Ventricular enlargement (appears to be associated with negative symptoms)
- Reduced brain size (frontal and temporal lobes, hippocampus, amygdala, parahippocampal gyrus)
- Reduced connectivity between brain regions (particularly frontal and temporal lobes)

Furthermore, people with schizophrenia demonstrate a wide range of cognitive abnormalities, particularly on tasks testing social cognition and memory. They also experience abnormalities of sensory integration leading to 'soft' neurological signs (e.g. abnormalities of stereognosis or proprioception).

Neurotransmitter abnormalities

Abnormalities in a range of neurotransmitter systems have been found in schizophrenia, predominantly glutamate and dopamine. It is not yet known how such abnormalities interact to lead to disorder, and if some abnormalities are a consequence rather than a cause of the disorder. The glutamate hypothesis of schizophrenia suggests that N-methyl-D-aspartic acid (NMDA) receptor hypofunction contributes to the pathogenesis of schizophrenia. The main evidence for this hypothesis is that genetic variants in NMDA receptor and related genes are associated with schizophrenia, and that giving NMDA receptor blockers to healthy control subjects causes psychotic symptoms.

The dopamine hypothesis suggests that schizophrenia is secondary to overactivity of the mesolimbic dopamine pathway in the brain. The key evidence for this pathway is that the dopamine D_2 receptor has been genetically linked to schizophrenia, antipsychotics block dopamine D_2 receptors, and drugs that potentiate this pathway (e.g. amphetamines, antiparkinsonian drugs) are known to cause psychotic symptoms.

Adverse life events

Exposure to childhood trauma (e.g. sexual abuse, death of a parent, neglect) increases the risk for schizophrenia in adulthood around threefold. Stressful life events in adulthood occur more frequently in the months before a first psychotic episode or relapse and may, therefore, precipitate the illness. However, it may be that the early stages of the illness itself cause the stressful events.

COMMUNICATION

Between the 1940s and 1970s, the concept of the 'schizophrenogenic mother' was common and suggested that schizophrenia was caused by early life difficulties in the relationship between the patient and their family. Although it is true that childhood adversity including emotional abuse and neglect is associated with schizophrenia in adulthood, it is no longer thought that relationship difficulties alone can cause schizophrenia, and families can be reassured on this point.

Cannabis

Chronic cannabis use is associated with an increased risk for schizophrenia (use on more than 10 occasions associated with a twofold increase in risk). Although there may be a degree of 'self-medication' in that people who are becoming unwell try recreational substances in an attempt to normalize their mental state, there is also evidence that cannabis use contributes to the causation of schizophrenia: psychotic symptoms can occur during acute intoxication, an association even when use is several years prior to first presentation, and a dose–response effect. Although cannabis use increases the risk for psychotic disorders, the fact remains that the majority of people who use it do not become mentally unwell. This suggests that it may be particularly detrimental to those who are already predisposed to schizophrenia in some way, for example, through genetic risk.

HINTS AND TIPS

NICE (2014) recommends screening for posttraumatic stress disorder in anyone with a first presentation of psychosis, because of the link between adverse life events and psychotic symptoms.

Assessment, clinical features, investigations and differential diagnosis

Discussed in Chapter 9.

Management

As with many chronic medical conditions, schizophrenia cannot be cured. However, appropriate management can greatly reduce symptoms and relapse. Long-term medication is the mainstay of treatment, although psychosocial treatment is also very important.

Treatment setting

The initial treatment setting depends on the presentation and severity of illness. Home treatment is preferable, but hospitalization is often necessary in cases of first-episode psychosis and when there is a significant risk that psychotic symptoms may lead to harm to self or others, or self-neglect. Detention under mental health legislation may be necessary in patients with reduced insight and impaired judgement.

Long-term community management is provided by community mental health teams or assertive outreach teams with the help of a care coordinator and regular follow-up in a psychiatric outpatient clinic. Patients with schizophrenia who have symptoms that are stable and well controlled can be managed in primary care.

Pharmacological treatment

Antipsychotics are of benefit in reducing positive symptoms (e.g. delusions and hallucinations). However, they have little or no benefit on negative symptoms (e.g. apathy and social withdrawal).

First- or second-line antipsychotic

Differences in efficacy between antipsychotics are small, with the exception of clozapine, which is the most effective antipsychotic known, but is not used first line because of its side-effects. Therefore the main factor influencing choice of antipsychotic is tolerability. Antipsychotics commonly cause side-effects, and as they are generally long-term medications, it is important to find one whose side-effects the patient feels they can tolerate for the foreseeable future. National Institute for Health and Care Excellence (NICE; 2009) does not recommend a particular antipsychotic as first line, but rather suggests that patients should be involved as much as possible in the decision. See Table 21.1 for a comparison of some common antipsychotic side-effects and see Chapter 2 for more information on antipsychotic side-effects and classification.

Treatment-resistant schizophrenia

Around two-thirds of people respond to the first antipsychotic trialled. Treatment-resistant schizophrenia is defined as a lack of satisfactory clinical improvement despite the sequential use of at least two antipsychotics for 6–8 weeks, one of which should be a second-generation antipsychotic. If a patient appears treatment resistant, reassess the diagnosis, check concordance, check whether psychological therapies have been offered, and assess for comorbid substance use. If treatment resistance is confirmed, offer clozapine at the earliest opportunity, assuming there are no contraindications and the patient is in agreement with taking oral medication and attending for regular blood tests. Clozapine is not used as a first-line medication due to its significant side-effects including life-threatening agranulocytosis in just less than 1% of patients. Thus regular haematological monitoring is obligatory (initially weekly, then monthly) and patients are required to be registered with a monitoring service. Clozapine will benefit over 60% of treatment-resistant patients.

Concordance with medication is poor in schizophrenia, with around 75% of patients stopping antipsychotics within 2 years. This frequently leads to relapse. Concordance can be increased using depot intramuscular medication (administered 1–12 weekly), increased social support and patient education.

The length of treatment requires careful consideration as single episodes cannot be predicted and most patients with schizophrenia relapse. After a first episode, prophylactic treatment is recommended for 1–2 years but relapse rates are high upon discontinuation (80%–98%). Relapse is less likely if withdrawal of treatment is gradual, over a few weeks. For most patients, antipsychotics are a long-term, lifelong, treatment.

Table. 21.1 Side-effects of commonly used antipsychotics

Antipsychotic	Sedation	Extrapyramidal side-effects	Weight gain/ metabolic syndrome	Hyperprolactinaemia	Drug-specific important side-effects
First generation					
Chlorpromazine	**Very common**	Common	Common	Common	Photosensitivity
Haloperidol[a]	Common	**Very common**	Common	Common	QTc prolongation on average >20 ms (baseline ECG recommended)
Flupentixol (Depixol)[a]	Common	Common	Common	Common	
Zuclopenthixol (Clopixol)[a]	Common	Common	Common	Common	
Second generation					
Olanzapine[a]	**Very common**	Common	**Very common**	Rare	
Quetiapine	**Very common**	Common	**Very common**	Rare	
Risperidone[a]	Common	**Very common**	Common	**Very common**	
Aripiprazole[a]	Common	Common	Rare	Rare	
Clozapine	**Very common**	Common (tardive dyskinesia very rare)	**Very common**	Rare	Agranulocytosis Hypersalivation

[a] Can be given in long-acting intramuscular injection (depot) form.
ECG, Electrocardiogram.

Other pharmacological treatments

Benzodiazepines can be of enormous benefit in short-term relief of behavioural disturbance, insomnia, aggression and agitation, but they do not have any specific antipsychotic effect.

Antidepressants and lithium are sometimes used to augment antipsychotics in treatment-resistant cases, especially when there are significant affective symptoms, as is the case in schizoaffective disorders, or in postschizophrenia depression.

Electroconvulsive therapy is now rarely used in schizophrenia. The usual indication is the rare case with severe catatonic symptoms.

Physical health monitoring

Patients with schizophrenia are at increased risk for cardiovascular disease. This risk is increased further by using antipsychotics. Therefore NICE (2014) recommends that a health screen should be carried out prior to commencing treatment, then at least annually, focusing on cardiovascular risk factors and including enquiry as to diet and activity levels. An electrocardiogram (ECG) is needed prior to commencing an antipsychotic if the patient is in hospital, has a history of cardiovascular disease, a family history of sudden cardiac death or has evidence of cardiovascular disease on examination (e.g. hypertension). Pretreatment ECGs are also recommended for some antipsychotics at high risk for prolonging the QTc interval (e.g. haloperidol). During treatment initiation, NICE (2014) recommends weekly weights for the first 6 weeks, then again at 12 weeks alongside assessment of serum lipids, glucose, pulse and blood pressure.

Psychological treatments

Historically, psychotic disorders were thought to be unresponsive to psychological interventions, but increasing evidence points towards their value in augmenting drug treatments:

- Schizophrenia can be a devastating condition and is associated with significant social morbidity. Therefore the importance of support, advice, reassurance and education to both patients and carers cannot be overemphasized.
- Cognitive-behavioural therapy has been shown to be effective in reducing some symptoms in schizophrenia. It is also useful for helping patients with poor insight come to terms with their illness, thereby increasing concordance with medication. It can also help the patient become aware of early warning signs of relapse. It is recommended by NICE (2014) for all patients with schizophrenia.
- Family psychological interventions focus on alliance building, reduction of expressions of hostility and criticism (expressed emotion), setting of appropriate expectations and limits and effecting change in relatives' behaviour and belief systems. Family intervention has been shown to reduce relapse and admission rates. It is recommended by NICE (2014) for all patients with schizophrenia who live with or are in close contact with their family.

Social inputs

Issues beyond pharmacological and psychological treatment should be addressed to optimize community functioning; these include financial benefits, occupation, accommodation, daytime activities, social supports and support for carers. A variety of agencies can provide these services, notably health services, social services, local authorities, local support groups and national support groups (e.g. SANE, MIND).

All patients with schizophrenia should be assessed for the care programme approach to achieve optimum coordination in the delivery of services. Community psychiatric nurses, consultant psychiatrists, occupational therapists, psychologists or social workers are appointed as care coordinators. Their primary role is to coordinate the multifaceted aspects of patients' care and to monitor mental state and concordance with medication.

Acute behavioural disturbance

Severe psychomotor agitation or aggressive behaviours frequently occur in acutely ill psychotic patients. It is vital that the correct diagnosis is established, especially in patients who are not well known. Many other conditions, for example, mania, delirium, dementia and alcohol and substance intoxication or withdrawal, can present with acute aggression and agitation, all of which require special consideration. The algorithm in Fig. 21.2 describes the principles of acute management. Many regions also have local protocols.

HINTS AND TIPS

Lorazepam is the only benzodiazepine that has a reliable rate of absorption from muscle tissue and therefore should always be used, if at all possible, when benzodiazepines are given intramuscularly. Other advantages include its relatively short half-life (10–20 hours) and its lack of active metabolites during elimination (no accumulation).

Course and prognosis

The course of schizophrenia is highly variable and difficult to predict for individual patients. In general, the disorder is chronic, showing a relapsing and remitting pattern. About 15% have a single lifetime episode with no further relapses. However, the majority of patients have a poor outcome characterized by repeated psychotic episodes with hospitalizations, depression and suicide attempts.

About 10% of patients with schizophrenia will die by suicide. Those most at risk are young men who have attained a high level of education and who have some insight into their illness. The periods soon after the onset of illness and in the months following discharge from hospital are particularly high risk, although all patients with schizophrenia are at lifelong increased risk for suicide.

The lifespan for patients with schizophrenia is on average 15 years shorter than for the general population. Causal factors include suicide, smoking, socioeconomic deprivation, cardiovascular disease, respiratory disease and accidents.

The overall prognosis for schizophrenia appears to be better in low-income as opposed to middle- and high-income countries; the reasons are unclear but may reflect better extended-family social support or greater social acceptance once recovered. The factors associated with a good prognosis are:

- Female sex
- Married
- Older age of onset

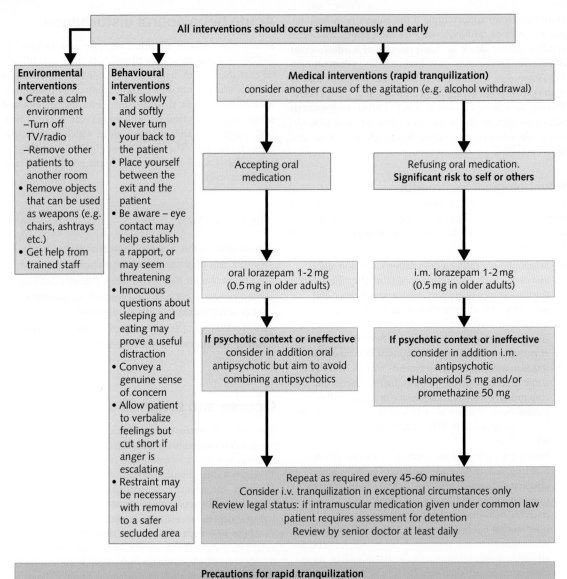

All interventions should occur simultaneously and early

Environmental interventions
- Create a calm environment
  - Turn off TV/radio
  - Remove other patients to another room
- Remove objects that can be used as weapons (e.g. chairs, ashtrays etc.)
- Get help from trained staff

Behavioural interventions
- Talk slowly and softly
- Never turn your back to the patient
- Place yourself between the exit and the patient
- Be aware – eye contact may help establish a rapport, or may seem threatening
- Innocuous questions about sleeping and eating may prove a useful distraction
- Convey a genuine sense of concern
- Allow patient to verbalize feelings but cut short if anger is escalating
- Restraint may be necessary with removal to a safer secluded area

Medical interventions (rapid tranquilization)
consider another cause of the agitation (e.g. alcohol withdrawal)

Accepting oral medication

oral lorazepam 1-2 mg
(0.5 mg in older adults)

If psychotic context or ineffective
consider in addition oral antipsychotic but aim to avoid combining antipsychotics

Refusing oral medication.
Significant risk to self or others

i.m. lorazepam 1-2 mg
(0.5 mg in older adults)

If psychotic context or ineffective
consider in addition i.m. antipsychotic
- Haloperidol 5 mg and/or promethazine 50 mg

Repeat as required every 45-60 minutes
Consider i.v. tranquilization in exceptional circumstances only
Review legal status: if intramuscular medication given under common law patient requires assessment for detention
Review by senior doctor at least daily

Precautions for rapid tranquilization
- If parenteral benzodiazepines are given, flumazenil must be available
- If haloperidol is given, procyclidine must be available (dystonias)
- After parenteral rapid tranquilization, frequently observe temperature, respiratory rate, hydration and level of consciousness until patient ambulatory

Fig. 21.2 Acute management of the agitated or aggressive patient (NICE, 2015).

- Abrupt onset of illness (as opposed to insidious onset)
- Onset precipitated by life stress
- Short duration of illness prior to treatment
- Good response to medication
- Paranoid subtype, as opposed to hebephrenic subtype (see Chapter 9)

- Absence of negative symptoms
- Illness characterized by prominent mood symptoms or family history of mood disorders
- Good premorbid functioning

Chapter Summary

- Schizophrenia occurs in around 1% of people worldwide.
- It arises from a combination of genetic and environmental factors influencing neurodevelopment and neurotransmission.
- Schizophrenia is treated with a combination of pharmacological (antipsychotics) and psychological therapy.
- Clozapine is an antipsychotic used for treatment-resistant schizophrenia.
- Acute behavioural disturbance should initially be managed with de-escalation techniques (behavioural and environmental) with medication (oral or parenteral) if required.
- Schizophrenia is associated with significantly reduced life expectancy: screening for and treating physical health problems are important.
- The majority of people with schizophrenia experience a relapsing and remitting course.

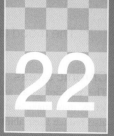

This chapter discusses the disorders associated with the presenting complaints in Chapters 6, 10 and 11, which you might find helpful to read first:

- Suicide and self-harm (Chapter 6)
- Depressive disorders (Chapter 10)
- Bipolar affective disorder (Chapter 11)
- Cyclothymia and dysthymia (Chapters 10 and 11)

Fig. 22.1 Simplified model of aetiology of mood disorder.

DEPRESSIVE DISORDERS

Epidemiology

Table 22.1 summarizes the epidemiology of the mood disorders.

Aetiology

Depression is a multifactorial disorder, with interacting risk factors from many aspects of a patient's make-up. Genetics, early upbringing and personality can increase vulnerability to depression, with episodes arising depending on the level of acute and chronic stress experienced (see Fig. 22.1).

Genetics

Twin studies show the heritability of depression as 40%–50%. The genetic risk is likely to be contributed to by multiple genes of individual small effect. Interestingly, recent genome-wide association studies have found that genetic variants that increase the risk for depression also increase the risk for other major mental disorders. The particular genes involved are only beginning to be identified, but so far include genes involved in calcium signalling, mitochondrial enzymes and regulation of growth of new neurons. To complicate matters further, some genetic influence may only manifest in particular circumstances (gene–environment interactions).

Early life experience

Parental separation (e.g. divorce) during childhood increases the risk for depression in adult life. This may partly relate to the loss of a parent, and partly to the disruption of care to the child. Other types of childhood adversity (e.g. neglect, physical and sexual abuse) increase the risk for depression and other psychiatric disorders. Postnatal depression in mothers can be associated with an indifferent early upbringing, leading to poor self-esteem and increased risk for depression in the child.

Personality

Genetics and early upbringing combine to shape personality, so it is unsurprising that some personality features are associated with increased risk for mood disorder. The personality trait 'neuroticism' (anxious, moody, shy, easily stressed) has consistently been found to increase the risk for unipolar depression. Certain personality disorders (e.g. borderline personality disorder, obsessive-compulsive personality disorder) also increase the risk for depression.

Acute stress

Adverse life events are common around the start of a depressive episode, particularly loss or humiliation events such as bereavement, relationship breakup or redundancy. The life event may not necessarily be causal, as being depressed—or at risk for depression—may also increase the risk for experiencing adverse life events. In recurrent depression, later episodes are less likely to be triggered by life events.

Table 22.1 Epidemiology of the mood disorders

	Lifetime risk	Average age of onset	Sex ratio (female:male)
Recurrent depressive disorder	10%–25% (women) 5%–12% (men)	Late 20s	2:1
Bipolar affective disorder	1%	20 years	Equal incidence
Cyclothymia	0.5%–1%	Adolescence, early adulthood	Equal incidence
Dysthymia	3%–6%	Childhood, adolescence, early adulthood	2–3:1

Chronic stress

The psychological and physiological effects of chronic stress may make someone vulnerable to depression and also reduce their ability to cope with more acute stressful life events. Chronic stressors such as poor social support (e.g. lack of someone to confide in), not having employment outside the home and raising young children are associated with depression. Chronic pain and any other chronic illness, particularly heart disease and stroke, are also associated with depression.

Neurobiology

The final common pathway of the multiple aetiological routes to mood disorder is abnormal brain structure and function. It is likely that mood disorders are due to malfunctioning communication between multiple brain regions involved in emotion regulation, rather than just one key abnormal area. Recurrent early onset depression is associated with reduced volume of the hippocampus, amygdala and some regions of frontal cortex. Depression with onset in later life is associated with white matter hyperintensities on neuroimaging, thought to represent small silent infarctions.

Neurochemically, multiple interacting neurotransmitter pathways are likely to be important. The two main abnormalities identified in depression are overactivity of the hypothalamic–pituitary–adrenal axis and deficiency of monoamines (noradrenaline (norepinephrine), serotonin, dopamine).

Assessment, clinical features, investigations and differential diagnosis

Discussed in Chapters 6, 10 and 11.

Management

A *biopsychosocial* approach is considered for the management of depression, which means that consideration should be given to treating biological, psychological and social aspects of the illness. See Fig. 22.2.

Treatment setting

Most patients with depression can be treated successfully in primary care, or in a psychiatric outpatient clinic. Day-hospital attendance may be helpful in patients with chronic or recurrent illness, especially if poor motivation or low self-esteem has led to a reluctance to go outside the home and make contact with others. Intensive support at home from crisis teams or inpatient admission may be advisable for assessment of patients with:

- Highly distressing hallucinations, delusions or other psychotic phenomena
- Active suicidal ideation or planning, especially if suicide has previously been attempted or many risk factors for suicide are present (see Chapter 6)
- Lack of motivation leading to extreme self-neglect (e.g. dehydration or starvation)

Detention under mental health legislation may be necessary for patients who need admission but are unwilling to accept inpatient treatment and lack capacity to make decisions regarding their treatment (see Chapter 4).

Lifestyle advice

All patients with low mood should be advised to avoid alcohol and substance use, eat a healthy diet, exercise regularly and practice good sleep hygiene (e.g. avoid caffeine and smoking in the evenings, do not sleep during the day, set regular sleep and wake times, do not use the bedroom for

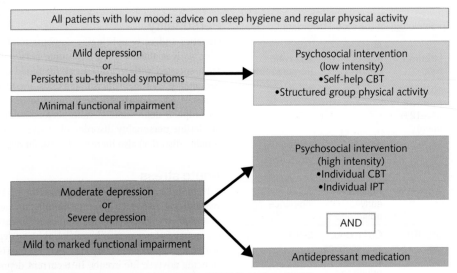

Fig. 22.2 Summary of first-line treatment for depression (NICE Guidelines 2009).

studying/watching TV). Patients can be referred to exercise groups; discounts may be available for those suffering from depression.

Psychological treatment

The National Institute for Health and Care Excellence (NICE; 2009) recommends that psychological treatments are used first line for mild depression, and in combination with drug treatments for moderate–severe depression. The severity of depression is determined in part by the number of symptoms (see Chapter 11) but mainly by the degree of functional impairment (i.e. whether the patient is still able to fulfil their normal social and occupational roles). Chapter 3 covers psychological treatments in detail. Modalities often used in depression are:

- Cognitive behavioural therapy (CBT)
- Interpersonal therapy
- Psychodynamic therapy
- Family and marital interventions
- Mindfulness-based cognitive therapy

COMMUNICATION

Patients reluctant to take medication may prefer the idea of 'talking therapies'. It is worth noting that cognitive-behavioural therapy can be as effective as antidepressants in treating moderate depressive episodes and that when used after medication it can reduce the rate of relapse up to 4 years later. You may want to discuss both options with the patient, encouraging the use of both but allowing the patient to make the final decision – this often aids concordance.

Pharmacological treatment

NICE (2009) recommends antidepressants only for patients with moderate–severe depression or for patients with persistent sub-threshold depressive symptoms or mild to moderate depression who have not benefited from a low-intensity psychosocial intervention. SSRIs (e.g. sertraline, paroxetine, citalopram, fluoxetine) are recommended by NICE (2009) as first-line antidepressants because they have the fewest side-effects. All antidepressants are similarly effective if prescribed at the correct dose and taken for an adequate length of time. Clinicians therefore tend to choose an antidepressant based not on efficacy, but on its side-effect profile (taking into account patient preference and comorbidity), and on which symptoms of depression are most troublesome. Table 22.2 summarizes some of the factors guiding the choice of an antidepressant. See Chapter 2 for more information on antidepressant mechanisms and side-effects.

Table 22.2 Factors influencing choice of antidepressant

Factor	Considerations
Side-effects	SSRIs, in general, are the best tolerated antidepressants. Side-effects should be matched to a patient's symptoms, lifestyle and preferences (e.g. the weight gain caused by mirtazapine may be preferable to the sexual dysfunction caused by the SSRIs); some patients benefit from the sedation caused by some antidepressants (e.g. amitriptyline, trazodone, mirtazapine (see Chapter 2)).
Previous good response	Prescribe previous drug.
Risk for overdose	SSRIs are safer in overdose than venlafaxine, which is safer than TCAs.
Severity of depression	For severe depression requiring hospitalization, antidepressants that affect both noradrenaline (norepinephrine) and serotonin may be preferable, that is, TCAs and high-dose venlafaxine (SSRIs may be slightly less effective in treating depression of severity sufficient to cause hospitalization).
Atypical depression	Atypical depression (i.e. hypersomnia, overeating and anxiety) may respond preferably to MAOIs.
Comorbid physical health problems	SSRIs can cause or worsen hyponatraemia. SSRIs should not normally be prescribed to people taking an nonsteroidal antiinflammatory drug, warfarin or heparin (as SSRIs increase risk for bleeding). SSRIs should be avoided in those taking 'triptan' drugs for migraine. TCAs are contraindicated in patients with a recent myocardial infarction, or arrhythmias. *See NICE (2009) Depression in Adults with a Chronic Physical Health Problem for further details.*
Comorbid mental health problems	Patients with obsessions or compulsions may respond preferably to high-dose SSRIs or clomipramine. A depressive episode with psychotic features usually requires the adjunctive use of antipsychotic medication.

MAOI, Monoamine oxidase inhibitor; NICE, National Institute for Health and Care Excellence; SSRI, selective serotonin reuptake inhibitor; TCA, tricyclic antidepressant.

Antidepressants are most effective in moderate–severe depression, where around 50% of patients will respond (compared with 30% on placebo), when prescribed at an adequate dose for a sufficiently long period (usually 4–6 weeks, longer in older adults), with appropriate patient education and encouragement. When an antidepressant has brought remission of symptoms, it should be continued at full dose (i.e. at the dose that induced the remission) for at least 6 months to reduce the relapse rate. Patients with a history of recurrent depressive disorder may benefit from taking antidepressants for a longer period, perhaps even lifelong in severe cases. The prophylactic effect of antidepressants in reducing relapse has been demonstrated for at least 5 years (with imipramine).

Treatment often fails due to inadequate dose of drug, duration of treatment or poor concordance; therefore these factors should always be ruled out. Box 22.1 describes the strategies

---

BOX 22.1 OPTIONS IF AN ANTIDEPRESSANT DOES NOT WORK

When an antidepressant does not work, management options include:

- Confirm concordance.
- Confirm duration of treatment and dose (at least 4 weeks at minimum therapeutic dose, longer periods may be required in older adults).
- Reassess the diagnosis: Is depression the cause of their low mood? Are they using alcohol or substances? Do they have a different psychiatric disorder? Is there an ongoing psychosocial stressor?
- Consider psychological therapy, if this is not already in place.
- Increase the dose of the current antidepressant (e.g. increasing fluoxetine from 20 mg to 40 mg).
- Change to another selective serotonin reuptake inhibitor (SSRI; e.g. from fluoxetine to sertraline).
- If trialled two SSRIs, or not appropriate to do so: change to another antidepressant from a different class (e.g. from sertraline (SSRI) to venlafaxine (selective serotonin-norepinephrine reuptake inhibitor) or mirtazapine).
- If adequately trialled at least two antidepressants, consider augmenting the current antidepressant with lithium or another antidepressant, for example, mirtazapine (usually done by a psychiatrist). Antipsychotics can also be used as augmenting agents in treatment-resistant depression. There are many other options.
- Consider electroconvulsive therapy if criteria met.

COMMON PITFALLS

- Patients may tell you that they have already taken antidepressants and that they do not work. People often respond to antidepressants from some classes but not others, so it can still be worth trialling a different antidepressant – you may want to explain this before prescribing.
- Remember that patients are often prescribed inadequate doses for inadequate lengths of time before the medication is changed – this does not represent treatment failure, for which a treatment dose needs to have been prescribed for 6–8 weeks without a response. You may find it useful to document dose and treatment period in your drug history.

---

that can be used when a patient has not responded to an antidepressant at the correct dose for the correct length of time.

Electroconvulsive therapy

See Chapter 2 for information on the administration and side-effects of electroconvulsive therapy (ECT). Indications for ECT in depression include:

- Poor response to adequate trials of antidepressants
- Intolerance of antidepressants due to side-effects
- Depression with severe suicidal ideation
- Depression with psychotic features, severe psychomotor retardation or stupor
- Depression with severe self-neglect (poor fluid and food intake)
- Previous good response to ECT

Course and prognosis

Depression is self-limiting, and without treatment a first depressive episode will generally remit within 6 months to 1 year. However, the course of depression is often chronic and relapsing and around 80% of patients have a further depressive episode, with the risk for future episodes increasing with each relapse.

Depression is one of the most important risk factors for suicide; rates of suicide are over 20 times greater in patients with depression compared with those in the general population.

BIPOLAR AFFECTIVE DISORDER

Epidemiology

Table 22.1 summarizes the epidemiology of the mood disorders.

Aetiology

Similar to depression, bipolar disorder is thought to arise from an interaction between genes and environmental stress, with genes being particularly important. Twin studies estimate heritability at 65%–80%. First-degree relatives of a patient with bipolar disorder have a roughly sevenfold increased risk for bipolar disorder (10%), a twofold to threefold increased risk for unipolar depression (20%–30%) and a higher risk for schizophrenia/schizoaffective disorder. Thus genetic susceptibility for severe mental disorder is not disorder specific: patients with a family history of any of bipolar, schizophrenia or schizoaffective disorder are at increased risk for bipolar disorder. Risk for most patients is likely contributed to by multiple alleles of small individual effect, although some rare high-penetrance alleles probably also exist. Many of the mutations identified so far that slightly increase the risk for bipolar disorder also increase the risk for schizophrenia, including genes related to neuronal development, neurotransmitter metabolism (dopamine and serotonin) and ion channels.

The most important environmental risk factor is childbirth. There is a 50% risk for mania postpartum in those with untreated bipolar affective disorder.

Neurobiologically, structural and functional abnormalities in brain regions linked to emotion and reward (particularly hippocampus, amygdala, anterior cingulate and corpus callosum) have been identified. Multiple neurotransmitter pathways have been implicated, with strongest evidence for dopaminergic pathway hyperactivity in mania and some evidence for dopaminergic hypoactivity in depression.

Assessment, clinical features, investigations and differential diagnosis

Discussed in Chapters 10 and 11.

Management

The main management scenarios are:

- Treatment of acute mania or hypomania
- Treatment of acute depression
- Maintenance treatment (prevention of relapse)

Treatment setting

The initial treatment setting depends on the presentation and severity of illness. A manic episode needs referral to secondary care. It may be managed by a crisis team, but may necessitate a period of hospitalization in cases of:

- Impaired judgement endangering the patient or others around them (e.g. sexual indiscretion, overspending, aggression)
- Significant psychotic symptoms
- Excessive psychomotor agitation with risk for self-injury, dehydration and exhaustion
- Thoughts of harming self or others

Detention under mental health legislation is often necessary in those lacking capacity to make decisions regarding treatment. Patients with bipolar disorder may also require hospital admission for depressive episodes for reasons outlined in the section on depression above.

Pharmacological treatment

The mainstays of acute and maintenance treatment of bipolar illness are mood stabilizers (lithium and some antiepileptics (sodium valproate/valproic acid, lamotrigine and carbamazepine)) and antipsychotics (which stabilize mood as well as reduce psychotic symptoms).

Treatment of acute mania or hypomania or mixed affective state

Antidepressants should be discontinued (this may need to be gradual if half-life is short, to avoid discontinuation symptoms). Short-term, benzodiazepines are often helpful in reducing severe behavioural disturbance. An antimanic agent should be started. NICE (2014) recommends an antipsychotic (haloperidol, olanzapine, quetiapine or risperidone), in part because of their benefits in reducing behavioural disturbance. If a different mood stabilizer is already being taken it can be continued, with consideration given to increasing the dose. If there is no improvement, augmentation is recommended with an antipsychotic. Because lithium can be harmful if taken for less than 2 years (discontinuation of lithium can precipitate mania), it is not advisable to start lithium in a manic patient who is unlikely to be concordant with long-term treatment.

Treatment of acute depression in context of bipolar disorder

Antidepressants need to be coprescribed with an antimanic agent, to avoid precipitating a hypomanic or manic episode. They should not be prescribed for mild depressive symptoms, only moderate–severe. Doses should start low and increase only gradually. Often, choice will be influenced by what medication someone is already taking. The first-line options are either quetiapine or a combination of fluoxetine and olanzapine (quetiapine and olanzapine have antidepressant properties in addition to antipsychotic effects). If these medications are not of benefit, lamotrigine alone can be given. If someone is already taking lithium or valproate, ensure the dose is providing a level at the upper end of the therapeutic window/is at maximum, and consider augmenting in turn with the three options as above. Long-term antidepressants should be avoided, with gradual discontinuation once depression has been in remission for 3–6 months.

Maintenance treatment

Not everyone who has suffered from a manic or hypo-manic episode needs long-term prophylactic treatment. Maintenance treatment is recommended in those who have had a manic episode associated with serious adverse risk or consequences, a manic episode and another disordered mood episode or repeated hypomanic or depressive episodes with significant functional impairment or risk. Treatment for at least 2 years is recommended but in practice is often required lifelong.

If maintenance treatment is indicated, NICE (2014) recommends lithium as first line. Lithium requires regular blood tests (usually three monthly) to monitor plasma level (see Chapter 3). Discontinuation of lithium can precipitate relapse, meaning net benefit is likely to be gained only after at least 2 years of treatment. Second line is to augment lithium with valproate. If someone is not able to take lithium (e.g. cannot tolerate, cannot attend for routine blood monitoring), alternatives are valproate (not in a woman of childbearing age as it is associated with a high risk for neural tube defects), olanzapine or quetiapine. Third-line options are lamotrigine (protects poorly against the manic pole) or carbamazepine (high risk for drug interactions due to induction of liver enzymes).

HINTS AND TIPS

Do not forget to take a comprehensive family history – including of treatment of psychiatric diagnoses. There is evidence to suggest that the level of response to lithium runs in families.

RED FLAG

Different preparations of lithium and valproate (which can mean sodium valproate, valproic acid or semisodium valproate) have different bioavailabilities so it is important to specify the preparation when prescribing.

Physical health monitoring

People with bipolar affective disorder are at increased risk for cardiovascular disease, regardless of whether they are taking medication with metabolic side effects or not. NICE (2014) recommends an annual physical health check including weight, pulse, fasting blood glucose, glycosylated haemoglobin, lipids and liver function. Any abnormalities should be proactively treated. Extra monitoring is required for those taking lithium (renal function, thyroid function and calcium).

Psychological treatment

A structured psychological intervention is recommended for all people with bipolar affective disorder to improve insight and awareness of early warning signs and identify strategies the patients can use themselves to stabilize their mood. If they are in close contact with family members, a family intervention is also recommended. In bipolar depression, a high-intensity psychological intervention is advised (cognitive behavioural therapy, interpersonal therapy or behavioural couples therapy). Psychological therapy is not recommended in hypomania or mania, when patients are generally unable to engage. Psychological therapies can harm as well as help, and therapists need to have training specifically to work with people with bipolar affective disorder.

Electroconvulsive therapy

Although ECT may precipitate a manic episode in bipolar patients, it can be an effective antimanic agent, especially in severe mania and mixed states. It can also be used in a severe depressive episode within bipolar affective disorder.

Course and prognosis

More than 90% of patients who have a single manic episode go on to have future episodes. The frequency of episodes varies considerably, but on average equates to four mood episodes in 10 years. Between 5% and 15% of patients have four or more mood episodes (depressive, manic or mixed) within 1 year, which is termed *rapid cycling* and is associated with a poor prognosis. Completed suicide occurs around 6 times more often in people with bipolar affective disorder than in the general population.

DYSTHYMIA AND CYCLOTHYMIA

Aetiology

The extent to which the aetiologies of dysthymia and cyclothymia resemble those of depression and bipolar affective disorder is unclear. There are biological similarities between dysthymia and depression; for example, rapid eye movement latency is decreased in both conditions. Genetic studies link cyclothymia and bipolar affective disorder, as up to one-third of patients with the former have a positive family history of the latter.

Epidemiology and course

Fig. 22.1 summarizes the epidemiology of the mood disorders. Both dysthymia and cyclothymia have an insidious onset and a chronic course, often beginning in childhood or adolescence. A significant number of patients with cyclothymia will go on to suffer more severe affective disorders, most notably bipolar affective disorder. Dysthymia may coexist with de-

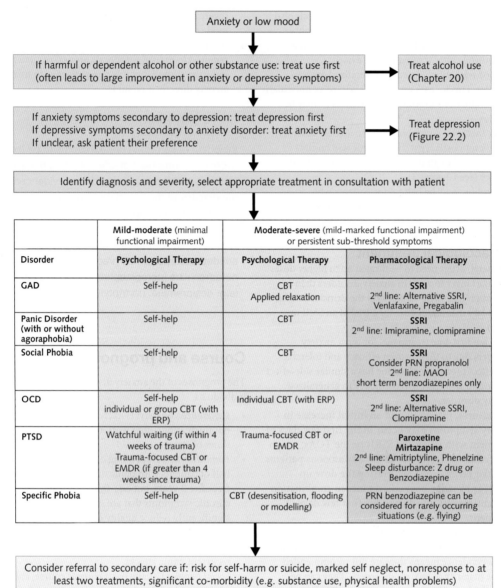

Fig. 23.1 Management of anxiety disorders. *CBT,* Cognitive-behavioural therapy; *EMDR,* eye movement desensitization and reprocessing therapy; *ERP,* exposure response prevention; *MAOI,* monoamine oxidase inhibitor; *SSRI,* selective serotonin reuptake inhibitor.

Psychological treatment

- There is strong evidence for the use of cognitive-behavioural therapy (CBT) in most anxiety disorders.
- CBT is the first-line treatment for specific phobias, mainly in the form of behaviour therapy, which may involve systematic desensitization, flooding or modelling (see Chapter 3).
- In panic disorder, CBT may help the sufferer to understand that panic attacks can start from a misinterpretation of a normal stimulus, leading to

a 'vicious cycle' of spiralling fear and sympathetic activation. When the patient understands this model, the therapist may encourage the patient to break the cycle by challenging the assumption that the original stimulus (e.g. palpitations) is indicative of an impending physical dysfunction (e.g. heart attack).
- Effective treatments in PTSD include trauma-focused CBT (CBT addressing thoughts and behaviours related to memories of the trauma) or eye movement desensitization and reprocessing therapy (where the

patient is asked to think about the trauma while also attending to another sensory stimulus (e.g. lights or beeps; see Table 3.4). Psychological debriefing immediately after trauma is not advised.

- Applied relaxation is used in generalized anxiety disorder. This focuses on being able to relax muscularly during situations in which the patient is or may be anxious.
- Other therapies commonly used in anxiety disorders include supportive, psychodynamic and family therapies, although there is less evidence for their efficacy (see Chapter 3).
- Counselling may be helpful for patients who are experiencing stressful life events, illnesses or bereavements (see Chapter 3).

Pharmacological treatment

- In general, drugs need to be titrated up to higher doses and take longer to work in anxiety disorders than in depression (e.g. up to 12 weeks at the British National Formulary maximum dose for a trial of an SSRI in OCD).
- SSRIs are first-line treatments for most anxiety disorders due to their proven efficacy and tolerable side-effect profile. Venlafaxine has a similar side-effect profile and also has proven efficacy in generalized anxiety disorder.
- Restlessness, jitteriness and an initial increase in anxiety symptoms may occur in the first few days of treatment with either the SSRIs or the TCAs, which may reduce concordance in already anxious patients. This can be managed by titrating the dose up slowly or by using benzodiazepines in combination with antidepressants during the first few days of treatment.
- Benzodiazepines are highly effective in reducing anxiety. However, the rapid development of tolerance and dependence means they are not recommended for the majority of anxiety disorders. They can be prescribed as a short-term hypnotic in PTSD, or for infrequent 'as required' use in social phobia (e.g. to allow a speech to be given) or specific phobias (e.g. to allow blood to be taken). They are not recommended for generalized anxiety disorder, panic disorder or OCD unless used short-term in a crisis.
- Pregabalin is licensed for treatment of generalized anxiety disorder (often used after an SSRI trial), epilepsy and neuropathic pain.
- TCAs are generally considered only after other treatments have been tried owing to their increased frequency of adverse effects (e.g. dry mouth, sedation, postural hypotension, tachycardia). Clomipramine, the most serotonergic of the TCAs, has proven efficacy in OCD.
- The monoamine oxidase inhibitors, despite being effective in some conditions, are not considered first-line treatment for anxiety owing to the possibility of severe side-effects and interactions with other drugs or food components (cheese reaction, see Chapter 2).
- A β-blocker such as propranolol can also be used as required to reduce autonomic arousal to anxiety-inducing stimuli, but it is more effective to treat the anxiety directly if possible.

HINTS AND TIPS

Inhibition of serotonin uptake seems to be the essential component of effective drug therapy for obsessive-compulsive disorder as evidenced by the efficacy of the selective serotonin reuptake inhibitors and clomipramine. Clomipramine, which predominantly inhibits serotonin reuptake, is more effective than the other tricyclic antidepressants, which predominantly inhibit noradrenaline (norepinephrine) reuptake inhibition (e.g. desipramine, nortriptyline).

Course and prognosis

The prognoses of the anxiety disorders vary greatly between individuals:

- *Generalized anxiety*: Is likely to be chronic, but fluctuating, often worsening during times of stress.
- *Panic disorder*: Depending on treatment, up to one-half of patients with panic disorder may be symptom free after 3 years, but one-third of the remainder have chronic symptoms that are sufficiently distressing to significantly reduce quality of life. Panic attacks are central to the development of agoraphobia, which usually develops within 1 year after the onset of recurrent panic attacks.
- *Social phobia*: Usually has a chronic course, although adults may have long periods of remission. Life stressors (e.g. a new job) may exacerbate symptoms.
- *Specific phobias*: Have an uncertain long-term prognosis, but it is thought that simple phobias that persist from childhood are less likely to remit than those that begin in response to distress in adulthood.
- *PTSD*: Approximately half of patients will recover fully within 3 months. However, a third of patients are left with moderate to severe symptoms in the long-term. The severity, duration and proximity of a patient's exposure to the original trauma are the most important prognostic indicators.
- *OCD*: The majority have a chronic fluctuating course, with worsening of symptoms during times of stress. About 15% of patients show a progressive deterioration in functioning.

Table 23.2 Epidemiology of somatization disorder and hypochondriacal disorder

Anxiety disorder	Lifetime prevalence	Usual age of onset	Sex ratio
Somatization disorder	0.2%–2%	Before 25 years of age, often in adolescence	Far more common in women (about 10:1)
Hypochondriacal disorder	1%–5%	Early adulthood	Equal
Body dysmorphic disorder	2%	Adolescence (declines with age)	Slight female excess
Functional/dissociative disorders		Varies between specific disorders	

DISSOCIATIVE AND SOMATOFORM DISORDERS

The dissociative disorders were described in Chapter 14. The common somatoform disorders (somatization disorder, hypochondriacal disorder, body dysmorphic disorder), factitious disorder and malingering were discussed in Chapter 15.

Epidemiology

Table 23.2 presents the epidemiological data for somatoform disorders. Functional or dissociative disorders are even more common – around a third of patients seen in hospital medical outpatient clinics. Functional seizures are found in around one in seven people attending a first fit clinic; functional paresis is as common as multiple sclerosis (affecting around 4 in 100 000 people per year), and up to half of presentations with 'status epilepticus' are in fact prolonged functional seizures.

Aetiology

The aetiology of dissociative and somatoform disorders is poorly understood. Childhood sexual abuse increases the risk for somatoform and dissociative disorders, although the majority of patients with the disorders have not been abused. Growing up in environments where physical distress is more readily acknowledged than psychological distress may have a role. Symptoms often (but not always) have onset or worsen after a stressor and this may be because emotional states influence the way pain and other bodily sensations are perceived. Symptoms also often follow an actual, minor, physical insult, for example, functional leg weakness following a sprained ankle or irritable bowel syndrome following a viral infection. Similarly, functional seizures occur most often in people who also experience epileptic seizures. There is no convergent pathophysiological explanation, but current theories include:

1. Abnormally intense self-directed attention interferes with normal 'automatic' cognitive processing, causing errors (much like thinking too long about how to spell a word)
2. Abnormal sense of agency or disrupted sensory prediction prevents patients from differentiating self-generated versus involuntary movements, or normal from abnormal sensory input

Assessment, clinical features, investigations and differential diagnosis

Discussed in Chapters 14 and 15.

Course and prognosis

Somatoform disorders tend to have a chronic episodic course, with waxing and waning symptoms often exacerbated by stress. Good prognostic features in hypochondriacal disorder include acute onset, brief duration, mild hypochondriacal symptoms, the presence of physical comorbidity and the absence of a comorbid psychiatric disorder. Functional/dissociative disorders vary widely in outcome. Some patients experience one acute episode, then make a full recovery; others become very disabled.

Management

NICE (2005) recommends CBT (including exposure with response prevention) for body dysmorphic disorder with any degree of functional impairment. SSRIs are recommended in addition for those with moderate to severe body dysmorphic disorder. Little research is available regarding the treatment of somatization and hypochondriacal disorders. Pharmacotherapy will only alleviate symptoms when the patient has a comorbid drug-responsive condition such as an anxiety disorder or depression. Both individual and group psychotherapy (mainly CBT) may be useful in reducing symptoms by helping patients to cope with their symptoms and develop alternative strategies for managing their emotions. Box 23.1 summarizes the role of the general practitioner in managing patients with somatoform disorders. A supportive relationship with an empathic doctor able to work with the patient to guide understanding of their condition is likely to be the most important intervention.

In functional/dissociative disorders, a clear and empathically delivered explanation that emphasizes reversibility can often be helpful (see Table 23.3). Treat comorbid psychiatric disorders, consider CBT, and consider physiotherapy for those who are deconditioned

BOX 23.1 ROLE OF THE GENERAL PRACTITIONER IN MANAGING PATIENTS WITH SOMATOFORM DISORDERS

- Arrange to see patients at regular fixed intervals, rather than reacting to the patient's frequent requests to be seen.
- Increase support during times of stress for the patient.
- Take symptoms seriously, but also encourage patients to talk about emotional problems, rather than just focusing on physical complaints.
- Limit the use of unnecessary medication, especially those that may be abused (e.g. benzodiazepines, opiates).
- Treat coexisting mental disorders (e.g. anxiety, depression).
- Limit investigations to those absolutely necessary, based on objective signs.
- Have a high threshold for referral to specialists.
- Communicate the diagnosis clearly and empathically.
- If possible, arrange that patients are only seen by one or two doctors in the practice to help with containment and to limit iatrogenic harm.
- Help patients to think in terms of coping with their problem, rather than curing it.
- Involve other family members and carers in the management plan.
- Consider referral to a psychiatrist or psychologist.

COMMUNICATION

A diagnosis of functional symptoms can be hard to explain. Phrases such as 'you are experiencing a functional, not a structural problem' or 'a software not a hardware problem' may help to reassure patients that you believe they are experiencing symptoms, but these are not driven by a disorder which requires specific treatment.

Table 23.3 Explanation and advice in dissociative/functional disorders

State what is wrong	'You have functional seizures'. 'You have irritable bowel syndrome'.
State what is not wrong	'You do not have epilepsy, coeliac disease, bowel cancer etc.'.
Describe the mechanism	'Your body is not damaged but it is not working properly'.
Try metaphor	'It's a software not a hardware problem'.
Explain how the diagnosis was made	Demonstrate tremor entrainment, Hoover sign, etc. Share normal investigation results. Point out other symptoms such as derealisation/depersonalization.
State you believe them	'I do not think you are making these symptoms up'.
Emphasize the problem is common	'Many people have similar symptoms'.
Emphasize the problem gets better	'There is no damage, so there is potential to make a full recovery'.
Emphasize self-help	'It's not your fault, but there are things you can do to make it better'.

● Chapter Summary

- Anxiety disorders are common, often chronic conditions, arising more frequently in women than men.
- Self-help is the first-line therapy for the majority of mild anxiety disorders.
- Psychological therapies are first line for moderate to severe anxiety disorders.
- Medication, usually selective serotonin reuptake inhibitors, can also be offered for moderate to severe anxiety disorders.
- Principles of treatment in somatoform and dissociative disorders are to take a holistic approach, give a clear explanation of diagnosis and minimize iatrogenic harm.

This chapter discusses the disorders associated with the presenting complaints in Chapter 16, which you might find helpful to read first.

ANOREXIA AND BULIMIA NERVOSA

Epidemiology

See Table 24.1.

Aetiology

As with the majority of mental disorders, both biological and psychosocial factors have been implicated.

Genetics

Estimates from twin studies suggest that around two-thirds of the variance in the liability to eating disorders is due to genetic factors. Genome-wide association studies in anorexia so far have not identified any common risk variants, but have been underpowered.

Early life experience

Premature birth and some perinatal complications increase the risk for a later eating disorder, potentially implicating epigenetic changes. Childhood adversity (physical, sexual or neglect) also increases the risk for an eating disorder. Relationship difficulties are often (but not always) found within families of patients with anorexia nervosa, including overprotectiveness, enmeshment (overinvolvement, with lack of differentiation between parent and child), conflict avoidance, lack of conflict resolution and rigidity (resistance to change).

Personality

It is possible that the inherited liability might be mediated by certain personality traits, including perfectionism (high attention to detail) and rigidity/obsessionality. High scores in these domains are seen in unaffected relatives of those with anorexia, and in those who have recovered and have a normal body mass index (suggesting that these findings do not simply reflect the substantial cognitive changes associated with starvation).

Cultural influences

In Western culture, the widely portrayed notion of the 'ideal body' influences perception of body image, meaning that unusual thinness is often valued more than natural curves. The increase in eating disorders seen in low- and middle-income countries supports the concept that idealized thinness may influence risk for eating disorder, but it is very hard to prove.

Neurobiology

The key neurobiological pathways underlying eating disorder remain to be clarified, but increased volume of the orbitofrontal cortex (involved in reward processing) has been found in anorexia and bulimia, both during and after an episode of illness (suggesting that the findings are not merely a consequence of starvation).

Assessment, clinical features, investigations, complications and differential diagnosis

Discussed in Chapter 16.

> **HINTS AND TIPS**
>
> Although depression and obsessive-compulsive disorder may coexist with anorexia nervosa, these symptoms can also result from the effects of starvation. It is helpful to ask, 'what happened first?', and aim to restore weight before treating any remaining mood or anxiety symptoms.

Table 24.1 Epidemiology of anorexia and bulimia nervosa

Disorder	Prevalence	Sex ratio	Age of onset
Anorexia nervosa	0.9% of women 0.3% of men	3:1 (10:1 in some studies)	Typically mid-adolescence
Bulimia nervosa	1.5% of women 0.5% of men	3:1	Typically late adolescence or early adulthood

Management

Anorexia nervosa

Ambivalence towards treatment coupled with the psychological consequences of starvation (poor concentration, depression, lethargy) means that anorexia nervosa is often difficult to treat. Treatment should be collaborative, with an early aim of establishing a therapeutic alliance. Fig. 24.1 gives an overview of management recommendations (National Institute for Health and Care Excellence (NICE) 2017). Suspected cases should be referred to a specialist eating disorder service for assessment.

Psychotherapy, preferably with familial involvement, is the treatment modality of choice for patients with anorexia nervosa. Table 24.2 lists the psychological interventions recommended by NICE (2017). The interventions for anorexia nervosa differ in detail but have common principles: they are long-term (20–40 sessions), they encourage regaining a healthy weight, they involve carers wherever possible and they seek to develop a positive therapeutic relationship. See Chapter 3 for more information about psychological therapies.

The only medication recommended by NICE (2017) in anorexia is a multivitamin. Previously, fluoxetine was often trialled, but this is now felt to be ineffective. A selective serotonin reuptake inhibitor may be of benefit in comorbid anxiety or depressive illnesses, but a return to a normal weight should be attempted first, as this is likely to improve mood and anxiety. When prescribing for anyone who is significantly malnourished, be aware of the additional risks of medications in this group, particularly QTc prolongation. Dose reductions and cautious titration are likely to be required.

Weight should be monitored, and physical complications (see Chapter 17) actively sought.

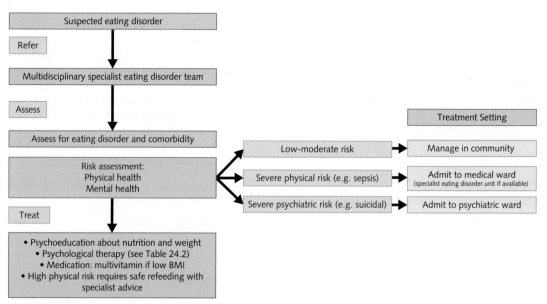

Fig. 24.1 Overview of management of eating disorders. *BMI,* Body mass index.

Table 24.2 Psychological interventions recommended in eating disorders (NICE 2017)

	Anorexia nervosa		Bulimia nervosa	
	First line	Second line	First line	Second line
Adult	One of: • CBT-ED • MANTRA • SSCM	• Different first-line therapy • Focal psychodynamic therapy	Guided self-help (CBT informed)	CBT-ED
Young person	Family therapy (anorexia focused)	One of: • CBT-ED • Psychotherapy (adolescent anorexia focused)	Family therapy (bulimia focused)	CBT-ED

CBT-ED, Individual eating-disorder-focused cognitive-behavioural therapy; MANTRA, Maudsley Anorexia Nervosa Treatment for Adults; NICE, National Institute for Health and Care Excellence; SSCM, specialist supportive clinical management.

Hospitalization is necessary in certain medical circumstances (e.g. body mass index less than 13.5 kg/m^2, rapid weight loss, severe electrolyte abnormalities, syncope) and psychiatric circumstances (risk for suicide, social crisis).

In severe cases, patients can lose insight into the severity of their illness, by virtue of both the psychopathology of the illness and the neuropsychological effects of starvation. Where a patient lacks capacity to make decisions regarding his/her care and treatment, it may be necessary to use mental health legislation (see Chapter 4) to effect compulsory admission to hospital, and to initiate life-saving treatment.

While mental health legislation in all UK countries only makes provision for the compulsory treatment of mental illness (not physical illness), food is considered to be treatment for mental illness because it leads to improvement in the psychological symptoms (impaired decision making) caused by starvation. Therefore, as a final resort, in certain cases patients may be force-fed under mental health legislation. In extreme cases, nasogastric or intravenous feeding may be necessary.

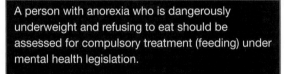

RED FLAG

A person with anorexia who is dangerously underweight and refusing to eat should be assessed for compulsory treatment (feeding) under mental health legislation.

Refeeding syndrome

When a patient starts eating after a prolonged (more than 5 days) period of starvation, care must be taken to avoid refeeding syndrome. This arises because of a rapid switch from gluconeogenesis (catabolic state) to insulin release stimulating glycogen, fat and protein synthesis (anabolic state), resulting in rapid intracellular uptake of the cofactors needed for this, such as potassium, phosphate and magnesium (Table 24.3). The associated electrolyte disturbances can be potentially fatal. Management hinges on replacement of fluid and electrolytes, which may need to be intravenous. To avoid it, refeeding is generally commenced cautiously,

Table 24.3 Clinical features of refeeding syndrome

Electrolyte abnormalities	Clinical manifestations
Hypophosphataemia	Muscle weakness
Hypokalaemia	Seizures
Hypomagnesaemia	Peripheral oedema
Hyponatraemia	Cardiac arrhythmias
Metabolic acidosis	Hypotension
Thiamine deficiency	Delirium

with frequent electrolyte monitoring for the highest risk period (first week of feeding) and with thiamine replacement.

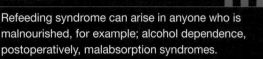

RED FLAG

Refeeding syndrome can arise in anyone who is malnourished, for example; alcohol dependence, postoperatively, malabsorption syndromes.

HINTS AND TIPS

Hypophosphataemia is the hallmark of refeeding syndrome. If you only remember one thing about it, remember to check for that. If it is significantly low, replace it, either orally or intravenously, depending on how low it is (check local guidelines).

Bulimia nervosa

Patients with bulimia nervosa tend to be more motivated to address their eating difficulties and are usually of a normal weight. Treatment is predominantly psychological, ranging from psychoeducation, self-help manuals and self-help groups in mild cases to individual cognitive-behavioural therapy in more serious cases (Table 24.2). Management by specialist eating disorder services may be necessary in severe cases. Inpatient treatment is not usually required; however, it may be necessary for the treatment of electrolyte disturbances resulting from purging (which can be fatal), or for management of the risk for suicide or self-harm. Antidepressants are no longer recommended to treat uncomplicated bulimia. However, comorbid substance abuse and depression are common and should be managed as standard. Unlike with anorexia, mood and anxiety symptoms are unlikely to be due to malnutrition.

Prognosis

Anorexia

Although weight and menstrual functioning usually improve, eating habits and attitudes to body shape and weight often remain abnormal. Recovery is slow; time to complete remission in anorexia nervosa is typically 5 years. Around a fifth of patients make a full recovery, a quarter develop bulimia nervosa and a fifth remain severely unwell. The remainder tend to follow a relapsing-remitting course. Risk for death in those with anorexia is increased sixfold relative to an age-matched population. Premature death is predominantly due to the complications of starvation (e.g. arrhythmia, sepsis), and around a fifth of deaths are due to suicide. Factors associated with a poorer prognosis are described in Box 24.1 and indicate that poorer outcomes are seen in more severe illness.

Bulimia

The course of bulimia is also variable, although generally better than anorexia, with 50%–70% of patients achieving either full or partial recovery after 5 years. Risk for death in those with bulimia nervosa is doubled compared with age-matched controls. Poor prognostic factors include severe bingeing and purging behaviour, low weight and comorbid depression.

● Chapter Summary

- Eating disorders arise due to a mixture of genetic and environmental risk factors.
- The mainstay of treatment for both anorexia and bulimia is structured psychological intervention.
- Anorexia nervosa is associated with a high mortality, mainly due to physical complications of starvation.
- Admission to hospital may be required to safely manage high-risk patients with eating disorders, potentially using mental health legislation.
- Recovery is typically slow, and many patients have a relapsing/remitting course.

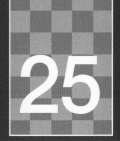

The sleep–wake disorders   25

Sleeping is intimately related to mental health. Not only can psychiatric illnesses such as depression and schizophrenia disturb the quantity and quality of sleep, but certain psychiatric drugs can also have the same effect. Furthermore, persistent primary sleep disturbances, which are common, can result in significant psychological consequences in an otherwise mentally healthy individual.

DEFINITIONS AND CLASSIFICATION

Sleep is divided into five distinct stages as measured by polysomnography (see discussion later): four stages of non-rapid eye movement (non-REM; stages 1, 2, 3 and 4) and an REM stage. Fig. 25.1 summarizes the key characteristics of the stages of sleep.

Sleep can be disrupted due to:

1. Primary sleep disorders
2. Sleep disorders secondary to another mental illness
3. Sleep disorders secondary to another medical condition
4. Sleep disorders secondary to the use of a substance

This chapter will focus principally on primary sleep disorders, which are not caused by another medical condition (e.g. arthritis) or mental illness (e.g. depression), and do not occur secondary to the use of a substance (e.g. alcohol). These disorders are presumed to arise from some defect of an individual's endogenous sleeping mechanism (the reticular activating system) coupled with unhelpful learned behaviours (e.g. worrying about not sleeping). The primary sleep disorders, in turn, are divided into the dyssomnias and the parasomnias:

1. The dyssomnias are characterized by abnormalities in the amount, quality or timing of sleep.
   They include:
   a. Primary insomnia
   b. Primary hypersomnolence
   c. Narcolepsy
   d. Circadian rhythm sleep disorders
   e. Sleep-related breathing disorders
   f. Sleep-related movement disorders (restless leg syndrome)
2. The parasomnias are characterized by abnormal episodes that occur during sleep or sleep–wake transitions. They include non-REM sleep arousal disorders (night terrors and sleepwalking), nightmares and REM sleep behaviour disorder.

Insomnia

Insomnia describes sleep of insufficient quantity or poor quality due to:

- Difficulty falling asleep
- Frequent awakening during the course of sleep
- Early morning awakening with subsequent difficulty getting back to sleep
- Sleep that is not refreshing despite being adequate in length.

In addition to daytime tiredness, persistent insomnia can have significant effects on mood, behaviour and performance. It has been shown that insomnia can also lead to an impairment of health-related quality of life similar to heart failure or depression.

HINTS AND TIPS

When considering sleep disturbance in mental illnesses you may find it useful to think in terms of 'altered sleep patterns' rather than of insomnia. While common in depression, it is only early morning wakening that is part of the somatic syndrome (see Chapter 11) and 20% of people with depression will have atypical symptoms (e.g. weight gain, increased appetite and hypersomnia.)

Primary insomnia is diagnosed when present for at least 3 months, and not attributable to medical or psychiatric illness, substance misuse or other dyssomnia or parasomnia. The numerous causes of insomnia as summarized in Box 25.1 include primary sleep disorders, medical and psychiatric illness and substance use.

Assessment of insomnia

Assessment involves excluding a medical, psychiatric or substance-related cause of insomnia. Many cases of primary insomnia are related to poor sleep hygiene (see Box 25.2 for advice to offer patients). Therefore it is essential to enquire about sleeping times and patterns, and caffeine consumption. It is also useful to obtain collateral information from the patient's sleeping partner regarding sleeping patterns, snoring and movements during the night.

The following questions might be helpful in eliciting the key symptoms of insomnia:

- Do you fall asleep quickly or do you find yourself tossing and turning for some time before dropping off?

Stage of sleep	Duration spent in this phase during night	Characteristics and electroencephalogram (EEG) findings
Stage 1	5%	• Transition from wakefulness to sleep **EEG: theta waves** Theta waves: low amplitude, spike-like waves, 4–7 Hz
Stage 2	45%	**EEG: sleep spindles and K-complexes** Sleep spindles: short rhythmic waveform clusters of 12–14 Hz K-complex: sharp negative wave followed by a slower positive component
Stage 3 and 4 (Slow wave sleep)	25%	• Deep sleep • Unusual arousal characteristics: disorientation, sleep terrors, sleepwalking • Occur in first third to half of night **EEG: delta waves** *Stage 3 – delta waves <50%* *Stage 4 – delta waves >50%* Delta waves: high amplitude, low frequency (<4 Hz)
REM	25%	• Occurs cyclically through the night, every 90 minutes alternating with non-REM sleep • Each episode increases in duration – most episodes occur in last third of night • Features penile erection, skeletal muscle paralysis, and surreal dreaming (including nightmares) **EEG: low amplitude, high frequency, with sawtooth waves** Saw-tooth pattern

Fig. 25.1 Stages of sleep. *REM,* Rapid eye movement.

- Do you wake up repeatedly in the night or can you sleep through once you have managed to get to sleep?
- Do you sometimes awaken too early in the morning and then find that you are unable to get back to sleep?
- Is your sleep refreshing or do you still feel tired in the morning?

If, after a full history, the cause of insomnia remains unclear, the National Institute for Health and Care Excellence (NICE; 2015) recommends a sleep diary. Refer the patient to a sleep specialist for further investigation if there is diagnostic uncertainty, or a suspicion of sleep apnoea, circadian rhythm disorders, parasomnias or narcolepsy. Further investigation is likely to include polysomnography: the simultaneous

BOX 25.1   COMMON CAUSES OF INSOMNIA

Primary sleep disorders

- Dyssomnias
  a. Primary insomnia
  b. Circadian rhythm sleep disorders (jet lag, shift work)
  c. Sleep-related breathing disorders (sleep apnoea syndromes)
  d. Sleep-related movement disorders (restless legs syndrome)
- Parasomnias (all)

Psychiatric disorders

- Anxiety
- Depression
- Mania
- Schizophrenia

Physical disorders

- Painful conditions (malignancies, arthritis, reflux disease)
- Cardiorespiratory discomfort (dyspnoea, coughing, palpitations)
- Nocturia (prostatic hypertrophy, urinary tract infections)
- Metabolic or endocrine conditions (thyroid disease, renal or liver failure)
- Central nervous system lesion (especially brainstem and hypothalamus)

Substances

- Caffeine and other stimulants
- Alcohol
- Prescribed drugs (e.g. selective serotonin reuptake inhibitors, some antipsychotics)
- Substance withdrawal syndrome

BOX 25.2   GOOD SLEEP HYGIENE

- Avoid sleeping during the day.
- Exercise during the day (but not within 4 hours of bedtime) and maintain a healthy diet.
- Eliminate the use of stimulants (e.g. caffeine, nicotine, alcohol) within 6 hours of bedtime.
- Condition the brain by only using the bed for sleeping and sex – not for reading, watching TV, etc.
- Go to bed and awaken at the same time each day.
- Avoid stimulating activities before bedtime (e.g. television, games). Instead, engage in relaxation techniques or reading.
- Try having a hot bath or drinking a cup of warm milk near bedtime.
- Avoid large meals near bedtime.
- Ensure that the bed is comfortable and that the bedroom is quiet.
- Do not lie in bed awake for longer than 15 minutes (but do not watch the clock!). Get up and do another relaxing activity and try sleeping later.

process of monitoring various physical parameters during sleep, including electroencephalogram, electrocardiogram, electromyogram, electrooculogram (eye movement), blood oxygen saturation, chest and abdominal excursion, mouth and nose air entry rates and the loudness of snoring.

COMMUNICATION

When considering insomnia, ask what the normal amount of sleep is for the patient in order for them to feel refreshed in the morning and what time they normally wake up. There is significant individual variation.

Management of primary insomnia

The most important aspect of management is providing education about correct sleep hygiene (see Box 25.3).

There is a limited role for medication in the treatment of primary insomnia. Hypnotics may help in the short-term, but the development of tolerance to their effects (usually within 2 weeks), possible dependence and their propensity to cause rebound insomnia limit their use. Therefore they should only be prescribed on a time-limited basis, ideally for use on alternate or occasional nights rather than every night. Drugs with a long half-life should be avoided, to prevent leaving patients feeling drowsy the next day (the 'chemical hangover') and to avoid accumulation with repeated doses. Commonly used agents include the 'Z-drugs' (zopiclone, zolpidem, zaleplon) and benzodiazepines with a short half-life (such as temazepam). NICE (2015) advises that if there is no response to one hypnotic, an alternative should not be prescribed.

Primary hypersomnolence

Hypersomnia describes excessive sleepiness that manifests as either a prolonged period of sleep or sleep episodes that occur during normal waking hours.

Primary hypersomnolence is diagnosed when patients present with hypersomnia for at least a month not attributable to a medical or psychiatric condition, substance use or other dyssomnia (especially narcolepsy and sleep apnoea) or parasomnia. The numerous causes of hypersomnia as summarized in Box 25.3 include primary sleep disorders, medical and psychiatric illness, substance use and sleep deprivation. The treatment of primary hypersomnia is usually with stimulants such as dexamphetamine, methylphenidate and modafinil.

Narcolepsy

Narcolepsy typically presents in young people aged 10–20 years who report an abrupt onset of pervasive daytime sleepiness. It affects around 1 in 2000 people. Symptoms of narcolepsy are the tetrad of:

1. Irresistible attacks of refreshing sleep that may occur at inappropriate times (e.g. driving)
2. Cataplexy (sudden, bilateral loss of muscle tone usually precipitated by intense emotion leading to collapse and lasting for seconds to minutes)

BOX 25.3 COMMON CAUSES OF HYPERSOMNOLENCE

Primary sleep disorders

Dyssomnias
  a. Primary hypersomnolence
  b. Narcolepsy
  c. Sleep-related breathing disorders (sleep apnoea syndromes)
  d. Sleep-related movement disorders (restless legs syndrome)
  e. Circadian rhythm sleep disorders (jet lag, shift work)
Parasomnias (all)

Psychiatric disorders

Depression with atypical features

Physical disorders

- Encephalitis and meningitis
- Stroke, head injury, brain tumour
- Degenerative neurological conditions
- Toxic, metabolic or endocrine abnormalities
- Kleine–Levin syndrome

Substances

- Alcohol
- Prescribed drugs (e.g. antipsychotics, benzodiazepines, tricyclic antidepressants)
- Substance withdrawal syndrome

Secondary to insomnia or sleep deprivation

---

3. Hypnagogic or hypnopompic hallucinations (see Chapter 9)
4. Sleep paralysis at the beginning or end of sleep episodes

The symptoms arise from elements of REM sleep intruding into wakefulness. Diagnosis is confirmed by observing rapid onset of REM on polysomnography during sleep latency studies.

In type 1 narcolepsy, cataplexy always occurs. It is due to a deficiency of hypocretin, a neuropeptide that regulates the initiation of REM sleep. Levels are low in cerebrospinal fluid obtained via lumbar puncture. It is thought to arise following autoimmune-mediated damage to hypocretin-producing cells in the hypothalamus, triggered following an infection. Over 98% of people with type 1 narcolepsy have a particular human leukocyte antigen haplotype. In type 2 narcolepsy (which is even rarer) cataplexy either does not occur or is atypical. Its aetiology overlaps with type 1 narcolepsy but in general is less well understood.

The treatment of narcolepsy includes taking naps at regular times and ensuring sufficient duration of night-time sleep. Typically, stimulants are needed to reduce daytime sleepiness (modafinil is first line). Cataplexy, sleep paralysis and hallucinations at the sleep–wake boundary can be improved by low-dose antidepressants (usually venlafaxine or clomipramine). Noradrenaline and serotonin suppress REM sleep, and so do antidepressants.

Circadian rhythm sleep disorders

Circadian rhythm sleep disorder (sleep–wake schedule disorder) is characterized by a lack of synchrony between an individual's endogenous circadian rhythm for sleep and that demanded by their environment, resulting in the individual being tired when they should be awake (hypersomnia) and being awake when they should be sleeping (insomnia). This disorder results from either a malfunction of the internal 'biological clock' that regulates sleep or from an unnatural environmental change (e.g. jet lag, night-shift work). Treatment comprises sleep hygiene, enhancing environmental cues regarding time of day (e.g. having a dark bedroom) and bright light therapy.

Sleep-related breathing disorders

Abnormalities of ventilation during sleep can cause repeated disruptions to sleep. This results in unrefreshing sleep and excessive sleepiness during the day. Obstructive sleep apnoea syndrome, the most common breathing-related sleep disorder, is characterized by obstruction of the upper airways during sleep, despite an adequate respiratory effort. Typically, an individual will have noisy breathing during sleep with loud snoring interspersed with apnoeic episodes lasting from 20 to 90 seconds, sometimes associated with cyanosis. It is an increasingly common condition, affecting around 10% of men, 5% of women and 1% of children. The prevalence is much higher in obese, elderly or hypertensive individuals and is also prominent in some patients with intellectual disabilities. The repeated stress of sudden arousals has significant cardiovascular and neuro-psychiatric morbidity and should be actively excluded when an at-risk patient presents with hypersomnia, impairment of concentration and memory or other psychiatric symptoms. Collateral history from a bed partner, who is often aware of the sleeping difficulties, is extremely useful.

The diagnosis is confirmed by polysomnography with concurrent monitoring of electroencephalogram and respiration. Treatment comprises lifestyle advice (weight loss, avoidance of alcohol, sleep on one's side, not back) and provision of nasal continuous positive airway pressure.

> **RED FLAG**
>
> Obstructive sleep apnoea increases the risk for road traffic accidents around sevenfold, and also increases the risk for systemic hypertension. It is a useful diagnosis to make as the majority of patients respond well to treatment with continuous positive airway pressure. However, most cases go undiagnosed.

> **HINTS AND TIPS**
>
> Medication and substances increase the risk for obstructive sleep apnoea, particularly opiates, benzodiazepines and alcohol. Always take a substance history in someone presenting with symptoms of sleep apnoea.

Sleep-related movement disorder

Restless legs syndrome is the commonest sleep-related movement disorder. Patients report uncomfortable sensations in their legs when at rest (typically crawling, burning, tingling or itching), which are relieved by movement. Because inactivity is required for sleep, restless leg syndrome can delay sleep onset and precipitate awakenings. The disorder arises most frequently in young adults and generally worsens slowly over time, affecting around 1 in 50 people. It runs in families, is twice as common in women, and often occurs transiently during pregnancy. Medication can cause it, particularly lithium, antidepressants, antihistamines and dopamine antagonists (e.g. metoclopramide, antipsychotics). Key differentials are peripheral neuropathy (not worse at night), vascular disease (worsened by movement, not relieved) and akathisia (movement driven by an inner restlessness, not a specific need to move legs). Ferritin levels should be checked, as restless legs are a rare presentation of iron deficiency, which impacts on dopamine metabolism.

Nonpharmacological management includes sleep hygiene, exercise and avoidance of agents which may worsen symptoms (e.g. alcohol, caffeine, medication). Pharmacological management is reserved for severe cases for short periods (e.g. 6 months) and includes dopamine agonists (e.g. pramipexole, ropinirole) or antiepileptics which bind voltage-gated calcium channels (gabapentin, pregabalin).

Non-REM sleep arousal disorders

Non-REM sleep arousal disorders are recurrent incomplete awakenings from sleep during sleep stages outwith REM, generally slow wave sleep and generally during the first third of the night. The duration of the incomplete awakening is generally 1–10 minutes but can be up to an hour. The two main subtypes are night terrors and sleep walking. They are thought to share a common pathophysiology. Management is to exclude other diagnoses, offer reassurance and advise good sleep hygiene. It is not necessary to attempt to terminate episodes, but it may be useful to remove potentially harmful objects or routes from around someone who sleepwalks frequently.

Sleep terrors (night terrors)

Sleep terrors are episodes that feature an individual (usually a child) abruptly waking from sleep, usually with a scream, appearing to be in a state of extreme fear. These episodes are associated with:

- Autonomic arousal, for example, tachycardia, dilated pupils, sweating and rapid breathing
- A relative unresponsiveness to the efforts of others to comfort the person, who appears confused and disorientated

Upon full awakening, there is amnesia for the episode and no recall of any dream or nightmare. Sleep terrors are seen in up to 6% of children aged 4–12 years and usually resolve by adolescence. Sleep terrors should be distinguished from nightmares, panic attacks and epileptic seizures. Panic attacks tend not to be associated with confusion, and amnesia is uncommon.

Sleepwalking (somnambulism)

Sleepwalking is characterized by an unusual state of consciousness in which complex motor behaviour occurs during sleep. While sleepwalking, the individual has a blank staring face, is relatively unresponsive to communication from others and is difficult to waken. When sleepwalkers do wake up, either during an episode or the following morning, they have no recollection of the event ever having occurred. Sleepwalking is not associated with impairment of cognition or behaviour, although there may be an initial brief period of disorientation subsequent to waking up from a sleepwalking episode. The peak prevalence of sleepwalking occurs at the age of 12 years, with an onset between the age of 4 and 8 years. About 2%–3% of children and about 0.5% of adults have regular episodes. Sleepwalking runs in families, with 80% of sleepwalkers having a positive family history for sleepwalking or sleep terrors.

Nightmares

Between 10% and 50% of children, aged 3–5 years, experience repeated nightmares, and they also occur occasionally in up to 50% of adults. Nightmares are characterized by an individual waking from sleep due to an intensely frightening dream involving threats to survival, security or self-esteem. Nightmares are distinguished from sleep terrors by the observation that not only is the individual alert and orientated immediately after awakening but is able to recall the bad dream in vivid detail. Furthermore, nightmares tend to occur during the second half of the night because they arise almost exclusively during REM sleep, which tends to be longer and have more intense, surreal dreaming during the latter part of the night. Nightmares can be precipitated by withdrawal from REM-suppressing agents (such as antidepressants or alcohol) or by commencing β-blockers or dopamine agonists. Management is to reassure, avoid medications that may precipitate nightmares and advise avoidance of stress.

REM sleep behaviour disorder

Unlike the other parasomnias, REM sleep behaviour disorder is more common in older adults, typically presenting in men in their 50s. There is a failure of muscle atonia during REM, allowing dreams to be acted out. The dream content is often of a negative and violent nature, so sufferers may jerk, punch, shout, get out of bed or attack their partner. This occurs regardless of whether the sufferer has a history of violence and aggression. When awakened, patients often report very vivid, intense, threatening dreams. Often, patients present because of injuries to themselves or their partner. The behaviours are more frequent in the last third of the sleep period and can occur cyclically (as REM sleep occurs approximately every 90 minutes).

There is a strong association between REM sleep behaviour disorder and neurodegenerative conditions involving abnormal deposition of synuclein protein (Parkinson disease, Lewy body dementia, multisystem atrophy). Over half of patients will go on to be diagnosed with Parkinson disease, potentially up to 10 years later. The sleep disorder can improve as the neurodegeneration progresses.

Management includes environmental modification to reduce injury (e.g. cushions around the bed, removal of potentially dangerous objects from the bedroom). Clonazepam is highly effective in reducing the behaviours (up to 90% of cases). Interestingly, tolerance does not seem to arise, so it can be continued long-term.

HINTS AND TIPS

Upon awakening from a rapid eye movement (REM) parasomnia, the patient is alert and recalls a dream. Patients who are woken from a non-REM parasomnia are disorientated and confused, with no recollection of a dream or their behaviour.

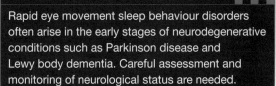

RED FLAG

Rapid eye movement sleep behaviour disorders often arise in the early stages of neurodegenerative conditions such as Parkinson disease and Lewy body dementia. Careful assessment and monitoring of neurological status are needed.

● Chapter Summary

- Sleep can be disrupted due to a primary sleep disorder, a psychiatric condition, a medical condition or substance use (prescribed medications or recreational).
- Dyssomnias are characterized by abnormalities in the amount, quality or timing of sleep.
- Parasomnias are characterized by abnormal episodes that occur during sleep or sleep–wake transitions.
- Good sleep hygiene, ensuring sufficient duration of sleep and avoiding recreational substances are recommended for all patients with sleep problems.
- Hypnotics can be helpful for short-term use in insomnia but lose effectiveness if continued long-term.

FURTHER READING

Sleep diary sample
http://yoursleep.aasmnet.org/pdf/sleepdiary.pdf

Epworth sleepiness scale
http://epworthsleepinessscale.com/about-the-ess/

The psychosexual disorders

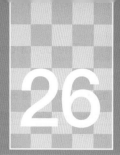

26

Healthy sexual functioning requires a healthy body and, perhaps more importantly, a healthy mind and relationship. Physical or psychological problems (or a combination of the two) can cause a wide variety of sexual problems. Mental health workers may be consulted about sexual problems that are largely due to psychological difficulties (not predominantly due to a biological problem) – that is, psychosexual problems.

The psychosexual disorders can be classified into three groups:

- Sexual dysfunction
- Disorders of sexual preference (paraphilias)
- Gender identity disorders

SEXUAL DYSFUNCTION

Clinical features

Sexual stimulation is summarized in a four-phase sexual response cycle (Fig. 26.1). Sexual dysfunction describes pain associated with intercourse or abnormalities of the sexual response cycle that lead to difficulties in participating in sexual activities. Although this chapter is focused on psychological dysfunction, the sexual response cycle

consists of both psychological and biological processes and it is rarely possible to identify cases of sexual dysfunction with a purely physiological or purely psychological aetiology. Nevertheless, both the International Statistical Classification of Diseases and Related Health Problems, 10th revision (ICD-10) and the Diagnostic and Statistical Manual of Mental Disorders, 5th Edition (DSM-5) stipulate that a sexual dysfunction disorder should only be diagnosed when the problem is not better explained by medication use, substance use or a physical medical condition. Table 26.1 summarizes the sexual dysfunction disorders.

HINTS AND TIPS

Women have a large interindividual variability in the type and duration of stimulation that results in orgasm. The diagnosis of female orgasmic disorder should only be made if the ability to achieve orgasm is less than would be reasonably expected for a woman's age, sexual experience and quality of sexual activity – and then only if the orgasmic dysfunction results in marked distress or relationship difficulties.

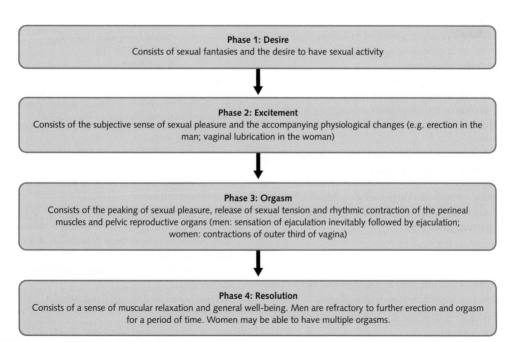

Phase 1: Desire
Consists of sexual fantasies and the desire to have sexual activity

Phase 2: Excitement
Consists of the subjective sense of sexual pleasure and the accompanying physiological changes (e.g. erection in the man; vaginal lubrication in the woman)

Phase 3: Orgasm
Consists of the peaking of sexual pleasure, release of sexual tension and rhythmic contraction of the perineal muscles and pelvic reproductive organs (men: sensation of ejaculation inevitably followed by ejaculation; women: contractions of outer third of vagina)

Phase 4: Resolution
Consists of a sense of muscular relaxation and general well-being. Men are refractory to further erection and orgasm for a period of time. Women may be able to have multiple orgasms.

Fig. 26.1 The four-phase sexual response cycle.

Table 26.1 Sexual dysfunction disorders

Phase of cycle	Dysfunction[a]	Description
Desire	Lack or loss of sexual desire (male hypoactive sexual desire disorder; female sexual interest/arousal disorder) Sexual aversion and lack of sexual enjoyment	Loss of desire to have, or to fantasize about sex – not due to other sexual dysfunction (e.g. erectile dysfunction, dyspareunia) Avoidance of sex due to negative feelings (fear, anxiety, repulsion) or lack of enjoyment
Excitement	Failure of genital response (male erectile disorder; female sexual arousal disorder)	Inability to attain or maintain sexual intercourse due to an inadequate erection in men, or poor lubrication–swelling response in women
Orgasm	Orgasmic dysfunction (female orgasmic disorder; delayed ejaculation) Premature ejaculation (premature ejaculation)	Recurrent absence, or delay, of orgasm or ejaculation despite adequate sexual stimulation Recurrent ejaculation with minimal sexual stimulation before the man wishes
Sexual pain	Nonorganic dyspareunia (genito-pelvic pain/penetration disorder) Vaginismus	Genital pain during sex in men or women – not due to other sexual dysfunction (e.g. poor lubrication–swelling response, vaginismus) or medical condition (e.g. atrophic vaginitis) Recurrent, involuntary spasm of the muscles that surround the outer third of the vagina, causing occlusion of the vaginal opening

[a] *The Diagnostic and Statistical Manual of Mental Disorders, 5th Edition (DSM-5) terms are in square brackets; the International Statistical Classification of Diseases and Related Health Problems, 10th revision (ICD-10) terms are not. In general, DSM-5 has simplified the classification of symptoms into fewer sexual dysfunction disorders. The current draft of ICD-11 (not yet published) is similar to DSM-5.*

Epidemiology

Sexual dysfunction is very common. A recent large UK survey found that 42% of men and 51% of women reported one or more problems with sexual response lasting at least 3 months, but only around 10% of people were distressed about their sexual function. The self-report cross-sectional prevalence (not clinical diagnoses) of specific sexual dysfunctions is shown in Table 26.2. The evidence suggests that:

- The prevalence of sexual problems in women tends to decrease with increasing age, except for those who report trouble lubricating.
- Men, by contrast, have an increased prevalence of erectile problems with increasing age.
- Sexual dysfunction is more likely among people with poor physical and emotional health (particularly depression).
- Sexual dysfunction is highly associated with negative experiences in sexual relationships.
- Sexual dysfunction is associated with relationship difficulties: being unhappy in a relationship, not being in a steady relationship and difficulties communicating with a partner about sex.

Aetiology

There are many, often interrelated, psychosocial factors that may result in psychogenic sexual dysfunction:

- Ambivalent attitude about sex or intimacy (e.g. anxiety, fear, guilt, shame)
- History of rape or childhood sexual abuse

Table 26.2 Reported frequency of sexual dysfunction in Britons aged 16–74 years

		(%)[a]
Men	Premature ejaculation	15
	Lack of sexual interest	15
	Erectile difficulties	13
	Unable to achieve orgasm	9
Women	Lack of sexual interest	34
	Unable to achieve orgasm	16
	Trouble lubricating	13
	Dyspareunia	8

[a] *Problem present for 3 or more months in those who have had sex within previous year (data from Sexual function in Britain: findings from the third National Survey of Sexual Attitudes and Lifestyles (Natsal-3). Mitchell KR et al., Lancet. 2013 Nov 30;382(9907):1817–29. Doi: 10.1016/S0140-6736(13)62366-1.)*

- Fears of consequences of sex (e.g. pregnancy, sexually transmitted diseases)
- A poor or deteriorating relationship (e.g. feeling undesirable, finding the partner undesirable, lack of trust, feelings of resentment or hostility, lack of respect, fear of rejection)
- Anxiety about sexual performance or physical attractiveness
- Fatigue, stress or difficult psychosocial circumstances

Frequently, there is more than one psychosocial problem that can affect more than one of the phases of the sexual response cycle. For example, the belief that sex is inherently sinful in the context of an abusive relationship may lead to a lack of desire, a poor lubrication–swelling response and difficulty in reaching orgasm.

Differential diagnosis

Other causes of sexual dysfunction should be excluded when assessing a patient with sexual dysfunction. These include:

- Medical conditions (e.g. diabetes mellitus, vascular disease, vaginitis, endometriosis, spinal cord injuries, pelvic fractures, prostatectomy, multiple sclerosis, thyroid disease, hyperprolactinaemia)
- Prescribed or recreational drugs (see Box 26.1)
- Psychiatric illness: mental disorders such as depression, anxiety and alcohol dependence are frequently associated with sexual dysfunction. In addition, psychiatric medication often results in sexual dysfunction as a side-effect. However, sexual functioning frequently improves as the patient's mental illness (e.g. depression) improves, even though the medication (e.g. antidepressants) may have adverse sexual effects.

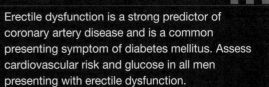

RED FLAG

Erectile dysfunction is a strong predictor of coronary artery disease and is a common presenting symptom of diabetes mellitus. Assess cardiovascular risk and glucose in all men presenting with erectile dysfunction.

HINTS AND TIPS

The clear presence of a biological cause of sexual dysfunction does not rule out a psychogenic sexual dysfunction, as the two are often interrelated. For example, a 55-year-old man with diabetes and advanced atherosclerosis notices a weakened erection; he subsequently becomes anxious during sex, fearing that he is losing his virility. This leads to a complete loss of his erectile potency.

BOX 26.1 PRESCRIBED AND RECREATIONAL DRUGS ASSOCIATED WITH SEXUAL DYSFUNCTION

Psychiatric drugs
- Antidepressants (tricyclics, SSRIs and MAOIs)[a]
- Antipsychotics (especially first-generation antipsychotics)
- Benzodiazepines
- Lithium

Recreational drugs
- Alcohol
- Amphetamines
- Cannabis
- Cocaine
- Opiates

Medical drugs
- Antiandrogens
- Anticonvulsants
- Antihistamines
- Antihypertensives (including β-blockers)
- Digoxin
- Diuretics

a The antidepressant least likely to be associated with sexual dysfunction is mirtazapine.
MAOI, Monoamine oxidase inhibitor; SSRI, selective serotonin reuptake inhibitor.

Assessment considerations

- The wide differential diagnosis requires a comprehensive history including medical, psychiatric, sexual and relationship histories as well as current medication and recreational substance use. Questions regarding sexual activities outside the problematic context (e.g. morning erections, masturbation, sexual fantasy) can be very helpful.
- A thorough physical examination, including genitalia, should be conducted. In addition, gynaecological examination may be needed for cases of dyspareunia or vaginismus in women.
- Blood tests should be performed to assess for medical causes of sexual dysfunction, particularly hyperprolactinaemia, hypotestosteronaemia and, in erectile dysfunction, glucose and lipids. Rarely, further investigations may be necessary to exclude medical causes of erectile dysfunction (e.g. monitoring of nocturnal penile tumescence (excludes physiological causes of impotence if able to have erection during rapid eye movement sleep) and monitoring penile blood flow with Doppler ultrasonography).

COMMUNICATION

Taking a sexual history can be embarrassing for both patients and doctors, and basic communication skills are very important. Privacy should be ensured, and nonverbal aspects of communication utilized (e.g. body language, use of silence). Straightforward terminology should be used (e.g. 'vagina', rather than 'down below'; 'condom', rather than 'protection'). Reassurance and acknowledgement of discomfort (e.g. 'I can see how difficult this is for you to talk about') can be very helpful.

Management considerations

- Many patients need no more than reassurance, advice and sexual education. Patients who have significant relationship difficulties may benefit from relationship counselling before attempting specific treatment for sexual dysfunction.
- Some couples with minor problems benefit from self-help materials, particularly those with no major relationship difficulties.
- Urology clinics deal mainly with physiological sexual dysfunction, particularly erectile problems.
- Sexual dysfunction clinics have multidisciplinary teams that focus on both psychological and physical aspects of sexual dysfunction and are best equipped to deal with cases that do not respond to nonspecific measures.
- Some couples benefit from sex therapy, in which partners are treated together and are taught to communicate openly about sex, in addition to receiving education about sexual anatomy and the physiology of the sexual response cycle. They also take part in graded assignments, beginning with caressing of their partner's body, without genital contact, for their own and then their partner's pleasure. These behavioural tasks progress through a number of stages with increasing sexual intimacy, with the focus remaining on pleasurable physical contact as opposed to the monitoring of sexual arousal or the preoccupation with achieving orgasm. Couples suitable for sex therapy include those with a significant psychological component to their problem, those with reasonable motivation and those with a reasonably harmonious relationship.
- Table 26.3 summarizes some of the specific exercises often used in the context of sex therapy that may be helpful with particular problems.
- Biological treatments may be very effective, especially for erectile problems (e.g. oral sildenafil (Viagra), intracavernosal injections, vacuum devices, prosthetic implants and surgery for venous leakage). See Box 26.2. Testosterone may increase sexual drive in patients with low levels of the hormone. For difficulties with premature ejaculation, selective serotonin reuptake inhibitors may delay ejaculation, but this is rarely a long-term solution.

Table 26.3 Specific exercises useful in sexual dysfunction

Sexual dysfunction	Exercise
Female orgasmic disorder	Exercises in sexual fantasy and masturbation, sometimes with a vibrator or dildo
Premature ejaculation	Squeeze technique: partner or individual squeezes the glans of penis for a few seconds when he feels that he is about to ejaculate Start–stop method: stimulation is halted and arousal is allowed to subside when the man feels that ejaculation is imminent. The process is then repeated Quiet vagina: man keeps penis motionless in vagina for increasing periods before ejaculating
Vaginismus	Desensitization, first by finger insertion followed by dilators of increasing size

---

BOX 26.2 MANAGEMENT OF MEN WITH ERECTILE DYSFUNCTION

- Check testosterone level.
- Calculate 10-year cardiovascular risk and manage appropriately.
- Lifestyle advice:
  - Weight loss, stop smoking, reduce alcohol, increase exercise.
  - If a man cycles more than 3 hours a week: advise a trial without cycling.
- Medication:
  - Consider substituting potentially contributory medication (see Box 26.1).
  - Consider a phosphodiesterase inhibitor (sildenafil, tadalafil or vardenafil), regardless of the cause.

Prognosis

Vaginismus has an excellent prognosis. Premature ejaculation and psychogenic erectile dysfunction also respond fairly well to treatment. Problems associated with low sexual desire, especially in men, seem more resistant to treatment.

DISORDERS OF SEXUAL PREFERENCE (PARAPHILIAS)

The essential features of a paraphilia are recurrent sexually arousing fantasies, sexual urges or behaviours involving: (1) nonhuman objects; (2) the suffering or humiliation of oneself or one's partner; or (3) children or other nonconsenting individuals. However, normal sexuality need not necessarily be focused on genitals with the aim of reproduction. To be a disorder, the paraphilia needs to be causing significant harm, or high risk for harm, to the individual or others. It is useful to divide the paraphilias into two groups:

1. Abnormalities of the object of sexual interest (e.g. paedophilia, fetishism, transvestic fetishism).
2. Abnormalities of the sexual act (e.g. exhibitionism, voyeurism, sexual sadism, sexual masochism).

Table 26.4 summarizes the specific paraphilias. The paraphilias are mainly confined to men (with the exception of sexual masochism) and usually begin in late adolescence or early adulthood. Paedophilia and exhibitionism are frequently seen in a forensic setting and account for the majority of sexual offenders referred for a psychiatric opinion (see Chapter 32). Prevalence of paraphilias in the general population has not been reliably assessed. The aetiology is unknown, but there is often an impaired capacity for affectionate sexual activity, and patients with paraphilia often have comorbid personality disorders.

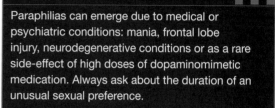

RED FLAG

Paraphilias can emerge due to medical or psychiatric conditions: mania, frontal lobe injury, neurodegenerative conditions or as a rare side-effect of high doses of dopaminomimetic medication. Always ask about the duration of an unusual sexual preference.

Table 26.4 The paraphilias

Abnormalities of the object of sexual interest	
Paedophilia	Sexual fantasies, urges or behaviours involving children
Fetishism	Sexual fantasies, urges or behaviours involving inanimate objects or parts of the body that are not directly erogenous
Transvestic fetishism	Sexual fantasies, urges or behaviours involving cross-dressing (wearing of clothes of the opposite sex). Rare in women.
Other	Many other abnormal objects of sexual interest are found more rarely (e.g. animals (*zoophilia* or bestiality), corpses (*necrophilia*), faeces (*coprophilia*), urine (*urophilia*))
Abnormalities of the sexual act	
Exhibitionism	Sexual fantasies, urges or behaviours involving the exposure of genitals to unsuspecting strangers
Voyeurism	Sexual fantasies, urges or behaviours involving the act of observing unsuspecting people engaging in sexual activity or undressing
Frotteurism	Sexual fantasies, urges or behaviours involving touching or rubbing against a nonconsenting person
Sexual sadism	Sexual fantasies, urges or behaviours involving the infliction of acts of physical or psychological suffering or humiliation on others
Sexual masochism	Sexual fantasies, urges or behaviours involving the infliction of acts of humiliation or suffering on oneself

Management options include behaviour therapy (covert sensitization, where patients attempt to pair paraphilic thoughts with humiliating consequences) and aversion therapy (pairing paraphilic thoughts with a noxious stimulus such as an unpleasant odour or taste). Individual psychodynamic and group therapies are also used. Cognitive-behavioural therapy programmes and antiandrogens (e.g. cyproterone acetate) have shown some efficacy in the treatment of some paedophiles and exhibitionists; however, there is little evidence that any treatment is consistently effective in either of these conditions. It should be noted that, dependent on risk for offending, management within a forensic setting may be required (see Chapter 32).

Paraphilias associated with a young age of onset, a high frequency of acts, no remorse about acts and a lack of motivation for change have a particularly poor prognosis.

GENDER IDENTITY

Gender identity describes an individual's inner sense of being male or female. This usually corresponds to the person's sexual identity which comprises all their biological and anatomical sexual characteristics (i.e. external and internal genitalia, chromosomes, sex hormones and secondary sex characteristics). Gender identity is thought to be fully formed by the age of 3 years.

There has been considerable debate over the years as to whether gender identity disorder (termed transsexualism in ICD-10) is a mental disorder. Many do not regard cross-gender feelings and behaviours as a 'disorder', and instead question what constitutes a normal gender identity or gender role. DSM-5 has replaced the term with the (less stigmatizing) term 'gender dysphoria' and the current draft of ICD-11 (not yet published) uses the term 'gender incongruence'.

Many areas provide multidisciplinary clinics for people whose biological gender is inconsistent with their gender identity. The role of the psychiatrist is to exclude the presence of mental disorder as a cause of gender dysphoria (e.g. a delusional belief in schizophrenia), and to assess and treat comorbid mental disorders which may be present.

Patients who are committed to gender change can be helped with hormones and surgery, usually after they have completed a 'real life test', which involves living as the opposite sex for at least a year.

HINTS AND TIPS

Transgenderism, transsexualism and transvestism are not the same.

- Transgenderism describes identifying with a gender different to the gender assigned at birth.
- Transsexualism describes a refusal to live as the gender assigned at birth.
- Transvestism describes dressing in clothes intended for members of the opposite sex.

Questions you may find useful are 'Do you wish to be accepted as the opposite sex?' 'Are you content with your gender?' 'Does cross-dressing cause sexual arousal?' The latter would suggest transvestic fetishism.

Chapter Summary

- Sexual dysfunction is common, particularly in those with poor physical or emotional health.
- It often arises due to a combination of physical and psychological factors.
- It is important to exclude potentially serious causes, particularly cardiovascular disease and diabetes in erectile dysfunction.
- Management of any psychological component hinges on reassurance, psychoeducation and graded intimate contact.
- Paraphilias are unusual sexual interests that are viewed as disorders when associated with significant harm, or risk for harm, to the individual or others.
- Gender dysphoria/incongruence is a mismatch between a person's initial gender assignment and experienced gender. Rarely, this arises due to mental disorder.

PREMENSTRUAL SYNDROME

Clinical features

The premenstrual syndrome (PMS) has been defined as the recurrence of symptoms during the premenstruum, with their absence in the postmenstruum. Symptoms tend to occur in the 10 days prior to menstruation, peaking 2 days before menses begin and remit in the 2 weeks following. Mental health symptoms include low mood, labile mood, irritability, concentration difficulties, anxiety and fatigue. Physical symptoms such as headache, abdominal bloating and breast tenderness are also fairly common. The timing of a given symptom relative to menstruation rather than its exact nature is what is diagnostically important.

The Diagnostic and Statistical Manual of Mental Disorders, 5th Edition (DSM-5) and the current draft of International Statistical Classification of Diseases and Related Health Problems, 11th edition (ICD-11; not yet published) describe *premenstrual dysphoric disorder* (PMDD), which in essence are the mental health symptoms of PMS combined with significant distress or functional impairment. Prospective evaluation of symptoms over at least two cycles is recommended prior to making the diagnosis, as retrospective recall is unreliable.

The National Institute for Health and Care Excellence (NICE; 2014) classifies PMS as mild, moderate or severe depending on its impact on personal, social or professional life. Mild PMS does not interfere with normal functioning in these domains, moderate PMS causes interference, and severe PMS causes withdrawal from these domains.

Epidemiology/aetiology

Up to 40% of women report experiencing some symptoms of PMS, however, only around a fifth seek medical help and only about 5% of women experience symptoms of a severity sufficient to interfere with their work or lifestyle. The prevalence is higher in women who experience significant degrees of psychosocial stress, have a history of trauma, are obese, have a family history of PMS or who have a history of depression or anxiety. In those who have a history of mental health problems it is important to confirm that the luteal phase symptoms are not merely an exacerbation of difficulties that are present continuously. If this is the case, management should focus on the primary mental health problem.

The principal theory of causation is that the rise in progesterone during the luteal phase is responsible for symptoms of PMS. Although women with and without PMS do not differ in levels of reproductive hormones, there is some evidence that those with PMS are more sensitive to a given level of progesterone. The responsiveness to progesterone is probably influenced by serotonin (which normally dampens the behavioural consequences of progesterone) and possibly also influenced by γ-aminobutyric acid.

Management

Management is informed by aetiology, with the principles being stress reduction, ovulation suppression (which prevents the luteal rise in progesterone) and central nervous system serotonin enhancement.

In mild PMS, NICE (2014) recommends advice on healthy eating, stress reduction, regular sleep and regular exercise. In moderate PMS, NICE (2014) recommends a new-generation combined oral contraceptive (first-line treatments are those containing the progestogen drospirenone). If pain is a prominent symptom, paracetamol or a nonsteroidal antiinflammatory drug is recommended. If the patient is interested in psychological intervention, refer for cognitive-behavioural therapy (CBT). In severe PMS (which would include anyone with a diagnosis of PMDD), the strategies for moderate PMS should be trialled first, and a selective serotonin reuptake inhibitor (SSRI) tried if these are ineffective. This can be given either continuously or during the luteal phase only (days 15–28, stopping on first day of menses). Standard doses of common SSRIs are recommended (e.g. fluoxetine 20 mg). If these treatment options do not work, further treatments can be initiated under specialist supervision including gonadotropin-releasing hormone analogues with add-back hormone replacement therapy (HRT) or even surgical treatment with add-back HRT.

MENOPAUSE

There is little evidence that the menopause itself leads to an increased incidence of mental illness. Psychological symptoms may understandably accompany the changes that occur with the menopause; however, it should be remembered that this is a time associated with other psychosocial stressors, such as children leaving home and a growing awareness of ageing. There is no clear psychiatric indication for HRT and its use for psychological symptoms remains controversial. HRT should never substitute treatment with recognized antidepressants for the treatment of a depressive illness.

PSYCHIATRIC CONSIDERATIONS IN PREGNANCY

- The development of new psychiatric illnesses during pregnancy is no more common than in the general population. However, both psychosocial stressors and changing or stopping maintenance medications in women with a history of major mental illnesses carry a degree of risk, and the puerperium is a high-risk period for relapse in major mental illness, particularly bipolar affective disorder. Domestic violence is more common during pregnancy, and this can impair mental health and resilience.
- Women with a major mental illness (bipolar affective disorder, schizophrenia, severe depression) or a history of puerperal psychosis who are pregnant or planning pregnancy should be referred to perinatal psychiatry services, even if they have been stable for some years. Box 27.1 summarizes the indications for referral to a specialist perinatal mental health team.
- For patients prescribed psychotropic medication during pregnancy, a judgement needs to be made – in conjunction with the patient – regarding the risk for relapse against the risk for medication-induced teratogenic or adverse effects for the mother or child. Risks associated with various psychotropic medications are summarized in Table 27.1. Decisions should be made prior to conception (if possible). Up-to-date information on the use of medications during pregnancy should always be sought.
- There is an increased incidence of adverse life events in the weeks prior to a spontaneous abortion (miscarriage).
- Following miscarriage and termination of pregnancy, there is an increased risk for adjustment and bereavement reactions (see Chapter 14). In addition, the risk for puerperal psychosis remains.

BOX 27.1   INDICATIONS FOR REFERRAL TO PERINATAL MENTAL HEALTH SERVICES

Preconceptual counselling (e.g. for women with bipolar disorder).

Pregnant women who are severely psychiatrically unwell.

Pregnant women who are at high risk for significant puerperal illness.

Women who are psychiatrically unwell and are the main carers of babies under 6 months of age.

Pregnant women with harmful or dependent use of substances including alcohol should be referred to a specialist substance misuse team.

Table 27.1 Psychiatric medication during pregnancy and breastfeeding[a]

Drug group	Pregnancy	Breastfeeding
Selective serotonin reuptake inhibitors	Can be associated with withdrawal symptoms in neonates, which are generally mild and self-limiting. Rarely associated with persistent pulmonary hypertension when given after first trimester.	Paroxetine and sertraline: very small amounts excreted in breast milk; short half-life fluoxetine and citalopram are excreted in relatively larger (but still small) amounts. Fluoxetine has a long half-life and thus may accumulate.
Tricyclic antidepressants	Have been used during pregnancy for many years. Commonly result in mild and self-limiting withdrawal reactions in neonates.	Tricyclics are excreted in small amounts only but avoid doxepin (accumulation of metabolite).
Mood stabilizers	All are associated with teratogenicity. Valproate and carbamazepine increase the risk for neural tube defects and should be avoided in pregnancy. Valproate also increases the risk for developmental disorders (30%–40% of babies). Lithium increases the risk for cardiac defects but may be taken during pregnancy.	Risk for neonatal lithium toxicity as breast milk contains 40% of maternal lithium concentration. Avoid if possible. Consider the use of valproate or carbamazepine if necessary, but bear in mind risk for infant hepatotoxicity.
Antipsychotics	Most antipsychotics have no established teratogenic effects but may cause self-limiting extrapyramidal side-effects in neonates. Olanzapine increases risk for gestational diabetes.	Only small amounts excreted but possible effects on developing nervous system. Avoid high doses due to risk for lethargy in infant.
Benzodiazepines and other hypnotics	Associated with floppy infant syndrome (hypotonia, breathing and feeding difficulties) and neonatal withdrawal syndrome.	May cause lethargy in infant. Choose drugs with short half-lives (e.g. lorazepam) if necessary.

[a] *Information on the risks of medication during pregnancy and breastfeeding is constantly evolving. Seek up-to-date advice (see box below).*

PUERPERAL DISORDERS

Any mental disorder can arise during or be exacerbated by pregnancy, delivery or new motherhood. These experiences are anxiety provoking, stressful and potentially life-threatening. They can be difficult for anyone to deal with, even without previous mental health problems, and can worsen symptoms or maladaptive behaviours in those with existing mental health problems. This chapter covers the most common and important perinatal psychiatric disorders, but all the other mental disorders can and do occur in the perinatal period.

In general, the symptoms of a mental disorder are the same within and without the perinatal period, but management can be different as treatment decisions involving medication during pregnancy or breastfeeding require a careful risk–benefit analysis.

Postnatal 'blues'

Also known as 'maternity blues' and 'baby blues', this occurs in up to 50% of postpartum women. It presents within the first 10 days postdelivery, symptoms peak between days 3 and 5 and it resolves within 2 weeks. It is characterized by episodes of tearfulness, mild depression or emotional lability, anxiety and irritability. There appears to be no links with life events, demographic factors or obstetric events, which is suggestive of an underlying biological cause (e.g. a sudden fall in progesterone postdelivery). Postnatal blues is self-limiting, resolves spontaneously and usually only requires reassurance. However, an apparent bad case of postnatal blues may mark the onset of postnatal depression. Symptoms lasting longer than 2 weeks should raise suspicion of a depressive episode.

Postnatal depression

Clinical features

Postnatal depression usually develops within 3 months of delivery (and can start during pregnancy), with peak time of onset at 3–4 weeks. A depressive episode arising more than 6 months after delivery is not generally viewed as postnatal depression. The symptoms are similar to a nonpuerperal depressive episode: low mood, loss of interest or pleasure, fatigability and suicidal ideation (although suicide is rare). Note that sleeping difficulties, weight loss and decreased libido can be normal for the first few months following delivery. Additional features of postnatal depression may include:

- Anxious preoccupation with the baby's health, often associated with feelings of guilt and inadequacy
- Reduced affection for the baby with possible impaired bonding
- Obsessional phenomena, typically involving recurrent and intrusive thoughts of harming the baby (it is crucial to ascertain whether these are regarded as distressing (ego-dystonic), as obsessions usually are, or whether they pose a potential risk).
- Infanticidal thoughts (thoughts of killing the baby) require urgent psychiatric assessment. True infanticidal thoughts are different from obsessions in that they are not experienced as distressing (ego-syntonic as opposed to ego-dystonic), and (worryingly) may involve active planning.

Epidemiology and aetiology

In high-income countries, postnatal depression is the most common complication of childbirth, with rates of around 12%. Evidence suggests that biological factors are not as important as they are in postnatal blues and postpartum psychosis. Psychosocial factors are strongly linked to the development of postnatal depression, with the lack of a close confiding relationship, intimate partner violence, low income and young maternal age all implicated. A previous history of depression is an important risk factor. In women with a history of depression, obstetric complications during delivery are associated with an increased rate of postnatal depression.

Management

The diagnosis and management of postnatal depression are often undertaken within primary care. Psychological and social measures, such as mother-and-baby groups, relationship counselling and problem solving, are often helpful. Midwives and health visitors can be very helpful. In mild cases, NICE (2014) recommends facilitated self-help. For more severe illness, NICE (2014) recommends a high-intensity psychological intervention (e.g. CBT) or antidepressant medication (a tricyclic, SSRI or serotonin-norepinephrine reuptake inhibitor). Antidepressants may be transmitted in small quantities to the baby via breast milk, and a judgement needs to be made, in conjunction with the patient, of the risks versus benefits of medication. It should be noted that (with the exception of doxepin) there has never been evidence to suggest that antidepressants transmitted via breast milk have caused

long-term harm to a baby, but there are significant risks for the baby's cognitive and emotional development if the mother has untreated depression. Table 27.1 provides information on the use of psychotropic medication in breastfeeding mothers. Mothers with severe postnatal depression with suicidal/infanticidal ideation may require hospital admission, with admission with the baby to a mother-and-baby unit usually being preferable. Electroconvulsive therapy may be indicated and usually results in a rapid improvement, which is important to allow the woman to resume contact with the baby as soon as possible. Remember that the assessment of the infant's well-being is an additional part of the comprehensive psychosocial and risk assessment.

HINTS AND TIPS

If a woman has been on an antidepressant during pregnancy, do not change after delivery to a different antidepressant that is 'better for breastfeeding'. Doing this means the child is exposed to two medications, instead of one. The foetus is exposed to far greater levels of antidepressant *in utero* than levels transmitted in breast milk, so if they are healthy at delivery they are unlikely to be harmed by further, lower, exposure.

Prognosis

Most women respond to standard treatment and episodes resolve within 3–6 months; however, some patients have a protracted illness and may require long-term treatment and follow-up. Woman who develop postnatal depression have around a 40% increased risk for developing a similar illness following childbirth in the future. Postnatal depression is associated with disturbances in the mother–infant relationship, and this can lead to problems with the child's cognitive and emotional development.

RED FLAG

Suicide is a leading cause of maternal death, even though it is fortunately rare (1 in 100,000 pregnancies). About 60% of cases were experiencing a severe affective or psychotic illness at the time of death. Always ask about thoughts of suicide in a new mother who is mentally unwell.

Perinatal anxiety disorders

Clinical features
Anxiety disorders in the perinatal period present very similarly to anxiety disorders outside the perinatal period and can include generalized anxiety disorder, obsessive-compulsive disorder, phobias and posttraumatic stress disorder, which may have onset following a highly distressing delivery. Tokophobia is a specific phobia of childbirth and can be primary (nulliparous) or secondary (often following a difficult first delivery). Anxiety disorders can occur on their own or comorbidly with depression.

Epidemiology and aetiology
Anxiety disorders occur in around 13% of women who are pregnant or postpartum. Many of these disorders arise prior to pregnancy rather than being triggered by it, however, there is some evidence that the risk for new-onset obsessive-compulsive disorder is increased postpartum (approximately doubled). Risk factors for perinatal anxiety disorders are unclear but are probably similar to those for anxiety disorders outside the perinatal period (see Chapter 23), combined with the natural increase in anxiety that responsibility for a vulnerable new infant brings.

Management
The diagnosis and management of perinatal anxiety are often done within primary care. As with postnatal depression, midwives and health visitors can be very helpful in identifying psychosocial supports such as community groups and classes. The first-line intervention in all cases is a psychological therapy (NICE 2014). The nature of the therapy depends on the type of anxiety disorder and its severity, following the general NICE guidance for adults (see Chapter 23). Medication may also be required, particularly if a woman is already taking this or has required it in the past.

Prognosis
With the exception of posttraumatic stress disorder, anxiety disorders tend to be chronic, relapsing/remitting conditions. Anxiety disorders during pregnancy are a risk factor for postnatal depression. Prenatal maternal anxiety is associated with altered stress-induced cortisol responses in 7-month-old infants and subsequently in adolescence, potentially influencing the child's own risk for anxiety and depression.

Failure to bond
Some women struggle to form a loving bond with their baby. Mothers at particular risk include those whose own mother–infant attachment was insecure (see Table 30.1), women who experienced childhood neglect or sexual abuse and women with perinatal psychiatric difficulties (e.g. postnatal depression). The woman may seek help, or difficulties may be identified by a health visitor. Management is to involve an early years service who can provide guidance to the mother regarding positive infant interactions.

Postpartum (puerperal) psychosis

Clinical features
The postpartum period is an extremely high-risk period for the development of a psychotic episode. Postpartum (puerperal) psychotic episodes characteristically have an abrupt onset with rapid deterioration. About 50% of symptoms begin on postnatal days 1–3 and the vast majority within 2 weeks of delivery. Episodes typically begin with insomnia, restlessness and perplexity, later progressing to suspiciousness and marked psychotic symptoms (often with content related to the baby). The symptoms can be polymorphic, and frequently fluctuate dramatically in their nature and intensity over a short space of time. Mood symptoms are prominent, and can comprise elation, depression or both (mixed affective state). Patients often retain a degree of insight, and may not disclose certain bizarre delusions or suicidal/homicidal thoughts.

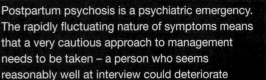

RED FLAG
Postpartum psychosis is a psychiatric emergency. The rapidly fluctuating nature of symptoms means that a very cautious approach to management needs to be taken – a person who seems reasonably well at interview could deteriorate rapidly. Admission is required in all cases.

Epidemiology and aetiology
Postpartum psychosis develops in about 1 in 500 childbirths. It occurs more frequently in primiparous women, and those who have a personal or family history of bipolar affective disorder or postpartum psychosis. If a close family member has bipolar affective disorder, the risk can be as high as 15 in 500 childbirths. Psychosocial factors seem less important, unlike in postnatal depression. Occasionally, a postpartum psychosis may be precipitated by an obstetric complication (e.g. preeclampsia, puerperal infection) or medication. Delirium secondary to such complications is an important differential. Box 27.2 summarizes the risk factors for postpartum psychosis.

Management
Postpartum psychosis is a psychiatric emergency. The assessment of the risk for infanticide and suicide is crucial. Concerning symptoms include:

BOX 27.2   RISK FACTORS FOR POSTPARTUM PSYCHOSIS

Previous postpartum psychosis

History of mood disorder (particularly bipolar affective disorder)

Family history of postpartum psychosis or bipolar affective disorder

Primiparous mother

Delivery associated with caesarean section or perinatal death

---

HINTS AND TIPS

The prevalence of postnatal blues, postnatal depression and puerperal psychosis is inversely related to their severity:

- Postnatal blues develops after 1 in 2 childbirths.
- Postnatal depression develops after 1 in 10 childbirths.
- Puerperal psychosis develops after 1 in 500 childbirths.

- Thoughts of self-harm or harming the baby
- Severe depressive delusions (e.g. belief that the baby is, or should be, dead)
- Command hallucinations instructing the mother to harm herself or her baby

Hospitalization is invariably necessary, with joint admissions to a mother-and-baby unit being preferable when the mother is able to look after her infant under supervision. Detention under mental health legislation may be necessary. Depending on presentation, antipsychotics, antidepressants and mood-stabilizing medications are indicated. Benzodiazepines may be needed in cases of severe behavioural disturbance. All psychotropic drugs should be used with caution in breastfeeding mothers (see Table 27.1), but many women are too unwell to breastfeed in any case.

Electroconvulsive therapy can be particularly effective in severe or treatment-resistant cases. Psychosocial interventions are similar to those for other psychotic episodes, but also include providing support for the father.

Prognosis

Most cases of puerperal psychosis will have recovered by 3 months (75% within 6 weeks). Around one in six women who have a first episode of mood disorder following delivery will go on to develop bipolar disorder. There is about a 50% chance of experiencing a recurrence of postpartum psychosis after future childbirths, which can be reduced by prophylactic therapy. Women who have had both puerperal and nonpuerperal depressive or manic episodes (i.e. have an established mood disorder) have up to an 85% chance of future puerperal psychotic episodes.

● **Chapter Summary**

- Premenstrual dysphoric syndrome describes mood and anxiety symptoms during the luteal phase only, which are severe enough to cause functional impairment.
- Treatment of premenstrual dysphoric disorder includes lifestyle advice, preventing ovulation via oral contraception, cognitive-behavioural therapy and selective serotonin reuptake inhibitors.
- Postnatal blues is a common and self-limiting episode of mood and anxiety symptoms, which resolve within 2 weeks of delivery.
- Postnatal depression is a common and potentially serious episode of depression arising within 6 months of delivery.
- Management of postnatal depression is very similar to standard management of depression, but in severe cases admission to a mother-and-baby unit may be required and electroconvulsive therapy is recommended at an early stage.
- Postpartum psychosis is a rare but very serious illness generally arising within 2 weeks of delivery.
- In all cases of postpartum psychosis admission to a mother-and-baby unit is required for risk management.

This chapter discusses the disorders associated with the presenting complaints in Chapter 17, which you might find helpful to read first.

THE PERSONALITY DISORDERS

Epidemiology

There is a lack of consensus about the definition of personality disorders. Although the Diagnostic and Statistical Manual of Mental Disorders, 5th Edition (DSM-5) and International Statistical Classification of Diseases and Related Health Problems, 10th revision (ICD-10) classification systems have produced definitions, it is rare for a patient with a personality disorder to neatly match with only one discrete category. It is also unclear whether there is any correlation between diagnostic criteria and the subjective experiences of people identified as having disordered personality. While a number of structured interview schedules and diagnostic instruments have been validated, the level of correlation between these is generally poor. Mental health professionals also remain divided as to how personality disorders should be conceptualized, with some clinicians questioning whether the diagnosis is of any clinical benefit.

Patients with personality disorders have a significantly increased mortality, as well as physical and psychiatric morbidity. Relationships with relatives and friends are adversely affected, and there is a strong association between some types of personality disorder and involvement with health care and criminal justice services.

Community studies have shown the prevalence of any personality disorder to be 4%–13%, with an increased prevalence in younger age groups (particularly 25–44 years), and an equal distribution between the sexes. This varies according to the population group sampled. It is higher in patients frequently consulting general practitioners (GPs; 10%–30%), even higher in psychiatric outpatient clinics (30%–40%) and higher still in psychiatric inpatients (40%–50%), self-harming patients (40%–80%) and prisoners (50%–80%).

Table 28.1 describes the prevalence of the individual disorders and their relevant epidemiology. Note the broad ranges of prevalence from different studies, highlighting the lack of correlation in the current literature.

Aetiology

Different environmental and biological/genetic factors are implicated in the aetiology of different personality disorders, supporting their heterogenicity.

Genetics

- Monozygotic twins show a higher concordance for personality disorders than dizygotic twins, suggesting a heritability of 30%–60%.
- Cluster A personality disorders (see Table 17.1; especially schizotypal) are more common in the relatives of patients with schizophrenia.
- Some authors have suggested that schizoid and schizotypal personality disorders may be a neurodevelopmental disorder, possibly within the autistic spectrum.
- Depressive disorders are more common in the relatives of patients with emotionally unstable (borderline) personality disorder.

Early life experience

- Early adverse social circumstances (such as parental alcoholism, physical or emotional neglect, violence, sexual abuse) are associated with the development of cluster B personality disorders (see Table 17.1).
- There is a strong association between borderline personality disorder and childhood sexual abuse, although this is not universal.
- Various psychoanalytical theories suggest that disordered attachment between infants and their caregivers lead to difficulties in relationships throughout the rest of life, which may manifest as personality disorders.

Assessment, clinical features, classification and differential diagnosis

Discussed in Chapter 17.

Management

In the past, there has been considerable debate concerning how (and by whom) patients with personality disorders should be managed. Previously, personality disorders were generally considered to be untreatable. However, advances in diagnosis, psychotherapy and psychopharmacology have equipped clinicians with a variety of treatment options that can be useful in maximizing engagement with services, reducing distress, managing comorbid mental illness and substance misuse, improving relationships and optimizing quality of life.

Patients with emotionally unstable (borderline) personality disorder are frequently encountered in clinical practice, and the most is known about what treatments do, and do not, help people with this diagnosis. This will therefore be the focus of this section.

Table 28.1 Epidemiology of personality disorders

Personality disorder	Prevalence in general population (%)	Comments
Paranoid	0.7–4.4	More common in males and lower socioeconomic classes More common in relatives of patients with schizophrenia
Schizoid	0.7–4.9	More common in males and offender populations May be more common in relatives of patients with schizophrenia
Schizotypal	1.6–3.9	More common in relatives of patients with schizophrenia May be slightly more common in males
Emotionally unstable (borderline)	1.2–5.9	More prevalent in younger age groups and females Aetiological link with childhood sexual abuse Most contact with services in mid-20s 40-fold increase in suicide rate Associated with poor work history and single marital status Often comorbid with depression, substance abuse, bulimia and anxiety
Antisocial (dissocial)	0.6–4.5	Much more common in men Highest prevalence in 25–44 year olds Associated with school dropout, conduct disorder and urban settings Very high prevalence in prisons and forensic settings Highly comorbidity with substance abuse
Histrionic	0.4–2.9	Recent research shows equal gender ratio (previously thought to be more common in women)
Narcissistic	0.1–6.2	More common in males and forensic settings
Dependent	0.3–0.6	Often comorbid with borderline personality disorder
Avoidant (anxious)	1–5.2	Equal gender ratio Comorbid with social phobia
Obsessive compulsive (anankastic)	1.2–7.9	More common in white, male, highly educated, married and employed individuals

Principles of managing patients with emotionally unstable personality disorder

Patients with emotionally unstable personality disorder should not be excluded from health or social care services because of their diagnosis or because they have self-harmed. A consistent and tolerant approach should be taken. Autonomy and choice should be encouraged, with the patient being actively involved in deciding treatment options and in finding solutions to their problems. An optimistic, trusting and nonjudgemental relationship should be developed. Endings and transitions may evoke strong emotions and reactions in patients with emotionally unstable personality disorder, and as such should be carefully planned and structured to minimize distress. A multidisciplinary approach to care should be considered, as psychological, social and biological treatment modalities all have an important role. A comprehensive assessment should be made of sources of distress to self and others (thoughts, emotions, behaviour and relationships), other comorbid mental illness and specific impairments of functioning at work or home.

PRINCIPLES OF CARE IN MANAGING EMOTIONALLY UNSTABLE PERSONALITY DISORDER

- Be positive, kind and nonjudgemental (many are victims of abuse).
- Be accessible, consistent and reliable (do what you say you will do).
- Encourage autonomy; facilitate the patient to find his/her own solutions to problems.
  - What is the problem right now?
  - What has worked in the past?
  - What would you like to do?
  - What is an achievable change?
- Manage transitions and changes carefully, in a planned way.
- Monitor for comorbid mental illness (e.g. depression or substance use)

Crisis management

It can be useful to develop a crisis management plan in conjunction with the patient, detailing self-management strategies, sources of support (family, friends, telephone-based services) and details on how to access emergency care. This should be shared with the patient and other relevant professionals (GPs, assessment and crisis teams).

EXAMPLE CRISIS PLAN IN EMOTIONALLY UNSTABLE PERSONALITY DISORDER

Triggers that might lead to a crisis
e.g. Losing job, drinking too much alcohol, argument with partner

Things I can do to help myself
e.g. Talk to my friend, go to a movie, exercise, get enough sleep, avoid drugs and alcohol

When I should seek help
e.g. If I injure myself badly, if I am having very strong thoughts of suicide, if I feel so sad that I can't go to work, if my friend advises me to

Who I should contact and how
e.g. Samaritans, general practitioner, community psychiatric nurse, crisis team, NHS24, best friend, mother

---

Short-term drug treatments can be useful to alleviate distress during a crisis. If possible, this should be agreed in advance with the care team and the patient. Drugs with acceptable side-effects and low dependence profiles are preferable, and should be dispensed in small quantities if there is a risk for overdose. Drugs should not be used in place of other more appropriate interventions.

Before admission to acute in-patient psychiatric care, crisis resolution or home treatment teams should be considered. Admission may be necessary if the management of the crisis involves significant risk to self or others that cannot be managed within other services. If possible, actively involve the patient in the decision, and ensure that it is based on an explicit, joint understanding of the potential benefits (and likely harm) that may result from admission. Agree the length and purpose of the admission in advance. If the patient is detained under mental health legislation, ensure that this is regularly reviewed and that management on a voluntary basis is resumed at the earliest opportunity.

After a crisis has resolved, ensure that the care plan is updated. If drug treatment was started, review this and discontinue if possible. If this is not possible, ensure that it is regularly reviewed to monitor effectiveness, side-effects, misuse and dependency.

Short-term management

While treatment of emotionally unstable personality disorder should be considered to be a long-term process, various biological, psychological and social management strategies can be employed in the shorter term, with the aim of facilitating trust, building a positive relationship with health and social care services and identifying and alleviating sources of distress.

Psychopharmacology

There are no medications that are currently recommended specifically for the treatment of emotionally unstable personality disorder (National Institute for Health and Care Excellence (NICE) 2009). However, drugs can be useful to treat comorbid mental illness, or to manage cases of behavioural disturbance and suicidal behaviour during the more severe phases. In addition, there is some evidence that some drugs may be efficacious in targeting specific symptoms. For instance, antipsychotics may be of some use in treating the pseudo-psychotic symptoms that are sometimes experienced, in reducing agitation and in stabilizing mood. Antidepressants may be useful in treating depressive symptoms. Selective serotonin reuptake inhibitors may help with obsessive-compulsive symptoms as well as impulsivity and self-harming behaviour. Mood stabilizers such as lithium, sodium valproate and lamotrigine may be useful in treating aggression, impulsivity and mood instability. Benzodiazepines should be used with caution due to the potential for abuse, dependence and diversion.

Psychosocial

Supportive psychotherapy provides patients with an authority figure during times of crisis. Regular contact with a health care professional can also provide the patient with a sense of containment. Members of the multidisciplinary team can provide psychoeducation, as well as facilitating development of coping strategies, relaxation and distraction techniques, improving disturbed relationships and development of skills and hobbies. In cooperation with social services, issues such as housing, finances and employment can be addressed.

COMMUNICATION

People with emotionally unstable personality disorder by definition have difficulties forming and maintaining relationships, and that includes doctor–patient relationships! Misunderstandings and frustration are common on both sides. Remember to be calm, clear and consistent and try to take the long view; do not let one difficult encounter dominate your relationship with the patient.

Longer-term management

The long-term management of patients with emotionally unstable personality disorder involves addressing and modifying maladaptive traits of personality. This generally involves psychological therapy. Because traits and behaviours tend to be deeply engrained, this process can take many years. Around 40% of people with emotionally unstable personality disorder disengage with psychotherapy, and so it is important to build a trusting relationship and to be prepared for therapeutic change taking a long time.

There is evidence suggesting the efficacy of various modalities of psychotherapy in the treatment of emotionally unstable personality disorder. It may be that the consistency of therapy, the maintenance of boundaries and the empathic and nonjudgemental stance of the therapist allows for the successful development of a therapeutic relationship, which may in itself be more important than the specific type of therapy. For more information on psychotherapy, see Chapter 3. The following psychological treatments can be helpful in emotionally unstable personality disorder:

- Dialectical behaviour therapy uses a combination of cognitive and behavioural therapies, with relaxation techniques and mindfulness. It involves both individual and group therapy, and can be helpful in reducing self-harming and improving functioning. It is recommended by NICE (2009).
- Mentalization-based therapy focuses on allowing patients to better understand what is going on in both their minds and in the minds of others. It can utilize both individual and group components.
- Cognitive behavioural therapy has been adapted for use as 'schema-focused therapy'.
- Cognitive analytical therapy.
- Psychodynamic psychotherapy, as both individual and group therapy, which focuses on the relationship with the therapist.

Therapeutic communities are a residential form of therapy, where the patient may stay for weeks or months. The community tends to run as a 'democracy', with patients often having as much say as the staff. Most of the therapeutic work is done in groups, and patients learn from getting on (or not getting on) with others. It differs from 'real life' in that any disagreements or upsets happen in a controlled and safe environment. These placements tend to be reserved for those with severe functional impairment or very high service usage, because of their high cost.

HINTS AND TIPS

Remember that personality disorders involve long-standing personality traits. While they are 'treatable', pharmacotherapy is not the mainstay, but is used to alleviate specific symptoms (e.g. comorbid depression, anxiety or impulsivity). Medications are unlikely to affect maladaptive personality traits. With appropriate psychosocial interventions, these may significantly improve with time. You may want to consider this when discussing management with patients.

Course and prognosis

The course of personality disorders, and the prognosis of sufferers, is not as dire as was once thought. Some 78%–99% of patients with emotionally unstable personality disorder will show signs of sustained symptomatic remission at 16-year follow-up. Patients with antisocial personality may also improve with time, especially if they have formed a relationship with a therapist. Schizotypal and obsessive-compulsive personality disorders tend to be stable over time, although schizotypal patients may go on to develop schizophrenia.

Patients with personality disorder have a greater incidence of other mental illnesses such as depression, bipolar affective disorder, anxiety and schizophrenia. Furthermore, these tend to be more severe and have a worse prognosis than if the personality disorder was not present. Patients with personality disorder (especially cluster B) also have far higher rates of suicide and accidental death than the general population.

● **Chapter Summary**

- Personality disorders are common, particularly in users of health services.
- Comorbid mental illnesses are more frequent and difficult to treat in those with personality disorder.
- When managing emotionally unstable personality disorder:
  - Take a consistent, nonjudgemental approach.
  - Help the patient to make a crisis plan and share it with everyone involved in the patient's care.
  - Symptoms can be improved by long-term psychological treatments such as dialectical behavioural therapy.
  - Medication is only recommended in crises and for comorbid mental illnesses.
- Personality disorders generally gradually improve over decades.

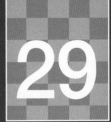

Neurodevelopmental disorders are a large and diverse group. This chapter covers those that most commonly present to psychiatry: intellectual disability, autism spectrum disorders (ASDs), attention deficit hyperactivity disorder (ADHD) and Tourette syndrome.

INTELLECTUAL DISABILITY

Epidemiology and aetiology

Key epidemiology is shown in Table 29.1. Some common causes of intellectual disability are shown in Table 29.2. No clear aetiology can be determined in at least a third of patients with mild intellectual disability, suggesting they may represent the lower end of the normal distribution curve for intellectual functioning. Specific causes are more likely to be found in people with severe or profound intellectual disabilities.

Assessment, clinical features, investigations and differential diagnosis

See Chapter 18.

Table 29.2 Causes of intellectual disability

Genetic	Trisomies or large structural variants (e.g. Down syndrome, fragile X syndrome, Prader–Willi syndrome) Inherited point mutations (e.g. phenylketonuria, neurofibromatosis, tuberous sclerosis, Lesch–Nyhan syndrome, Tay–Sachs disease, other enzyme-deficiency diseases) *De novo* (sporadic) point mutations have been identified in over 700 genes, potentially all with the capacity to contribute to intellectual disability
Prenatal	Congenital infections (e.g. TORCH infections (toxoplasmosis, rubella, cytomegalovirus, herpes simplex and zoster (chicken pox)), also syphilis and human immunodeficiency virus (HIV)) Substance use during pregnancy (e.g. foetal alcohol syndrome, prescribed drugs with teratogenic effects) Complications of pregnancy (e.g. preeclampsia, intrauterine growth retardation, antepartum haemorrhage)
Perinatal	Birth trauma (e.g. intracranial haemorrhage, hypoxia) Prematurity (e.g. intraventricular haemorrhage, hyperbilirubinaemia (kernicterus), infections)
Environmental	Neglect, malnutrition (e.g. iodine deficiency in developing countries), poor linguistic and social stimulation
Medical conditions in childhood	Infections (e.g. meningitis, encephalitis) Head injury Toxins (e.g. lead, other heavy metals)

Table 29.1 Epidemiology of neurodevelopmental disorders

Disorder	Population prevalence[a]	Sex ratio (female:male)
Intellectual disability	1%	1:1.5
Autism spectrum disorders	1%	1:3
Attention deficit hyperactivity disorder	5% in children 2.5% in adults	1:2
Tourette syndrome	0.3%	1:3

[a] These estimates are approximate but taken from meta-analysis where possible. Different diagnostic systems give different prevalence estimates

Management and prognosis

Prevention and detection

Primary prevention includes genetic screening and counselling for higher risk groups, prenatal testing (e.g. amniocentesis, rhesus incompatibility), improved perinatal and neonatal care and early detection of metabolic abnormalities that may contribute to intellectual impairment (e.g. phenylketonuria, neonatal hypothyroidism). Milder intellectual disabilities may be less obvious, and early detection requires the ability of teachers and family doctors to be able to identify difficulties as soon as possible.

Secondary prevention aims to prevent the progression of disability, by providing compensatory education and early attempts to reduce behavioural problems. If you suspect a child has an intellectual disability, this should be discussed with either a paediatrician or a child and adolescent mental health specialist, who will be able to provide guidance on local services. If you suspect an adult has an undiagnosed mild intellectual disability, this should be discussed with the local intellectual disabilities team, who may suggest an initial referral for neuropsychological assessment.

Help for families

Families require information, advice and both psychological and practical support from the time that the diagnosis is first made. Adequate time should be devoted to this, and should aim to involve the parents in helping their child achieve their full potential. Support should be ongoing, and should focus on education, practical matters and psychological support. This may need to be increased at the more challenging times, such as puberty, starting or leaving school, times of stress (e.g. bereavement or illness) and the transition to adult services.

Education, training and occupation

If the needs of a child with intellectual disability can be met by mainstream education, this should be encouraged due to the benefits of societal inclusion and mutual understanding. However, many children with intellectual disabilities have complex needs that are better addressed in specialist schools. Later, vocational guidance should be offered: most people with mild intellectual disabilities are able to take mainstream or supported employment (e.g. Remploy).

Housing and social support

Most people with mild intellectual disabilities are able to live independently, with varying degrees of social and familial support. Assessment of tasks of daily living will be necessary to ensure that people are appropriately placed. For people with more severe difficulties, residential care may be necessary. In such cases, development of social skills should be encouraged as far as is practical.

Medical care

People with intellectual disabilities should have the same access to medical services as everyone else, although communication difficulties and false attribution of symptoms to the intellectual disability (diagnostic overshadowing) mean care is often suboptimal. Extra medical care is often required due to comorbidities such as physical disability or epilepsy. Many general hospitals have specialist nurses who are experienced in the management of individuals with intellectual disabilities admitted for medical treatment or surgery.

HINTS AND TIPS

Epilepsy is a common comorbidity in individuals with intellectual disabilities and can often complicate assessment and management. Remember that a number of different psychotropic medications can lower seizure threshold, and that 'mood stabilizers' (with the exception of lithium) are antiepileptic medications.

COMMUNICATION

Collateral histories are invaluable when assessing someone with an intellectual disability. When a change in behaviour occurs, it is useful to ask about what else has changed in the patient's life or their daily routine. However, the prevalence of other psychiatric disorders is three to four times higher and so these must be excluded.

Psychiatric care

Given the higher prevalence of comorbid mental illness in this group, people with intellectual disabilities should have access to specialist care (usually on an outpatient, community or day-patient basis) as and when required. Because the assessment and management of psychiatric illness and behavioural disturbances in individuals with intellectual disability can be difficult, most areas have multidisciplinary specialist teams. These teams can address not only major mental illnesses (e.g. schizophrenia, bipolar affective disorder, depression), but can also help manage autism and challenging behaviours. Psychotropic medication may be indicated; however, given the common difficulties with unusual presentations, polypharmacy, comorbidities and sensitivity to medication, there should be a low threshold for seeking advice from, or referral to, a specialist doctor. Behavioural therapy may be useful in the management of maladaptive or otherwise difficult behaviours (e.g. self-injury, aggression, destructiveness).

AUTISM SPECTRUM DISORDERS

Epidemiology and aetiology

Key epidemiology is shown in Table 29.1. Autism is a highly heritable condition (heritability of around 80%). A substantial proportion of this genetic risk is not inherited but arises from sporadic mutations – *de novo* (sporadic) variants occur four times as often in people with autism as their unaffected siblings. Rare variants in over 800 genes have been linked to autism in this manner and are thought to be the cause in around one in five cases. Common genetic variants of small effect are also thought to exist, but these have not yet been conclusively identified. Analyses of common biological processes influenced by the numerous implicated genes have highlighted a range of core cellular functions underlying synaptic formation and signalling: cell adhesion, chromatin remodelling and regulation of transcription and translation. It seems likely that what is currently referred to as 'autism spectrum disorder' is made up of many different sorts of disorder influencing distinct but related basic neuronal functions.

Although genetics may seem far removed from clinical practice at present, it can provide clinically relevant information. For example, if parents have one child with autism, the overall risk for having a second child with autism is 10%–15%. However, if genetic testing identifies a causative genetic variant as *de novo* or inherited, this risk can be much more accurately estimated at 1% or 50%, respectively (if the variant is 100% penetrant).

HINTS AND TIPS

Many of the genes linked to autism have also been associated with intellectual disability, epilepsy, schizophrenia and attention deficit hyperactivity disorder: the same genetic variants can influence risk for many neurodevelopmental disorders.

COMMUNICATION

There is no evidence to support the claim that the measles, mumps, rubella (MMR) vaccine results in autism. The small study that did suggest there was a link has since been conclusively discredited.

Assessment, clinical features, investigations and differential diagnosis

See Chapter 18.

Management and prognosis

No pharmacological treatments are recommended for the core symptoms of autism (National Institute for Health and Care Excellence (NICE) 2012, 2013). Instead, the emphasis is on psychosocial interventions (see Box 29.1, adults). In

---

BOX 29.1   PSYCHOSOCIAL INTERVENTIONS IN ADULTS WITH AUTISM (NICE 2012)

Everyone:
- Self-help or support groups – for individuals, and for their families, partners or carers.
- Social learning program (group or individual). Should include modelling of useful social behaviour, explicit statement of social rules and strategies for difficult social situations.

If appropriate to individual:
- Supported employment programme
- Structured leisure activity, with a facilitator
- Anger management
- Antivictimization intervention
- Crisis plan

---

children, a social–communication intervention that is play based and designed to maximize joint attention and reciprocal communication between the child and their parents, carers or teachers is recommended (NICE 2013). Comorbid mental health problems (e.g. anxiety or depression) should be treated as normal, except that psychological interventions should focus more on changing behaviour rather than cognitions and avoid the use of metaphor and hypothetical situations.

ASDs are lifelong conditions for which there is no cure. The functional impact of symptoms fluctuates in response to stressors such as change (school, relationships, employment) and physical illness. The prognosis is extremely variable, reflecting the great variability between those with a diagnosis. An intelligence quotient (IQ) above 70, communicative language by age 5 years and absence of epilepsy are predictors of better long-term outcome. Some people can learn to develop strategies to work around their difficulties and make use of their strengths; however, many continue to have difficulty in finding employment or friendship and require family support into adulthood. Those with a comorbid intellectual disability are unlikely to be able to live independently in adulthood.

ATTENTION DEFICIT HYPERACTIVITY DISORDERS

Epidemiology and aetiology

Key epidemiology is shown in Table 29.1. Twin studies have shown that ADHD has one of the highest heritabilities of all psychiatric illnesses, at around 80%.

A first-degree relative of someone with ADHD has a 20% chance of also having ADHD. Replicated candidate gene studies and genome-wide association studies of copy number variants implicate variants in genes encoding dopaminergic, serotonergic and glutamatergic pathways as influencing risk.

Prenatal, perinatal and postnatal environmental factors also modestly increase risk: maternal smoking, alcohol consumption and heroin use during pregnancy; very low birth weight; foetal hypoxia; perinatal brain injury and prolonged emotional deprivation during infancy.

Assessment, clinical features, investigations and differential diagnosis

See Chapter 18.

Management and prognosis

Children

Psychosocial interventions are recommended in all cases and are used first line in children and young people with mild to moderate ADHD, and in all preschool children (NICE 2008). The choice of treatment naturally depends on the developmental stage of the child or adolescent. Useful strategies include parental education or training, cognitive-behavioural therapy (CBT) and social skills training.

Pharmacological management is the first-line treatment in school-age children with severe ADHD and is second line for those with moderate ADHD in whom psychosocial interventions have been of insufficient benefit (NICE 2008). The central nervous system stimulant methylphenidate (Ritalin, Concerta, Equasym) is normally tried in the first instance. Atomoxetine (Strattera) and dexamfetamine are also licensed in the UK for the management of ADHD: these tend to be used in cases where methylphenidate is ineffective or poorly tolerated. In treatment-resistant cases, the (unlicensed) use of bupropion, clonidine, modafinil and guanfacine, as well as some antidepressant drugs, may be considered; however, this should only be done following referral to a tertiary centre.

Improvement usually occurs during adolescence, particularly in hyperactivity. Unstable family dynamics and coexisting conduct disorder are associated with a worse prognosis. Around two-thirds of patients have symptoms persisting into later life, although most do not require ongoing management from adult mental health services. Children with ADHD are at increased risk for substance use and imprisonment in adult life. However, many people with ADHD go on to have successful and enjoyable lives, with professional athletes, doctors, journalists and actors publicly stating they have ADHD.

COMMUNICATION

Parents' concerns need to be addressed as well as the patient's. Treatment of attention deficit hyperactivity disorder has received much media interest, especially potential side-effects – be aware of this. Methylphenidate is associated with growth suppression with prolonged use. It is only prescribed in specialist settings with regular weight and height monitoring. Drug holidays can be used to allow children to make-up growth gains. Rarely, atomoxetine is associated with liver dysfunction and suicidality.

RED FLAG

Before starting attention deficit hyperactivity disorder drug treatment, assess height, weight, blood pressure and heart rate and personal or family history of cardiovascular disease. Then monitor these parameters during treatment. Stimulants are sympathomimetic and can suppress appetite.

COMMUNICATION

One way to sum up management of severe childhood attention deficit hyperactivity disorder (ADHD), or adult ADHD, is to tell patients they need both 'pills and skills'. 'Pills' can provide a window of opportunity to allow people to develop organizational 'skills' they struggled to achieve before.

Adults

Pharmacological management is first line for adults with moderate or severe ADHD. Psychological interventions such as CBT may have benefit, but little research is available yet. Methylphenidate is recommended first, with dexamfetamine and atomoxetine second line.

Diversion of stimulant medication is a risk in young people and adults. If someone is actively using recreational substances, advise them that they should stop doing so before a trial of ADHD medication. If fears remain regarding diversion, try atomoxetine or lisdexamfetamine (Elvanse). Lisdexamfetamine is a prodrug that is metabolized to dexamfetamine by an enzyme in red blood cells. This limits the rate at which dexamfetamine is generated, reducing its potential for abuse.

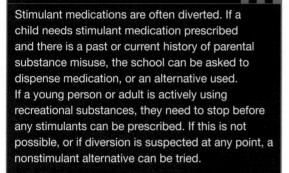

RED FLAG

Stimulant medications are often diverted. If a child needs stimulant medication prescribed and there is a past or current history of parental substance misuse, the school can be asked to dispense medication, or an alternative used. If a young person or adult is actively using recreational substances, they need to stop before any stimulants can be prescribed. If this is not possible, or if diversion is suspected at any point, a nonstimulant alternative can be tried.

Little research has been done on the persistence of ADHD symptoms across the lifespan. It seems reasonable that symptoms might become more tolerable as people learn additional coping strategies (e.g. diaries, reminders), or modify their environment to minimize functional impairment (e.g. get a job that requires brief bursts of sustained attention only). 'Drug holidays' every couple of years to assess whether medication is still of benefit are probably worth trying.

ADHD is often comorbid with other psychiatric disorders (bipolar disorder, depression, anxiety disorders, substance use), so ensure these are assessed and treated also.

TOURETTE SYNDROME

Epidemiology and aetiology

Key epidemiology is shown in Table 29.1. Aetiology is unclear but abnormalities in dopaminergic neurotransmission have been found.

Assessment, clinical features, investigations and differential diagnosis

See Chapter 18.

Management and prognosis

Often tics do not require treatment, particularly if they are not interfering with daily life. Tourette syndrome is very commonly comorbid with other conditions (anxiety, obsessive-compulsive disorder, ADHD), and these should be treated first, according to standard guidelines. If tics remain problematic after other disorders are treated, psychological treatments should be tried first (psychoeducation, habit reversal and exposure and response prevention). If tics persist, clonidine (an agonist) is recommended first. Antipsychotics can also help (haloperidol, pimozide, risperidone or aripiprazole). Risk for side-effects should always be balanced against benefits on an individual basis.

Around two-thirds of children and young people with Tourette syndrome go on to have no or very mild tics in adulthood.

● **Chapter Summary**

- Neurodevelopmental disorders are common, particularly attention deficit hyperactivity disorder (ADHD).
- Neurodevelopmental disorders are often comorbid with other mental disorders and epilepsy. It is important to treat comorbid conditions.
- Intellectual disability and autism spectrum disorders are managed primarily with psychosocial interventions.
- ADHD is managed with a combination of psychosocial and pharmacological interventions.

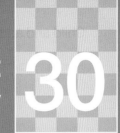

This chapter covers the assessment and management of problems with mood, anxiety or conduct in children and young people. Neurodevelopmental disorders, including intellectual disability, can cause similar symptoms or be comorbid with these disorders, but are covered separately in Chapters 18 and 29. Mental illnesses that commonly affect adults such as eating disorders, bipolar affective disorder and schizophrenia can also present in adolescence; these are predominantly covered in their own chapters but also briefly here. Finally, this chapter briefly covers child abuse. Mental disorders in children can both be caused by child abuse and increase the risk of experiencing abuse, and it is important to always be alert to this possibility.

CHILD AND ADOLESCENT MENTAL HEALTH SERVICES

Child and Adolescent Mental Health Services (CAMHS) provide emotional and mental health support, diagnosis and treatment to individuals up to the age of 18 years.

Children often find it difficult to explicitly verbalize psychological distress. Instead, the presenting problem is most commonly a nonspecific concern about a child's abnormal behaviour or performance (e.g., 'being disruptive in the classroom'), often raised by someone other than the young person (e.g., parent, schoolteacher, paediatrician). This means the ability to take a good history and synthesize information from multiple sources is particularly important in CAMHS.

Family and wider community are important in assessing and maintaining a young person's well-being and this is reflected in the broad composition of multidisciplinary teams in CAMHS, which are likely to include psychiatrists, psychologists, occupational therapists, community mental health workers, social workers, community psychiatric nurses, family therapists and creative therapists. Fig. 30.1 shows an overview of the tiered approach to CAMHS services common in the UK.

ATTACHMENT

Attachment refers to the bond between an infant and their primary caregiver. How the primary caregiver responds to a young child's needs during their early years sets the tone for that child's expectations for the rest of their life: how others are likely to behave towards them and how they should behave in return. Put simply, if a child is shown kindness and understanding, they are likely to become a kind and empathic adult. If a child is ignored and neglected, they are less likely to be social or caring towards others. If a child is treated inconsistently, sometimes with love, sometimes with disdain, they will expect the world to be unpredictable and chaotic, people in authority to be untrustworthy and themselves as unable to be in control. Disrupted attachment during early childhood can often lead to behavioural difficulties in children and potentially personality disorders in adulthood (see Table 30.1).

Importantly, not everyone who has a difficult upbringing will have a difficult adulthood; many individuals are resilient, and behaviour and thinking patterns can be changed (sometimes with the help of psychological therapy). It is also important to note that primary caregivers do not always provide an optimal early environment for a range of reasons, some within and some outwith their control (e.g., postnatal depression, substance use, poverty, bereavement, war). Nonetheless, encouraging parents and care providers to provide a loving and responsive environment for infants and young children has become a key governmental priority.

HINTS AND TIPS

As you meet children, young people and adults who seem to be behaving in harmful ways, it can often be helpful to try to understand how their early experiences have shaped them. Often thoughts or behaviours that are helpful during times of adversity (e.g., not trusting others when experiencing abuse) can become unhelpful in other times and contexts (e.g., difficulty forming close relationships).

EPIDEMIOLOGY

Mental health problems affect around 1 in 10 children. See Table 30.2 for individual disorders.

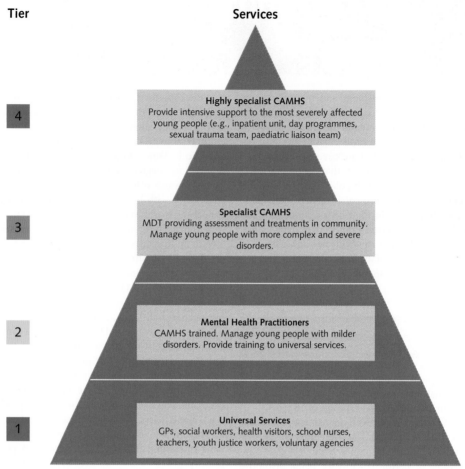

Fig. 30.1 Tiered structure of CAMHS. *CAMHS,* Child and Adolescent Mental Health Services; *GP,* general practitioner; *MDT,* multidisciplinary team.

Table 30.1 Attachment styles

Child attachment style	Caregiver behaviour	Child behaviour	Adult attachment style	Adult behaviour
Secure (two-thirds)	Responsive, understanding, consistent	Happy, curious	'Autonomous'	Able to self-soothe, but also able to maintain relationships.
Insecure (a third)				
'Avoidant' (21%)	Aloof, unresponsive, ridiculing	Emotionally distant, withdrawn	'Dismissive'	Desire to be independent. Avoidance of intimacy.
'Ambivalent/resistant' (16%)	At times sensitive, at times ignores	Anxious, uncertain, angry	'Preoccupied'	Hypersensitive to rejection, care-seeking.
'Disorganized' (rare)	Abusive, scary, scared	Sad, angry, fearful	'Disorganized'	Fearful, abusive, dissociative.

Table 30.2 Epidemiology of mental disorders in childhood and adolescence

Disorder	Typical age of presentation	Prevalence in under 18-year-olds (post-typical age of onset)
Intellectual disability	Infancy or preschool	3%
Autism spectrum disorder	Preschool or primary	1%
Attention deficit hyperactivity disorder	Preschool or primary	5%
Anxiety disorders	Primary or older	5% (up to 20% have a phobia)
Conduct disorder	Primary or older	8% males, 4% females
Oppositional defiant disorder	Primary or older	4%
Eating disorders	Adolescence	1%
Depression	Adolescence	4%
Bipolar affective disorder	Late adolescence	Rare
Schizophrenia	Late adolescence	Rare
Personality disorder	Late adolescence	Characteristic traits common, but not usually diagnosed in adolescence

MENTAL ILLNESS IN CHILDREN AND ADOLESCENTS

Anxiety disorders

The anxiety disorders in childhood are often thought to be exaggerations of normal developmental trends rather than discrete illnesses in themselves. They rarely persist into adulthood and tend to have a good prognosis. The treatment of these disorders is focused on behavioural and family therapy. In late adolescence common anxiety disorders of adulthood (generalized anxiety disorder, panic disorder and obsessive-compulsive disorder (OCD)) emerge; diagnosis and management are very similar to adulthood (see Chapters 12, 13 and 23) but with an even stronger emphasis on psychological therapy.

Separation anxiety disorder

Normal separation anxiety usually occurs in children from 6 months to 2 years of age. However, some children experience inappropriate and excessive anxiety about separation from attachment figures. This disorder is only diagnosed when the anxiety is of such a severity that it is markedly different from other children of a similar age or when it persists beyond the usual age period (e.g., a 6-year-old girl becoming incredibly distressed when her mother drops her off at school).

Phobic anxiety disorder

Minor phobic symptoms are common in childhood, and the object of the phobia varies with developmental stage (e.g., fear of animals or monsters in preschool children). Phobic anxiety disorder is diagnosed when the phobic object is age inappropriate (e.g., a 9-year-old boy who is afraid of monsters under the bed), or where levels of anxiety are clinically abnormal. Nondevelopmental phobias (e.g., agoraphobia) do not fall under this category, but under the adult phobia category (see Chapters 12 and 23).

Obsessive-compulsive disorder

Median age of onset is 10 years, but can be from age 5 years. About two-thirds of young children have various rituals/habits (e.g., lining up toys, specific stories before bed) that parents may be concerned is OCD. What is important to bear in mind is the developmental stage of the child. Rituals/habits help children to make sense of the world around them as they grow and develop. OCD is suggested if the ritual/habit is very intense or frequent, impairs the child's ability to function or causes them distress. Another key difference between diagnosis in adults and children is that children are not required to recognize their thoughts as abnormal. Treatment is largely psychological.

Social anxiety disorder

Normal stranger anxiety occurs in well-adjusted children from 8 months to 1 year of age. Social anxiety disorder is a persistent and recurrent fear and/or avoidance of strangers. This disorder is only diagnosed when the anxiety is of such a severity that it is markedly different from other children of a similar age or when it persists beyond the usual age period.

HINTS AND TIPS

Social anxiety is common in children with neurodevelopmental disorders. Remember to screen for autism and attention deficit hyperactivity disorder (see Chapter 18) in a child presenting with anxiety.

Disorders of social behaviour

Conduct disorder

Conduct disorder is one of the commonest reasons for referral to CAMHS. The disorder is characterized by a repetitive and persistent pattern of aggression to people and animals, destruction of property (including fire-setting), deceitfulness or theft and major violations of age-appropriate societal expectations or rules (e.g., truancy, staying out at night, running away from home). Rates among populations in young offender institutions have been estimated to be as high as 87%. The male-to-female ratio is approximately 2:1. Aetiological factors include genetics, parental psychopathology (mental illness, substance abuse, antisocial personality traits), child abuse and neglect, poor socioeconomic status and poor educational attainment. Many adolescents improve by adulthood; however, a substantial proportion go on to develop antisocial personality disorder and substance-related problems, especially those with an early age of onset. Management is predominantly psychosocial. The National Institute for Health and Care Excellence (NICE; 2013) recommends parental skills training programmes for parents/carers, cognitive-behavioural problem-solving programmes for young people and multimodal interventions (e.g., multisystemic therapy) aiming to influence how the young person interacts with their family, school, community and criminal justice system. Input from social work is often required as the young person can be outwith parental control.

Oppositional defiant disorder

A persistent pattern of negative, defiant, hostile and disruptive behaviour *in the absence of* behaviour that violates the law or the basic rights of others as occurs in conduct disorder (e.g., theft, cruelty, bullying, assault). Children with this disorder deliberately defy requests or rules, are angry and resentful and annoy others on purpose. Management is very similar to conduct disorder.

Reactive attachment disorder

Occurs in children under 5 years of age who have been severely neglected and unable to form a secure attachment to a primary caregiver. Manifests with abnormal social relationships, for example, fearfulness and hypervigilance, withdrawal, listlessness, aggression, not seeking or responding to comfort, no interest in play. Paradoxically, some children may be indiscriminately warm and disinhibited towards strangers, showing no preference for their primary caregiver.

Elective mutism (selective mutism)

Elective mutism is a selectivity in vocal communication depending on the social circumstances. The child speaks normally in some situations (e.g., at home), but is mute in others (e.g., at school). These children have adequately developed language comprehension and ability (although a minority may have slight speech delay or articulation problems). It usually presents before the age of 5 years, is slightly more common in girls and is associated with psychological stress, social anxiety and oppositional behaviour.

Disorders of elimination

Nonorganic enuresis

This condition is characterized by the involuntary voiding of urine in children who, according to their developmental stage, should have established consistent bladder control (therefore ordinarily not diagnosed before the age of 5 years). It may occur during the day or night and is not directly caused by any medical condition (e.g., seizures, diabetes, urinary tract infection, constipation, structural abnormalities of the urinary tract) or use of a substance (e.g., diuretic). Two types of enuresis have been described: primary enuresis means that urinary continence has never been established; and secondary enuresis means that continence has been achieved in the past. Nonorganic enuresis occurs in around 7% of 5 year olds; 4% of 10 year olds and around 1% of adolescents over 15 years. Gender distribution is equal in younger patients; however, cases that persist into adolescence tend to be males. Aetiological factors include genetics, developmental delays, psychosocial stressors (moving house, birth of a sibling, start or change of school, divorce, bereavement) and inadequate toilet training. About 75% of children with nonorganic enuresis have a first-degree biological relative who has had the same problem. Management (NICE 2010) involves exclusion of physical cause, parental education about toilet training (especially in primary enuresis), behavioural therapy (pad and buzzer apparatus, star chart, bladder training) and—as a last resort—pharmacotherapy (imipramine, nasal desmopressin). Most cases of nonorganic enuresis resolve by adolescence.

Nonorganic encopresis

This condition is characterized by the deposition of normal faeces (i.e., not diarrhoea) in inappropriate places, in children who—according to their developmental stage—should have established consistent bowel control (therefore ordinarily not diagnosed before the age of 4 years). It may be due to unsuccessful toilet training where bowel control has never been achieved (primary encopresis) or may occur after a period of normal bowel control (secondary encopresis). Encopresis may result from a developmental delay; coercive or punitive potty training; emotional, physical or sexual abuse; a disturbed parent–child relationship; parental marital conflict or can feature as a symptom of a neurodevelopmental disorder (e.g., autism or intellectual disability). About 1% of 5 year olds have the condition and it is more common in males. Management includes ruling out an organic cause (constipation with overflow incontinence, anal fissure, gastrointestinal infection), assessing and treating disturbed family dynamics (ruling out child abuse), parental guidance regarding toilet training and behaviour therapy (e.g., star chart). Stool softeners may be used for constipation. The prognosis is good with 90% of cases improving within a year.

Disorders arising in adolescence and adulthood

Eating disorders

Eating disorders (see Chapter 16 and 24) often commence in adolescence. Symptomatology and diagnosis are the same as in adulthood. The management is very similar to that recommended for adults except the first-line treatment is always psychological therapy (family-based therapy is the gold standard in young people), not medication. When assessing physical risk from eating disorder in adolescents it is important to refer to age-specific guidelines (e.g., the Junior Management of Really Sick Patients with Anorexia Nervosa (MARSIPAN) guidelines).

Depression

Depression also arises frequently in adolescence. The treatment is similar to adults, but psychological therapies are first line and a far smaller range of antidepressants are recommended. NICE (2005) suggests watchful waiting for mild depression and an individual psychological treatment (cognitive-behavioural therapy, interpersonal therapy, family therapy or psychodynamic psychotherapy) for moderate-to-severe depression. This can be combined with fluoxetine from the start, or fluoxetine trialled if no improvement is seen with psychological therapy. Second-line antidepressants are sertraline and citalopram.

RED FLAG

Selective serotonin reuptake inhibitors should be started at lower doses in adolescents than adults. Young people should be monitored closely for thoughts of self-harm or suicide weekly for the first month of commencing treatment or after a dose increase.

Bipolar affective disorder and schizophrenia

Severe and enduring mental illnesses such as bipolar affective disorder and schizophrenia often begin to manifest in adolescence (60% of bipolar disorder has onset before age 20) but are uncommonly fully symptomatic or diagnosed until late adolescence. Suspected cases are generally managed in early intervention for psychosis teams. Classification is the same as in adulthood. Treatment follows the same principles as in adults but focusses on psychological treatments and family interventions rather than pharmacological treatments, with a smaller range of medications used in young people. Management of acute mania remains pharmacological.

Personality disorder

The concept of diagnosing personality disorder in CAMHS is somewhat controversial. By definition, personality disorders are stable and enduring patterns of maladaptive behaviour (see Chapter 17). Young people are still developing their ways of responding to the world, and have had limited life experience, making it hard to predict whether any maladaptive behaviours will persist or not. However, core aspects of personality are evident from infancy onwards, and it is to be expected that someone who will later have a personality disorder will show evidence of these traits from childhood onwards. Certainly, adolescents exhibit characteristic behaviours and symptoms identical to those seen in adults with personality disorders.

It can be harmful to label a young person with a personality disorder diagnosis which turns out to be incorrect, but it can also be harmful to misattribute problems due to personality traits to a different mental disorder, or to minimize them. Pragmatically, if a diagnosis is helpful (e.g., in young person or carer understanding, to access appropriate treatment, to avoid inappropriate treatment, to access other supports), it is useful to make. Treatment of personality disorder in CAMHS is very similar to that in adulthood (see Chapter 28). Psychological therapies in CAMHS offer a particularly powerful opportunity to allow the young person to adjust their trajectory.

CHILD ABUSE

Child abuse includes the overlapping concepts of physical, sexual and emotional mistreatment, as well as neglect or deprivation of the child. Child abuse is very common: around 1 in 4 adults report severe abuse of some kind as a child, with 1 in 20 children in the UK experiencing sexual abuse. Table 30.3 lists the risk factors associated with child abuse. In addition to the physical manifestations, victims of abuse may present with failure to thrive and symptoms of depression, anxiety, aggression, age-inappropriate sexual behaviour and self-harm. They are also at an increased risk for the development of a substantial range of psychiatric problems in later life.

All National Health Service Trusts in the UK have specific child protection guidelines which should be easily accessible and consulted before they are needed. Box 30.7 provides some general principles. All healthcare staff (not just child psychiatrists and paediatricians) have a duty to protect children from harm, and the safety of a child should always take priority. If a child discloses abuse (of any sort), or if you suspect that they are being abused or neglected, confidentiality cannot be maintained, and this should (if appropriate) be explained to the child. Comprehensive notes should be kept, and care taken to allow the child to make the disclosure in their own words without suggestion from others (either family or healthcare staff). Concerns should be reported as soon as practically possible. While local procedures vary slightly, the police, social workers and the duty paediatrician should be able to offer guidance. In some cases, the child may be in imminent danger (e.g., being taken home by the alleged perpetrator). It may be necessary to involve the police to prevent further harm and to remove the child to a place of safety.

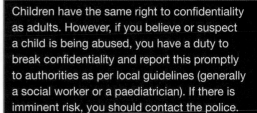

RED FLAG

Children have the same right to confidentiality as adults. However, if you believe or suspect a child is being abused, you have a duty to break confidentiality and report this promptly to authorities as per local guidelines (generally a social worker or a paediatrician). If there is imminent risk, you should contact the police.

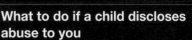

RED FLAG

What to do if a child discloses abuse to you

Listen carefully – do not interrupt or express surprise or your own views

Say

- 'You've done the right thing to tell me'
- 'It's not your fault'
- 'I believe you'

Share

- Tell a senior doctor
- Share the information with authorities
- Consider if the child is safe to go home
- Tell the child what you plan to do, if age appropriate
- Document carefully using child's own words
- Do not challenge the alleged abuser

Table 30.3 Risk factors for child abuse

Parent/environmental factors	Child factors
Parents who were abused	Low birth weight or prematurity
Parental substance abuse	Early maternal separation
Parental mental illness (intellectual disability, depression, schizophrenia, personality disorders) Step-parent	Unwanted child Intellectual or physical disability Challenging behaviour Hyperactivity
Young, immature parents	Excessive crying
Parental criminality	
Poor socioeconomic status and overcrowding	

ASSESSMENT CONSIDERATIONS IN YOUNG PEOPLE

- Problems need to be considered in the context of a child's developmental stage; for example, 'temper tantrums' are normal for a 2-year-old child but should have subsided by age 5 years.
- Parents or carers usually accompany children and young adolescents. It is often useful to first interview them—with or without the child present—to obtain a full description of the current concerns, as well as a complete history (psychiatric, neurodevelopmental, educational and medical). An indirect evaluation of the parents' personalities, marital relationship and style of parenting often creates another perspective from which to understand the context of the presenting complaint.

- An interview with the young person usually follows. The ability of youngsters to provide a candid account of their difficulties varies dramatically. The assessment style should be tailored to the individual abilities of the young person rather than to their age. In children who are unable to articulate their inner experiences (usually younger children), it is often necessary to observe them in play situations.
- The child's own understanding of their difficulties should (if possible) be taken into consideration, as this can affect their management (in terms of motivation to engage with psychosocial interventions, and concordance with medication).
- It may be useful to change the order of the assessment to build rapport. For example, start with open and general questions about school and home rather than the presenting complaint.
- The importance of obtaining collateral information cannot be overstated. This is extremely important in fully understanding the development of the presenting problem, and the young person's premorbid functioning. It includes obtaining academic, educational or psychological reports as well as discussions with teachers and any other agencies involved. Remember to obtain consent from the parent/carer (and the child, if they are able).

- Further information can be obtained from structured and semistructured interviews [e.g., Kiddie Schedule for Affective Disorders and Schizophrenia (K-SADS-P), Diagnostic Interview Schedule for Children (NIMH-DISC-IV)], objective assessment instruments [Autism Diagnostic Observation Schedule (ADOS)] and parent/teacher/self-rating scales [strengths and difficulties questionnaire (SDQ), attention deficit hyperactivity disorder rating Scale IV].

FURTHER READING

Junior MARSIPAN guidelines for management of eating disorders in under 18-year-olds http://www.rcpsych.ac.uk/usefulresources/publications/collegereports/cr/cr168.aspx

Summary of multisystemic therapy http://mstservices.com/files/overview_a.pdf.

Website with useful resources for carers of young people with mental health problems https://www.minded.org.uk/.

Website with information about psychotropic medication for young people Headmeds.org.uk.

> ● **Chapter Summary**
>
> - Mental health problems are common in children and adolescents.
> - Collateral histories and multidisciplinary working are particularly important in Child and Adolescent Mental Health Services.
> - Anxiety disorders in childhood often resolve by adulthood.
> - First-line treatment of mental health problems in young people is generally psychological, not pharmacological.
> - Child abuse is common. Communicating concerns is key.

Older adult psychiatry

The most common psychiatric disorders in older adults are dementia and delirium (see Chapter 19). This chapter considers other psychiatric disorders in older adults.

Ageing is associated with an increased prevalence of both mental and physical health problems. Older adults may also face new social challenges such as coming to terms with retirement; income reduction; living alone or being separated from family; death of spouse, siblings and peers and coping with deteriorating physical health and mobility.

Patients used to arbitrarily come under the care of older adult psychiatrists at the age of 65 years. However, concerns were raised that an automatic transfer to older adult services at a given age resulted in age-based discrimination. Instead, a 'needs-based' approach is now being taken in the majority of areas, whereby patients with problems that older adult services are expert in are transferred, with everyone else remaining under the care of general adult services, whatever their age. This also has the advantage of maintaining continuity of care. Examples of patients that older adult services are best placed to manage are:

- People with dementia of any age.
- People with a mental disorder and significant physical problems or frailty which cause or complicate the management of their mental illness (e.g., delirium, or someone with both schizophrenia and chronic obstructive pulmonary disease requiring nursing home care).
- People with mental health problems closely related to the ageing process (e.g., a grief reaction or depression triggered by social isolation).

Regardless of which services care for them, the number of people aged over 65 years is set to increase substantially over coming decades. Currently, one in five of the UK population is over 65 years of age but by 2040 one in four people are projected to be aged over 65 years. The number of 'very old' (aged over 85 years) is also continuing to increase.

MENTAL ILLNESS IN OLDER ADULTS

Epidemiology

The prevalence of all mental illness tends to increase with age and tends to be higher in residential homes. Fig. 31.1 summarizes the prevalence of the individual psychiatric disorders in older adults.

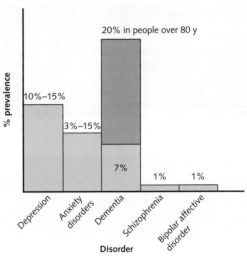

Fig. 31.1 Prevalence of mental illness in people over the age of 65 years.

Depression

- Depression in older adults presents similarly to that in younger people, but a slightly different symptom set needs to be focused on. Symptoms such as fatigue, insomnia and anorexia are more likely to arise in older adults for reasons other than depression and so are less specific in supporting the diagnosis. Similarly, poor concentration and memory are very common in older adult depression but could also reflect a cognitive disorder (see Chapter 7). Instead, negative cognitions such as guilt, hopelessness and suicidality are given more diagnostic weight. There are also certain features of depression that are more common in older adults:
- Severe psychomotor agitation or retardation.
- Cognitive impairment (sometimes called 'depressive pseudodementia').
- Poor concentration.
- Generalized anxiety.
- Excessive concerns about physical health (hypochondriasis).
- When psychotic, older adults are particularly likely to have hypochondriacal delusions, delusions of poverty and nihilistic delusions (see Table 9.1).

Depression is often underdiagnosed in older adults, so a high index of suspicion is needed. Older adults are also less likely to be referred to mental health services regarding depression. This may reflect a perception that low mood is part of normal ageing: it is not. Effective management of depression is important not least because older adults are at high risk for completed suicide, even though the prevalence of self-harm in this group is lower than in younger adults.

> **RED FLAG**
>
> Always think about depression in an older adult presenting with abnormal illness behaviour: hypochondriasis is a common presenting symptom.

> **RED FLAG**
>
> Self-harm in an older adult should be considered to be with suicidal intent until proven otherwise.

The principles of treatment are the same as for younger adults, taking a stepwise approach guided by severity of illness. In addition, it is particularly important to check for physical problems or medication that can cause low mood as the likelihood of these is higher in older adults (see Tables 11.1 and 11.2).

Mild depression and subthreshold symptoms may respond well to psychosocial interventions alone (e.g., befriending, assistance in accessing community supports such as lunch clubs, structured exercise programmes).

Psychological therapies for depression (mainly cognitive-behavioural therapy) are just as effective in older adults as in younger adults and are recommended in those with moderate-to-severe depression. Psychological therapies are particularly useful for patients whose comorbidities place them at high risk of side-effects from medications.

The National Institute for Health and Care Excellence (NICE) also recommends antidepressant medication for those with moderate-to-severe depression, although medication should be introduced cautiously as older adults have an increased risk of developing adverse side-effects and generally need lower doses. Selective serotonin reuptake inhibitors are first line. Tricyclic antidepressants should be avoided if possible as postural hypotension and cognitive impairment are very common side-effects in older adults. Response to antidepressants is often slower in older adults, with benefits taking 6–8 weeks to emerge. Lithium augmentation may be used in treatment-resistant cases, although the dose is generally lower than that used in younger adults.

> **HINTS AND TIPS**
>
> Some selective serotonin reuptake inhibitors side-effects are more likely to occur in older adults than younger adults: hyponatraemia (consider monitoring sodium), gastrointestinal bleeding (consider proton pump inhibitor) and drug interactions (least likely with citalopram and sertraline).

Electroconvulsive therapy (ECT) is a very effective treatment for severe depression in older adults and should be considered for severe symptoms of psychosis, suicidality or life-threatening food and fluid refusal. Dementia is not a contraindication.

Poor prognostic factors include comorbid physical illness, severity of illness and poor concordance with antidepressant medication. The median duration of an episode is 18 months, longer than in younger adults. Having depression reduces life expectancy in older adults by on average 3 years, even when physical illness is taken into account. It also doubles the person's risk of developing dementia.

> **HINTS AND TIPS**
>
> Cotard syndrome describes the presence of nihilistic and hypochondriacal delusions as part of a depressive psychosis and is typically seen in older adults

> **HINTS AND TIPS**
>
> A common triad in older adults is depressive symptoms, cognitive impairment and functional impairment. It is often difficult to tease out whether someone is experiencing depression manifesting with cognitive impairment or an early dementia leading to comorbid depression. Ideally, depression is treated first, then cognition reassessed once mood is euthymic.

Anxiety disorders

Studies that have assessed prevalence of anxiety disorders in older adults alongside younger adults have found that anxiety disorders reduce with age. Generalized anxiety disorder is the commonest specific anxiety disorder in those aged over 65 years (affecting 2%–7%), specific phobias affect around 3% and social phobia, obsessive-compulsive disorder and panic disorder are all uncommon, each occurring in less than 1%. It is rare for anxiety disorders to arise for the first time in older adults. Importantly, anxiety (particularly health related) is a common presenting symptom of depression in older adults, so anyone presenting for the first time with anxiety in later life should be carefully assessed for depression.

Treatment of anxiety disorders in older adults is broadly similar to that in younger adults, with evidence supporting benefits from both medication and psychological therapies (although psychological therapies appear to be not as beneficial as in younger adults). Benzodiazepines should be avoided where at all possible because of the risks of cognitive impairment and falls in older adults.

Mania

Unlike depression, the incidence of bipolar affective disorder does not increase with age, although late-onset cases seem to be less influenced by genetic factors (fewer of these patients have positive family histories for mood disorders). In a fifth of cases, mania is precipitated by an acute medical condition (e.g., stroke or myocardial infarction), making it particularly important to screen for physical or medication causes (see Box 10.2). Hyperactive delirium is an important differential. The presentation and treatment are similar to those of younger adults.

Late-onset schizophrenia (late paraphrenia)

Older adult psychiatrists in the UK use the term *late-onset schizophrenia* or *late paraphrenia* to denote a group of patients who develop their first psychotic symptoms late in life, usually over the age of 60 years. Late-onset schizophrenia is characterized predominantly by delusional thinking, usually of a persecutory or grandiose nature. These delusions tend not to be as bizarre as they sometimes are in earlier-onset schizophrenia (e.g., rather than believing that secret agents are monitoring them by satellite, a patient with paraphrenia may assert that the neighbours have been poisoning their water supply). Hallucinations may occur, but disorganized thinking, inappropriate affect and catatonic features are rarer than in younger adults. The key differentials are dementia, delirium or medication-induced psychotic symptoms.

The aetiology of late-onset schizophrenia seems different to early onset schizophrenia in that affected patients are less likely to have a family history of schizophrenia. In addition, late-onset schizophrenia is far more common in women than men – unlike early onset schizophrenia, which is slightly more likely to arise in men. Sensory deprivation, particularly hearing loss, and social isolation are also implicated in its aetiology.

The treatment is with antipsychotics, but some work is needed in building up a therapeutic relationship as these patients are often difficult to engage and poor concordance is associated with a poor treatment response. Note that although late-onset schizophrenia does seem to be a distinct entity, it is not a term used by the International Classification of Diseases, 10th edition (ICD-10) or the Diagnostic and Statistical Manual of Mental Disorders, 5th edition (DSM-5); here, these patients would be classified as having schizophrenia or delusional disorder.

HINTS AND TIPS

'Diogenes syndrome' is the term used to describe a self-isolated person who lives in a state of significant self-neglect, which may include hoarding and lead to squalid living conditions. This is purely a descriptive term and may occur in individuals who misuse alcohol or have frontal lobe dysfunction, personality disorder and chronic psychotic illness. It may also occur at a younger age.

ASSESSMENT CONSIDERATIONS IN OLDER ADULTS

- Home assessments are a very important part of older adult psychiatry. Patients can be assessed in their normal environment and collateral information can be obtained from family members. It is important to ascertain whether the patient can be managed at home (i.e., risk of harm to self and others; ability to carry out activities of daily living, drive, manage financial affairs), or whether additional community support or hospitalization is needed.
- Collateral information from the patient's general practitioner (GP), family and carers is an important part of history taking.
- Ensure the patient has any aids they require to optimize their communication (e.g., glasses, hearing aids, dentures).
- Mental state examination follows the same format as for all adults, although extra consideration should be given to the assessment of cognitive functioning and it is advisable to always do a standardized test (see Table 7.6 for examples).
- A thorough physical assessment is very important – this may be best done by the patient's GP. Do not forget to consider hearing and vision as well as tremors and involuntary movements.

- Routine investigations in newly diagnosed or hospitalized older adults include: full blood count, urea and electrolytes, liver function tests, thyroid function tests, calcium, glucose, urinalysis (with midstream urine microscopy and culture if indicated), chest X-ray, electrocardiogram and consideration of serum magnesium, phosphate, vitamin B_{12} and folate and a computed tomography or magnetic resonance imaging of the head. Remember that the chances of a physical illness causing or aggravating a mental disorder are significant in older adults.

TREATMENT CONSIDERATIONS IN OLDER ADULTS

Physiological changes with ageing

There are a number of physiological changes that occur with ageing, which may affect the way the body handles certain drugs. Table 31.1 describes the most important changes and their effects. The net result of these changes is that the tissue concentration of a drug may be increased by over 50%, especially in malnourished, dehydrated and debilitated patients. Therefore, the adage, 'start low and go slow' applies especially to the use of psychotropic drugs in the older adult.

Polypharmacy

In 2012–2013, around 80% of those aged over 65 years in the UK were taking at least one prescribed medication, with around two-thirds taking three or more and a quarter taking six or more. Polypharmacy increases the risk of adverse reactions, drug interactions and poor concordance. Therefore, prescribing psychotropic drugs for common, self-terminating symptoms such as insomnia and headache should be avoided wherever possible. When psychotropic drugs are recommended, follow-up arrangements should include a timely assessment of response and discontinuation of any ineffective treatments. Medication should not be a substitute for adequate social care, the lack of which often underlies many nonspecific symptoms.

Concordance

Concordance is often a problem in older adults, especially with those who are visually impaired, cognitively impaired, take numerous drugs and live alone. This may be improved by simplifying medication regimens, taking time to explain dosing schedules, using large font prescription labels or concordance aids such as dosette boxes. Organizing supervision of medication by a relative, friend or support worker may be necessary.

Psychosocial interventions

Psychological treatments, such as cognitive-behavioural therapy, can be used with success in older adults as with younger adults. Reality orientation and reminiscence therapies have been used to reduce disorientation and stimulate remote memories in patients with dementia. Practical psychosocial interventions such as memory aids (e.g., notebooks, calendars) and assistance with mobility and daily activities by a support worker should not be underestimated. Occupational therapy assessment of activities of daily living, which assess skills such as washing, dressing, eating, shopping, give carers an indication of patients' strengths and weaknesses and enable a care package to be tailored that caters specifically for these.

Table 31.1 Age-related changes in drug handling and effects

Physiological changes	Effects
Reduction in renal clearance (glomerular filtration rate and tubular function)	Drugs excreted by filtration (e.g., lithium) need lower doses. Drug concentrations may rise rapidly with dehydration, heart failure, etc.
Decreased lean body mass and total body water and increased body fat	Volume of distribution increases for lipid-soluble drugs (most psychotropic drugs), and reduces for water-soluble drugs (e.g., lithium). Half-life of lipid-soluble drugs prolonged.
Decreased plasma albumin	Reduced drug binding resulting in increased physiologically active unbound fraction.
Reduced hepatic metabolism and first-pass metabolism	May increase the bioavailability and elimination of some drugs.
Increased sensitivity to central nervous system drugs	Sedating drugs may result in drowsiness, confusion, falls and delirium. Tricyclics are more likely to be associated with anticholinergic and postural hypotensive effects. Antipsychotics are more likely to be associated with parkinsonism and increased risk of cerebrovascular accident.
Decreased total body mass	Lower doses of drugs needed (think in terms of milligram/kilogram as opposed to standard dose for all).

Chapter Summary

- Mental illness in older adults is overall similar in presentation and management to younger adults.
- Depressive episodes in older adults often have prominent features of cognitive impairment, agitation and health-related anxiety.
- Self-harm in an older adult should be considered to be with suicidal intent until proven otherwise.
- New-onset mood, anxiety and psychotic illnesses are rare but do occur.
- Be cautious with psychotropic medication use in older adults.
- Psychological interventions are effective in older adults.

act, the party accused was labouring under such a defect of reason, from disease of the mind, as to not know the nature and quality of the act he was doing, or, if he did know it, that he did not know what he was doing was wrong.' It is a defence that is rarely successful due to the high threshold of the legal definition of insanity.

- Diminished responsibility: In English law, a defence of diminished responsibility is only available in relation to charges for murder. If successful, this will lead to the accused being found guilty of manslaughter rather than murder, which allows for flexible sentencing (murder carries a mandatory life sentence). It depends upon the presence of 'an abnormality of mind (whether arising from a condition of arrested or retarded development of mind or any inherent causes or induced by disease or injury)'. An 'abnormality of mind' is not a psychiatric term and is open to wide interpretation, leading to successful defences such as 'emotional immaturity' and 'premenstrual tension'.
- Automatism: An act committed without presence of mind (e.g., during sleepwalking or epileptic seizure) may warrant this rare defence.

HINTS AND TIPS

Self-induced (voluntary) intoxication with alcohol or other drugs cannot be used as a defence on the grounds of insanity or diminished responsibility.

HINTS AND TIPS

It is the responsibility of the Court (taking into consideration advice from expert witnesses) to decide upon sentencing or 'disposal' (i.e., what happens to the individual after trial). In cases where psychiatric defences are successfully used, the Court may utilize mental health legislation to transfer the individual to a secure hospital. In other cases, the Court may decide to impose a custodial sentence, or to place conditions upon the individual (e.g., to adhere to a drug treatment programme).

● Chapter Summary

- Forensic psychiatrists assess and treat mental disorders in people who have committed serious offences.
- Mental disorders are more common in offenders, but usually do not directly cause offending.
- Misuse of drugs and alcohol is a major risk factor for offending.
- Assessment of risk of future violence is imprecise, but is aided by a structured approach.
- Forensic psychiatrists act as expert witnesses regarding the impact of mental disorder on criminal responsibility.

SELF-ASSESSMENT

Single best answer (SBA) questions

Chapter 2 Pharmacological therapy and electroconvulsive therapy

1. Nurses ask for urgent review of a 24-year-old man who is a psychiatric inpatient and is hypertensive, tachycardic and pyrexial. He is very drowsy and has rigid limbs. What action will most help distinguish between neuroleptic malignant syndrome and serotonin syndrome?
   A. Checking serum creatinine kinase levels.
   B. Looking at his prescription.
   C. Checking his past medical history.
   D. Formally assessing his cognition.
   E. Monitoring his condition over time.

2. Nurses ask for urgent review of a 24-year-old man who is a psychiatric inpatient and is hypertensive, tachycardic and pyrexial. He is very drowsy and has rigid limbs. He was admitted a week ago with a first episode psychosis and has received large doses of haloperidol since. What is the most appropriate first management step?
   A. Discontinue all antipsychotics.
   B. Work up for electroconvulsive therapy.
   C. Give dantrolene.
   D. Give bromocriptine.
   E. Assess ABC.

3. A 37-year-old woman with treatment-resistant schizophrenia is considering commencing clozapine. What should she be advised regarding the monitoring that is initially required?
   A. Weekly blood pressure checks.
   B. Weekly liver function tests.
   C. Weekly full blood counts.
   D. Weekly lipid profiles.
   E. Weekly fasting glucose assays.

4. A 45-year-old woman has recently started phenelzine. She is out for lunch with her friend who is a doctor. She asks her friend what she can eat from the menu.
   A. Broccoli and stilton soup.
   B. Pickled herring on a bed of salad.
   C. Marmite and sesame toast.
   D. Smoked mackerel pâté.
   E. Egg mayonnaise toastie.

5. A 37-year-old woman who takes lithium for bipolar affective disorder has recently completed a course of ibuprofen for a knee injury. She now feels very tired and weak. She is unsteady on her feet and has a coarse tremor. A random lithium level is assessed. What is the lowest result that would strongly suggest her symptoms are due to lithium toxicity?
   A. 0.2 mmol/L
   B. 0.4 mmol/L
   C. 0.8 mmol/L
   D. 1.0 mmol/L
   E. 1.8 mmol/L

Chapter 3 Psychological therapy

1. A 49-year-old man has been struggling to move on with his life after his son died in a car accident 6 months ago. Which of the following would be the most appropriate psychological therapy in the first instance?
   A. Psychodynamic therapy
   B. Cognitive-behavioural therapy
   C. Person-centred counselling
   D. Exposure and response prevention
   E. Mindfulness-based cognitive therapy

2. A 35-year-old man is undergoing psychodynamic psychotherapy, and a letter from his therapist describes his 'transference.' Which of the following is the most accurate description of transference?
   A. The level of trust in the patient-therapist relationship.
   B. Good eye contact throughout sessions.
   C. Patient response towards the therapist based on previous relationships.
   D. The level of empathy in the patient-therapist relationship.
   E. Therapist attitude towards the patient based on previous relationships.

3. A 25-year-old male student has a history of depression and has been referred for cognitive-behavioural therapy. He reports that 'my life is over because I failed my final exams.' Which of the following most accurately describes this cognitive distortion?
   A. Emotional reasoning
   B. Fortune telling
   C. Personalization
   D. Labelling
   E. Magnification

5. A 74-year-old man is admitted to hospital because he has acute cognitive impairment and is hypervigilant and agitated. Past medical history is of insomnia and ischaemic heart disease. His medications are amitriptyline 50 mg nocte, aspirin 75 mg mane, lisinopril 5 mg, omeprazole 20 mg mane, simvastatin 20 mg nocte. His daughter thinks he has recently started a new medication. Physical examination, blood tests, electrocardiogram, chest X-ray and head computed tomography are normal. What is the most likely cause of his presentation?
   A. Amitriptyline
   B. Aspirin
   C. Lisinopril
   D. Omeprazole
   E. Simvastatin

Chapter 8 The patient with alcohol or substance use problems

1. A 54-year-old man reports consuming a litre of vodka per day. Which of the following symptoms is not consistent with alcohol dependence?
   A. He feels compelled to drink
   B. After having a drink he feels shaky and sweaty
   C. He started off by drinking a quarter litre of vodka per day but now needs a litre to have the same effect
   D. He has noticed his mood has been low since he started drinking every day and thinks this might be due to alcohol
   E. He has stopped going to visit his family because they don't like him to drink

2. A 57-year-old woman described auditory hallucinations telling her that she was evil. These started a week ago, after several months of heavy alcohol use. She is socially isolated. Her mood, concentration and memory were normal. Other than slightly abnormal liver function tests, physical examination and investigations were normal, and breath alcohol was undetected. What is the most likely diagnosis?
   A. Delirium tremens
   B. Late-onset schizophrenia
   C. Hepatic encephalopathy
   D. Alcoholic hallucinosis
   E. Wernicke–Korsakoff syndrome

3. A 62-year-old salesman is admitted to an orthopaedic ward following a fractured neck of femur. Two days later (before surgery to repair his hip), he appears shaky, confused, and disorientated and tells you that he can see a small horse on the table. His wife discloses that he had been drinking a bottle of whisky per day in the 3 months prior to admission. Which of the following aspects of his management should be delayed?

   A. Benzodiazepines
   B. Parenteral thiamine
   C. Full physical exam
   D. Neck of femur repair
   E. Consistent nursing care

4. A 27-year-old man comes to your outpatient clinic and tells you that he has been injecting heroin on a daily basis for several months and wants you to restart his methadone to help him stop. What is the most appropriate initial step in patient care?
   A. Prescribe his previous dose of methadone
   B. Give him some dihydrocodeine to use first
   C. Obtain a urine sample for drug testing
   D. Refer him to the drug counselling service
   E. Give him advice on harm minimization

5. A 35-year-old woman asks you about 'safe' limits for drinking alcohol. You know the answer is 14 units per week; however, she asks you to explain this in terms of how many drinks she can safely take. What would you tell her?
   A. Six pints (568 mL) of continental lager (5.3% alcohol by volume (ABV)) per week
   B. A 'half bottle' (350 mL) of premium gin (40% ABV) per week
   C. Two bottles (2 × 750 mL) of red wine (12.5% ABV) per week
   D. A large (3 L) bottle of strong white cider (8.4% ABV) per week
   E. Six bottles (6 × 330 mL) of 'alcopops' (4.9% ABV) per week

6. A 24-year-old accountant confides in you that he has tried cocaine on a work night out. He experienced some strange feelings and wants to know whether these were likely to be due to cocaine, or whether he was sold something else. Which of the following symptoms is not suggestive of cocaine intoxication?
   A. Chest pain
   B. Fast heart rate
   C. Fever
   D. Hallucinations
   E. Drowsiness

Chapter 9 The patient with psychotic symptoms

1. A 78-year-old widow with macular degeneration is brought to her general practitioner by her daughter who is concerned that her mother has been asking her to move nonexistent dogs and cats off her couch. Her mother is otherwise alert, orientated and in good health. What is the most likely diagnosis?
   A. Brain tumour
   B. Charles Bonnet syndrome

C. Delirium
D. Dementia
E. Schizophrenia

2. A 62-year-old man with schizophrenia attends his general practitioner. He is dishevelled and smells strongly of tobacco. He reports feeling that someone is pressing on his chest, particularly when he approaches the church at the top of the hill. He wonders if it is the devil. What is the most probable cause of the sensation in his chest?
A. Delusion of control
B. Ischaemic heart disease
C. Persecutory delusion
D. Tactile hallucination
E. Thought disorder

3. A 43-year-old man tells his general practitioner, 'I think my wife is having an affair'. She has frequently been coming home late from work and 2 weeks ago he thought he saw her kissing another man. He is very upset by this and determined to get conclusive evidence to confront her with. He has quit his job to follow her and taken out a personal loan to purchase cameras to place in her car, workplace and handbag. What is the psychopathology described here?
A. Delusion
B. Erotomania
C. Hallucination
D. Obsession
E. Over-valued idea

4. A 19-year-old man is brought to accident and emergency by his flatmates because for the last fortnight, he has been complaining the neighbours are talking about him and tonight stated 'enough was enough' and picked up his cricket bat to go and confront them. His friends cannot hear the neighbours. The man has smoked cannabis every day for the last 6 months and has recently been experimenting with some 'stimulant medication' he bought online. What is the most likely diagnosis?
A. Delusional disorder
B. Depressive episode, severe, with psychotic features
C. Psychosis secondary to psychoactive substance use
D. Schizophrenia
E. Schizophrenia-like psychotic disorder

5. A 16-year-old boy is referred to psychiatry because he has not been able to attend school for 3 months and has lost contact with his friends. He is very difficult to understand because his words do not seem to follow on from each other. Sometimes he laughs or grimaces for no discernible reason. What subtype of schizophrenia does he have?
A. Catatonic
B. Hebephrenic
C. Paranoid
D. Simple
E. Undifferentiated

Chapter 10 The patient with elated or irritable mood

1. Reception staff ask the general practitioner to see a 29-year-old man with a history of bipolar affective disorder who has arrived 2 hours late for his appointment. He is speaking very quickly and the words don't make sense. What is the most likely cause for his presentation?
A. Manic episode
B. Hypomanic episode
C. Depressive episode
D. Cyclothymia
E. Schizophrenia

2. A 55-year-old man has had several admissions to hospital with elated episodes when he believes he is Jesus Christ but has never been depressed. What is the diagnosis?
A. Recurrent hypomania
B. Bipolar affective disorder
C. Schizoaffective disorder
D. Cyclothymia
E. Recurrent mania

3. A 25-year-old farmer is brought to accident and emergency by the police after he tried to steal a tractor. He is agitated, but shows no remorse, stating loudly that it rightfully belongs to him as he is the King of Tractors. He has no past psychiatric history, past medical history or previous criminal offences. Which investigation will be most important diagnostically?
A. Computed tomography (CT) scan
B. Electroencephalogram (EEG)
C. Full blood count
D. Urine drug screen
E. Thyroid function

4. A 24-year-old unemployed woman presents to her general practitioner asking to be treated for bipolar disorder. She has looked it up on the internet and thinks it may explain why she is always losing her temper with people. Her mood swings frequently, sometimes several times in a day. She often does things she later regrets and has never managed to maintain a long-term relationship or job. She has had

these mood swings from when she was a little girl. What is the most likely diagnosis?

A. Bipolar affective disorder
B. Dysthymia
C. Cyclothymia
D. Personality disorder
E. Substance use

Chapter 11 The patient with low mood

1. A 40-year-old woman who was started on a new medication a month ago presents with a 4-week history of depression. Which of the following might account for her presentation?

A. Paracetamol
B. Omeprazole
C. Salbutamol
D. Verapamil
E. Prednisolone

2. A 35-year-old woman presents with mild depression. On examination you notice a midline neck swelling. What is the most appropriate initial step in patient care?

A. Refer to psychiatry
B. Check thyroid function
C. Start an antidepressant
D. Request a neck ultrasound
E. Advise her to return if the symptoms persist

3. A 55-year-old man with no previous psychiatric history presents with low mood, anhedonia and fatigue. He has come for help as he believes his organs are rotting away. What is the most likely diagnosis?

A. Bipolar disorder
B. Schizoaffective disorder
C. Schizophrenia
D. Depressive episode with psychotic features
E. Dementia

4. A 25-year-old student turns up late for her appointment. She gives a 1-month history of low mood, anhedonia and fatigue. What is the most important area to cover in what remains of the appointment time?

A. Presence of biological symptoms of depression
B. Drug history
C. Family history of mood disorder
D. Suicidal ideation
E. Past medical history

5. A 19-year-old shop assistant presents in tears because her boyfriend broke up with her the day before. She did not sleep well last night and did not feel like having breakfast. She feels hopeless about the future and thinks she will never meet anyone else.

She says she feels really depressed. What is the most appropriate initial step in patient care?

A. Start an antidepressant
B. Refer to psychiatry
C. Ask her to complete a mood diary
D. Watchful waiting
E. Check full blood count, urea and electrolytes, liver function test and thyroid function test

Chapter 12 The patient with anxiety, fear or avoidance

1. A 21-year-old student calls an ambulance for the fourth time in a month because of chest pain, shortness of breath and a feeling she is about to die. This settles by the time she reaches the accident and emergency department. On all occasions, her examination, electrocardiogram and cardiac enzymes are normal. She has her final exams in a fortnight and admits she is very worried. What is the most likely diagnosis?

A. Acute coronary syndrome
B. Thyrotoxicosis
C. Hypoglycaemia
D. Panic attack
E. Asthma

2. A 57-year-old obese man keeps cancelling appointments with the practice nurse to have bloods taken for cholesterol and glucose. Although he is normally very cheerful and relaxed, he becomes pale, sweaty and tremulous when you offer to take his bloods during the consultation. What is the most likely diagnosis?

A. Myocardial infarction
B. Hyperglycaemia
C. Blood-injection-injury phobia
D. Panic disorder
E. Hypochondriasis

3. A 63-year-old woman with a history of depression presents to the accident and emergency department and tells you she has a dry mouth, a choking sensation, butterflies in her stomach, palpitations and shortness of breath. She tells you she had some bad news recently. What is the most appropriate first step in management?

A. Electrocardiogram (ECG)
B. Airway, breathing, circulation (ABC)
C. Psychiatry referral
D. Bloods: full blood count, urea and electrolytes, liver function tests and troponin
E. Arterial blood gas (ABG)

4. A 24-year-old man who was recently diagnosed with type 1 diabetes attends his general practitioner (GP). Over the last month he has experienced recurrent attacks of anxiety associated with sweating and

tachycardia. The episodes do not seem to have any triggers, last for about 20 minutes, and resolve when he sits down with his girlfriend and has a cup of tea and a biscuit. What should the GP advise the patient to do next time it happens?

A. Deep breathing exercises
B. Note it in a diary
C. Take diazepam
D. See a counsellor
E. Check blood sugar

5. A 44-year-old businessman presents to his general practitioner (GP) because for the last month he has felt anxious, sweaty and shaky in the mornings. He feels better when he has lunch and generally his mood is good. He admits to drinking a bottle of red wine every night, and usually having champagne during business lunches. What is the most likely diagnosis?

A. Depressive episode
B. Diabetes
C. Panic disorder
D. Alcohol withdrawal
E. Work phobia

Chapter 13 The patient with obsessions and compulsions

1. A 29-year-old woman mentions she is obsessed with a TV talent show. She watches each episode multiple times and has pictures of all the contestants on her bedroom wall. She called in sick the day of the final as her shift clashed with the showing. She enjoys watching and thinking about the show and thinks she might audition next year. What is the most likely diagnosis?

A. No mental illness
B. Social phobia
C. Obsessive-compulsive (anankastic) personality disorder
D. Obsessive-compulsive disorder
E. Delusional disorder

2. A 36-year-old man keeps thinking about his own death. He sees repetitive images of his body in a coffin. He tries to distract himself, but it does not work. The images started about 3 months ago, around the time he started to feel low in mood associated with fatigue, less pleasure in life, insomnia and anorexia. What is the most likely diagnosis?

A. Obsessive-compulsive disorder
B. Generalized anxiety disorder
C. Depressive episode
D. Hypochondriacal disorder
E. Nihilistic delusion

3. A 44-year-old man has had intrusive thoughts for several years regarding security. He keeps thinking his house is unlocked and has developed a routine of checking every door and window nine times before leaving the premises. This means he has to get up half an hour early and sometimes come home from work early to recheck. This has caused friction with a new manager at work and over the last month he has noticed his mood is lower. He no longer enjoys playing football, is very tired all the time, and is struggling to concentrate at work. What is the most likely diagnosis?

A. Depressive episode
B. Obsessive-compulsive disorder (OCD)
C. Generalized anxiety disorder
D. OCD with comorbid depressive episode
E. Obsessive-compulsive (anankastic) personality disorder

4. A 33-year-old graphic designer is driven to produce perfect images. She has always been very conscientious, even at primary school. The thought of a mistake in one of her designs makes her feel so anxious she often stays late at work checking them through. She is proud of the quality of work, and feels her colleagues are sloppy and should work harder. She had to leave her last company because she told the manager this. What is the most likely diagnosis?

A. Obsessive-compulsive disorder
B. Obsessive-compulsive (anankastic) personality disorder
C. No mental illness
D. Autistic spectrum disorder
E. Obsessive-compulsive disorder with subsyndromal depressive symptoms

5. A 23-year-old woman reports a voice inside her head telling her to harm herself. She is not sure where it comes from as no one is around when she hears it. What is the psychopathology she displays?

A. Obsession
B. Pseudohallucination
C. Rumination
D. Thought insertion
E. Hallucination

Chapter 14 The patient with a reaction to a stressful event

1. A 23-year-old man with a history of schizophrenia appears confused and withdrawn the morning after he was severely assaulted by a group of youths in the local park. He has no recollection of the event. Which of the following diagnoses should be initially considered?

A. Acute stress reaction
B. Adjustment disorder
C. Relapse of schizophrenia
D. Intracranial haemorrhage
E. Posttraumatic stress disorder

2. A 57-year-old woman has been referred urgently by her general practitioner for symptoms of low mood, weight loss and insomnia. These have been troublesome for the past 10 weeks, since she watched her husband drown while on a yachting holiday. Which of the following would be suggestive of a diagnosis of depression rather than a normal bereavement reaction?
   A. Thinking that she would be better off dead
   B. Difficulty concentrating on watching the television
   C. Inability to tend to her self-care or get out of bed
   D. Extreme guilt for not making her late husband wear a lifejacket
   E. Hearing the voice of her late husband while lying alone in bed

3. A 28-year-old woman was signed off her job in a call centre 2 weeks ago with 'work-related stress', a month after she was promoted to a supervisory position in a new department. She has no psychiatric history and denies substance misuse. At interview, she tells you she feels 'unable to cope' with the demands of her new role. She is sleeping well, and continues to enjoy jogging on a daily basis. Which of the following would be the most appropriate diagnosis?
   A. Depressive disorder
   B. Adjustment disorder
   C. Conversion disorder
   D. Acute stress disorder
   E. No mental illness

4. 19-year-old female asylum seeker is brought to hospital by a social worker regarding concerns with her memory. She recalls her entire life until 3 months ago when she received news that government militia were coming towards her former hometown in Sierra Leone. She has memory of the last 4 weeks of her life in the UK and is able to tell you about her current address, social circle and circumstances. You see from her medical notes that she had a termination of pregnancy 6 weeks ago; however, she has no recollection of either the conception or the procedure. Physical examination and investigations reveal no abnormalities, and she seems indifferent to her difficulties. Which ONE of the following is the most likely diagnosis?
   A. Dissociative amnesia
   B. Anterograde amnesia following head trauma
   C. Transient global amnesia
   D. Posttraumatic stress disorder
   E. Wernicke–Korsakoff's syndrome

Chapter 15 The patient with medically unexplained physical symptoms

1. A 26-year-old male teacher attends his general practitioner (GP) requesting tests to confirm that he is suffering from multiple sclerosis. He thinks that he has this because he had some stabbing pain in his upper arm last week. The pain has now resolved and examination is unremarkable. Which ONE of the following should the GP do?
   A. Watchful waiting
   B. Refer for urgent neurology appointment
   C. Organize magnetic resonance imaging scan and lumbar puncture
   D. Tell the patient that he is worrying too much
   E. Organize another appointment in 3 days

2. A 25-year-old woman insists that she wants plastic surgery on her nose, as she feels it is crooked and deformed. She has stopped leaving the house for fear of other people noticing. She cannot stop thinking about how ugly it is, and this often keeps her awake at night. On examination, her nose is entirely normal, and she does appear slightly reassured when told this. Which of the following is the most likely diagnosis?
   A. Somatic delusional disorder
   B. Factitious disorder
   C. Malingering
   D. Body dysmorphic disorder
   E. Hypochondriacal disorder

3. A 32-year-old former nurse complains of pelvic pain. Despite the apparent severity of the pain and the presence of multiple abdominal surgical scars, her physical appearance, examination and basic investigations are entirely normal. She tells you in detail about her previous diagnoses and invasive investigations, and requests pethidine and a diagnostic laparoscopy. She is visiting from a distant town. Which of the following should be the next step in her management?
   A. Urgent diagnostic laparoscopy
   B. Prescribe pethidine
   C. Tell her that she is lying
   D. Contact previous centres of care
   E. Refer to psychiatry

4. A 72-year-old man is referred to psychiatry because of dyspnoea and stabbing pain in his chest. He has not seen a general practitioner for years, and examination and routine blood tests are normal. The medical doctor feels that he has panic attacks. Which ONE of the following should be the next step in his management?
   A. Cognitive-behavioural therapy
   B. Further physical investigations

C. Explanation of functional illness
D. Antidepressant medication
E. Watchful waiting

5. A 41-year-old woman is a frequent visitor to her general practitioner (GP). She has had numerous investigations over several years for a multitude of physical symptoms, including abdominal pain, dysmenorrhoea, dysuria and difficulty swallowing. She refuses to accept her GP's explanation that there is no physical cause for her symptoms. She is now requesting a referral to a neurologist because she has a persistent tingling sensation in her legs. Which of the following is the most likely diagnosis?
A. Multiple sclerosis
B. Factitious disorder
C. Somatisation disorder
D. Hypochondriacal disorder
E. Generalised anxiety disorder

Chapter 16 The patient with eating or weight problems

1. A 22-year-old female medical student is brought to your clinic by her mother, who discovered she was making herself vomit after meals. Which of the following is suggestive of a diagnosis of anorexia nervosa rather than bulimia nervosa?
A. Body weight at least 15% below expected for height
B. A dread of fatness and a distorted image of being too fat
C. Use of herbal dieting medications
D. A tendency to exercise excessively
E. A preoccupation with being thin

2. The weight of a 13-year-old boy is 25% lower than expected, having previously been on the 50th percentile for both height and weight. He has not started puberty. He reports that he eats well and denies any concerns regarding body image. What is the most appropriate next management step?
A. Refer for psychiatric assessment
B. Refer for cognitive-behavioural therapy
C. Investigate for physical causes of growth restriction
D. Try to establish rapport to facilitate assessment
E. Ask him to keep a food diary

3. A 32-year-old barmaid is worried that she has lost a great deal of weight recently (body mass index 17). She describes feeling tired all the time and having no appetite. Her mood has been low for the last 3 months, and she is anhedonic. She drinks six vodkas and cokes when she is working, and three on her days off. If she doesn't have a drink she feels anxious and gets palpitations. She is sometimes sick, not always after meals. Physical examination and investigations reveal no abnormalities. What is the most likely diagnosis?
A. Bulimia nervosa
B. Depressive episode, severe
C. Panic disorder
D. Anorexia nervosa
E. Alcohol dependence

4. A 25-year-old female lawyer has a diagnosis of anorexia nervosa, with a body mass index of 14.5 kg/m^2. Which of the following investigation results requires urgent treatment?
A. Glucose 3.7 mmol/L
B. Haemoglobin 95 g/L
C. Total cholesterol 7 mmol/L
D. Phosphate 0.7 mmol/L
E. Potassium 2.1 mmol/L

5. A 19-year-old female accountant describes a dread of fatness, and feels that she is overweight despite having a body mass index of 13.6 kg/m^2. She describes a 1-year history of severely restricting her dietary intake. She reports amenorrhoea (secondary) and has lanugo hair. Which of the following is the most likely diagnosis?
A. Depressive episode, severe
B. Bulimia nervosa
C. Paranoid schizophrenia
D. Anorexia nervosa
E. Obsessive-compulsive disorder

6. A 17-year-old boy has anorexia nervosa and is receiving weekly weights and physical examination. Which of the findings below places him at high physical risk?
A. Blood pressure 95/65 mm Hg supine, 88/60 mm Hg erect
B. Capillary refill time <2 seconds
C. Heart rate 58 bpm, regular
D. Temperature 36.5°C
E. Unable to rise from squatting without assistance

Chapter 17 The patient with personality problems

1. A 20-year-old woman attends her general practitioner frequently reporting low mood. Which of the following symptoms would support a diagnosis of emotionally unstable personality disorder?
A. Chronic feelings of emptiness
B. Callous unconcern for the feelings of others
C. Perfectionism that interferes with task completion
D. Seeking others to make most of one's important life decisions
E. Takes pleasure in few, if any, activities

2. A 45-year-old male, single and living alone, seems indifferent to praise or criticism, appears aloof and prefers his own company. He is not depressed and there has been little change in his situation since he left school. Which of the following personality disorders is most likely?
   A. Narcissistic personality disorder
   B. Antisocial personality disorder
   C. Avoidant personality disorder
   D. Schizoid personality disorder
   E. Paranoid personality disorder

3. A 25-year-old male prisoner injured a fellow inmate by throwing him down the stairs. He states that he feels no guilt as the man 'was asking for it' after looking at him strangely. Which of the following personality disorders is most likely?
   A. Borderline personality disorder
   B. Schizoid personality disorder
   C. Antisocial personality disorder
   D. Paranoid personality disorder
   E. Anankastic personality disorder

4. A 19-year-old man has carved the name of his ex-partner on his chest. He reported feeling incredibly depressed since she separated from him and kicked him out of the house the day before. He is crying and tells you that he wants to die. He is intoxicated with alcohol. Which of the following is the most likely diagnosis?
   A. Acute severe depression
   B. Borderline personality disorder
   C. Adjustment reaction
   D. No mental illness or personality disorder
   E. Unable to say

5. A 22-year-old man has a long history of self-harm, explosive outbursts of anger, impulsive, reckless behaviour, feelings of emptiness and quickly forming intense and volatile 'love–hate' relationships. He reports hearing the voice of his uncle, who sexually abused him as a child, inside his head when he is feeling stressed. He has no history of mental illness. Which of the following would be the most appropriate diagnosis?
   A. Borderline personality disorder
   B. Schizoid personality disorder
   C. Dependent personality disorder
   D. Paranoid personality disorder
   E. Antisocial personality disorder

Chapter 18 The patient with neurodevelopmental problems

1. A 7-year-old boy keeps getting up at school and walking to the front of the classroom. His mother is worried he has attention deficit hyperactivity disorder (ADHD). He is not restless at home and sits calmly during the interview. What is the most appropriate initial step in management?
   A. Check thyroid function
   B. Collateral history from teacher
   C. Ensure he has an up-to-date eye test
   D. Genetic testing to exclude ADHD
   E. Refer for ADHD assessment

2. A 1-year-old girl has stopped crawling. She used to cry a lot but is now calm and placid. She had developed a social smile but has not done this for a few weeks. She also makes less eye contact than she used to. What is the most likely diagnosis?
   A. Autism spectrum disorder
   B. Heller syndrome
   C. Intellectual disability
   D. Muscular dystrophy
   E. Rett syndrome

3. A 23-year-old man reports he is very anxious in social situations. He recently lost his job because he talked too much in the office. Now he is worried about talking to others at all. He says he 'doesn't get the rules' and he thought his workmates were enjoying what he was telling them about the history of photocopiers. What is the most likely diagnosis?
   A. Anankastic (obsessive-compulsive) personality disorder
   B. Autism spectrum disorder
   C. Depressive episode
   D. Generalized anxiety disorder
   E. Social phobia

Chapter 19 Dementia and delirium

1. A 91-year-old nursing home resident with severe Alzheimer dementia frequently shouts unintelligible words. Physical examination and investigations are normal, and she does not seem low in mood. Staff can detect no pattern or triggers to her shouting. She appears mildly distressed by it. What option should be tried first to reduce her shouting?
   A. Aromatherapy
   B. Antipsychotic
   C. Antidepressant
   D. Cholinesterase inhibitor
   E. Referral to speech and language therapy

2. A 75-year-old man has Lewy body dementia. His carers are worried that he is not eating well. He tells his general practitioner that he is certain his carers are trying to poison him. What management strategy should be avoided if possible?
   A. Antipsychotics
   B. Nutritional supplements
   C. Cholinesterase inhibitors

D. Antibiotics

E. Antidepressants

3. A 77-year-old man was admitted 3 days ago with abdominal pain of uncertain aetiology. Initially he was alert and orientated but nurses are concerned that he is now acutely disorientated and agitated. Which medication is most likely to explain his behaviour?

A. Paracetamol

B. Metoclopramide

C. Co-codamol

D. Omeprazole

E. Cyclizine

4. A general practitioner (GP) is asked to visit a 71-year-old woman in her home. She is disorientated in time, does not recognize the GP (whom she has known for years) and is very drowsy. She is plucking at her bed clothes and refuses to let the GP examine her because she thinks he wants to hurt her. Her husband states she was fine until 2 days ago, but now he cannot cope with her. Where should the GP manage this lady with acute onset psychotic symptoms?

A. Her own home

B. Day hospital

C. Emergency respite via social work

D. Acute medical ward

E. Acute psychiatric ward

Chapter 20 Alcohol and substance-related disorders

1. A 29-year-old man with alcohol dependence syndrome tells you that he wants to give up drinking, but he is worried that he will lose all his friends from the pub. At which stage of the Prochaska and DiClemente Transtheoretical Model of Change would you consider him to be?

A. Precontemplation of change

B. Contemplation of change

C. Preparation for change

D. Action for change

E. Maintenance of change

2. A 21-year-old homeless woman tells you that she uses £20 of heroin per day via intravenous injection. She is keen to be prescribed methadone. Which of the following measures would be essential prior to starting methadone?

A. History from a friend to corroborate her usage

B. Viral serology for HIV and hepatitis B and C

C. Thorough physical examination with focus on injection sites

D. Admission to psychiatric hospital

E. Urine drug test to confirm presence of opioids

3. A 45-year-old man is being treated by the alcohol problems team. He has successfully been 'detoxified' using chlordiazepoxide. Which of the following is true regarding his future pharmacological treatment?

A. Trazodone can be prescribed to treat his alcohol dependence

B. Long-term, low-dose chlordiazepoxide is the treatment of choice

C. Naltrexone can be helpful even if he relapses to drinking

D. Acamprosate causes an unpleasant reaction when taken with alcohol

E. Disulfiram should control his cravings for alcohol

4. A 26-year-old woman asks you for help with her heroin dependence. She does not want to receive methadone, as she feels this is more addictive than heroin. Which of the following drugs might she prefer to try as substitution therapy?

A. Lofexidine

B. Diazepam

C. Buprenorphine

D. Clonidine

E. Naltrexone

Chapter 21 The psychotic disorders: schizophrenia

1. A pregnant woman with schizophrenia asks how likely her child is to develop schizophrenia? Her partner does not have a mental illness.

A. 1%

B. 12.5%

C. 2.5%

D. 37.5%

E. 50%

2. A pregnant woman with schizophrenia asks how likely her child is to develop schizophrenia? Her partner also has schizophrenia.

A. 1%

B. 12.5%

C. 25%

D. 37.5%

E. 50%

3. A 22-year-old man was started on olanzapine 4 months ago for a first episode of schizophrenia. He is now symptom free, but troubled by weight gain. He asks how long in total he needs to stay on an antipsychotic?

A. 6 months

B. 9 months

C. 1–2 years

D. 3–5 years

E. Lifelong

4. A 27-year-old woman has developed schizophrenia. She is interested in talking therapies. What type of psychological therapy does NICE (2014) recommend to her?
   A. Psychodynamic psychotherapy
   B. Interpersonal therapy
   C. Dialectical behaviour therapy
   D. Cognitive-behavioural therapy
   E. Cognitive analytic therapy

5. A 35-year-old woman experiencing a manic episode with psychotic features had been attempting to make the voices go away by repeatedly banging her head against her sink. De-escalation techniques had not worked, and she had refused oral medication, so in view of the significant risk to herself she received intramuscular rapid tranquillization. She has no past medical history. It is now 30 minutes postadministration and she is sitting dozing peacefully in the quiet room. What monitoring does she now require?
   A. No monitoring is required
   B. General observations
   C. Temperature, pulse, blood pressure, respiratory rate, hydration status and consciousness level every hour
   D. Temperature, pulse, blood pressure, respiratory rate, hydration status and consciousness level every 15 minutes
   E. Continuous monitoring of pulse, blood pressure and respiratory rate with regular temperatures

6. A 35-year-old woman has received intramuscular rapid tranquillization. Which of the following complications is least important to monitor for?
   A. Respiratory depression
   B. Inability to protect her own airway
   C. Hyperglycaemia
   D. Acute arrhythmia
   E. Life-threatening hypotension

Chapter 22 The mood (affective) disorders

1. Which of the following patients with depression would be the highest priority for electroconvulsive therapy (ECT)?
   A. Someone who is not eating or drinking
   B. Someone who believes they are already dead, so there is no point taking medication
   C. Someone who has experienced no benefit from two antidepressants
   D. Someone who has benefited from ECT in the past
   E. Someone who has experienced no benefit from several antidepressants but does not want ECT

2. A 24-year-old man is brought to accident and emergency by the police. He has a 1-week history of irritable mood, insomnia and grandiose delusions that he has super powers. The police found him about to jump off some scaffolding to prove he is invincible. He does not believe he is unwell and says there is no way he is coming into hospital. What is the best initial step in management?
   A. Appointment with general practitioner later that day
   B. Informal admission
   C. Admission under mental health legislation
   D. Urgent outpatient psychiatric review
   E. Police custody after arrest for breach of the peace

3. A 45-year-old man is admitted to hospital with a 6-week history of low mood. He plans to kill himself at the first opportunity because he believes the world is going to end soon and wants to die quickly. He is not currently on any medication. What would be the best management option?
   A. Citalopram
   B. Amitriptyline
   C. Quetiapine
   D. Citalopram and quetiapine
   E. Amitriptyline and quetiapine

4. A 29-year-old postgraduate student with a diagnosis of bipolar affective disorder is admitted with a manic episode after stopping medication. She is very agitated on the ward, pacing, being verbally aggressive to staff and fellow patients, and punching her wardrobe. What is the best medication to commence?
   A. Lithium
   B. Olanzapine
   C. Citalopram
   D. Valproate
   E. Lamotrigine

5. A 36-year-old lecturer with moderate to severe depression wants to try a psychological therapy for depression. Which of the following should be offered?
   A. Self-help cognitive-behavioural therapy (CBT)
   B. Structured group physical activity
   C. Individual CBT
   D. Dialectical behaviour therapy
   E. Graded exposure therapy

Chapter 23 The anxiety and somatoform disorders

1. A 35-year-old woman has been recently diagnosed with somatization disorder. How should this diagnosis change her management by her general practitioner?
   A. She should not be allowed access to urgent appointment slots
   B. She should be seen on a planned, regular schedule

C. She should not be investigated for physical complaints
D. She should never be prescribed benzodiazepines
E. She should be reassured that her symptoms do not really exist

2. A 17-year-old school pupil has a phobia of bodily fluids but aspires to be a nurse. What treatment can she be offered?
A. None – she should change her career plans
B. Cognitive-behavioural therapy (CBT) with desensitization
C. CBT focused on trauma
D. Diazepam when necessary (PRN) – to be taken before any possible contact with bodily fluids
E. Selective serotonin reuptake inhibitor (SSRI)

3. A 29-year-old chemist has obsessive-compulsive disorder (OCD) regarding orderliness. She has been tidying up her colleagues' laboratory benches and spoilt some experiments. She has been threatened with dismissal. She does not want to try any talking therapies. What treatment can she be offered?
A. Clomipramine
B. Mirtazapine
C. Selective serotonin reuptake inhibitor (SSRI)
D. Pregabalin
E. Self-help

Chapter 24 Eating disorders

1. A 17-year-old boy has a body mass index of 16 kg/m^2, wears baggy clothes, and states that he is worried about being overweight. He is diagnosed with anorexia nervosa, although he does not feel that he has a problem. However, he is agreeable to meeting a therapist, mainly to please his mother. Which of the following modalities of psychotherapy would be recommended in the first instance?
A. Maudsley model of anorexia treatment for adults
B. Family therapy
C. Focal psychodynamic psychotherapy
D. Cognitive-behavioural therapy
E. Specialist supportive clinical management

2. A 20-year-old man has a body mass index of 16 kg/m^2, wears baggy clothes, and states that he is worried about being overweight. He was diagnosed with anorexia nervosa as a 17-year old. After a period of treatment and remission his symptoms have returned. Which of the following modalities of psychotherapy would be recommended in the first instance?
A. Exposure-response prevention therapy
B. Family therapy
C. Focal psychodynamic psychotherapy
D. Interpersonal therapy
E. Specialist supportive clinical management

3. A 29-year-old female actuary is diagnosed with anorexia nervosa. Which of the following factors is associated with a poor prognosis?
A. Early age of onset
B. Rapid weight loss
C. Binge–purge symptoms
D. Family history of anorexia
E. Slow to engage with psychotherapy

4. A 17-year-old woman has been diagnosed with anorexia nervosa. Which medication should she be advised to take until she regains a healthy nutritional intake?
A. Citalopram
B. Fluoxetine
C. Multivitamin
D. Paroxetine
E. Sertraline

5. A 21-year-old woman with severe anorexia nervosa was found collapsed in the street secondary to heart failure due to malnutrition. She has subsequently been admitted to a specialist eating disorder unit to receive nasogastric feeding under mental health legislation. Which of the following blood test results raises concern that she is experiencing refeeding syndrome?
A. Calcium 2.4 mmol/L
B. Magnesium 1.7 mEq/L
C. Phosphate 0.3 mmol/L
D. Potassium 3.7 mmol/L
E. Sodium 141 mmol/L

Chapter 25 The sleep–wake disorders

1. A 33-year-old woman describes creeping, burning sensations in her legs which keep her awake at night. She finds getting up and walking around eases them. Her mother had the same problem. She has tried nonpharmacological management and would like to try medication. Which medication is recommended first line?
A. Fluoxetine
B. Haloperidol
C. Lithium
D. Metoclopramide
E. Pramipexole

2. A 33-year-old woman describes creeping, burning sensations in her legs which keep her awake at night. The pain also affects her throughout the day. She finds getting up and walking around makes little difference. She has poorly controlled type one diabetes. What is the most likely diagnosis?
A. Akathisia
B. Intermittent claudication
C. Iron deficiency
D. Neuropathy
E. Restless legs syndrome

3. A 33-year-old woman describes trouble sleeping at night, with early morning wakening. She has recently been diagnosed with depression and started on fluoxetine (20 mg) 2 weeks ago. Her mood is slightly better, but she is worried that her sleep is not. What is the next best management step?
   A. Increase fluoxetine dose
   B. Keep a sleep diary
   C. Refer for polysomnography
   D. Sleep hygiene advice
   E. Short course of temazepam

Chapter 26 The psychosexual disorders

1. A 24-year-old woman presents to her general practitioner concerned that she achieves orgasm infrequently during penetrative sex with her partner. What should she be advised?
   A. Caressing without genital contact can improve sex
   B. Sexual dysfunction is rare in young people
   C. She is likely to have a physical problem preventing orgasm
   D. She should stop any medication which could be contributing
   E. Talking about sexual problems with her partner is likely to increase anxiety in the bedroom

2. A 57-year-old man tells his general practitioner he is unable to have an erection, even when masturbating. He occasionally found it hard to achieve an erection as a younger man but it has got much worse recently. He was previously obese but has lost weight recently. What is the most important next management step?
   A. Advise to lose more weight and return if problem persists
   B. Check blood glucose
   C. Direct to self-help resources regarding sexual dysfunction
   D. Prescribe sildenafil
   E. Refer to urology

3. A 63-year-old man with Parkinson disease has recently started making obscene phone calls. He becomes sexually aroused during this. He has been working his way through his wife's address book and several of her friends have been very distressed. Which of the medications below is least likely to have caused this behaviour?
   A. Levodopa
   B. Olanzapine
   C. Pergolide
   D. Pramipexole
   E. Selegiline

4. A 22-year-old man tells his general practitioner that he enjoys dressing as a woman during sex with his partner. What is he describing?
   A. Gender dysphoria
   B. Transgenderism
   C. Transsexualism
   D. Transvestic fetishism
   E. Transvestism

Chapter 27 Disorders relating to the menstrual cycle, pregnancy and the puerperium

1. A 27-year-old schoolteacher reports increased irritability in the week prior to menstruation. This quickly resolves within a day of starting her period. Most of the time the irritability does not cause her any problems apart from when recently she had an argument with her boyfriend. What is the best management option?
   A. Encourage exercise
   B. Prescribe combined oral contraceptive pill
   C. Prescribe ibuprofen
   D. Prescribe selective serotonin reuptake inhibitor (SSRI)
   E. Refer for cognitive-behavioural therapy (CBT)

2. A 53-year-old company director reports low mood, increased fatigability and early morning wakening for the past 2 months, accompanied by increased suicidal thoughts. She has had to take some time off work. She attributes her symptoms to her menopause. What is the best management option?
   A. Hormone replacement therapy
   B. Dietary and lifestyle advice
   C. Omega-3 fish oils
   D. Counselling
   E. Psychological therapy

3. A 25-year-old artist has a history of bipolar affective disorder. She has been taking lithium and has been well for the past 3 years. She wants to start a family with her partner and has heard that lithium can cause problems with fetal malformations. What is the most appropriate management?
   A. Switch to semisodium valproate
   B. Switch to carbamazepine
   C. Discontinue lithium and continue without treatment
   D. Switch to olanzapine
   E. Refer to perinatal mental health team

4. A 33-year-old woman previously experienced a protracted episode of postnatal depression following the birth of her first child, which necessitated admission to a mother-and-baby unit. The episode responded well to antidepressant medication. She has recently become pregnant and is incredibly anxious

that she will become unwell again postnatally. What is the most appropriate management?

A. Reassure that becoming unwell again would be unlikely
B. Restart antidepressant treatment immediately
C. Referral to psychologist to identify relapse signature
D. Watchful waiting
E. Referral to perinatal mental health team

5. A 22-year-old lady is found by the police. She was knee-deep in a river with her 2-week-old baby boy. She reported that the infant was possessed by the devil, and that she needed to drown him to save humanity. At interview, she appears perplexed and is openly responding to auditory hallucinations. She does not want to be admitted to hospital as she does not think she is unwell. She has a very supportive family who are keen to look after her at home. What is the most appropriate management option?

A. Detention in hospital under mental health act
B. Treatment at home under care of crisis team
C. Transfer to police cells and charge with attempted murder
D. Urgent referral for outpatient follow-up by perinatal mental health team
E. Urgent referral to social work

Chapter 28 The personality disorders

1. A 19-year-old hairdresser has a diagnosis of emotionally unstable personality disorder, and requests information on drug treatment that may be beneficial. What should she be advised?

A. Sodium valproate is effective for reducing interpersonal problems
B. Omega-3 fatty acids are effective in reducing impulsivity
C. Risperidone is effective for reducing anger
D. Amitriptyline reduces chronic feelings of emptiness
E. Drug treatment is not the main intervention

2. A 34-year-old man has a diagnosis of emotionally unstable personality disorder, and requests information on different types of psychotherapy that may be beneficial. Which of the following psychological treatments does NICE (2009) recommend?

A. Dialectical behaviour therapy
B. Mentalization-based therapy
C. Psychodynamic
D. Cognitive-analytical therapy
E. Therapeutic communities

3. A 27-year-old female postgraduate student has a diagnosis of emotionally unstable personality disorder. She reported low mood and insomnia for the past month and has subsequently been absent from

university (which is unusual for her). Normally, she is easily angered, but relatively cheerful. At assessment she reports increased thoughts of suicide, but no immediate plans. What is the most appropriate next step in management?

A. Refer for dialectical behaviour therapy
B. Request a urine drug screen
C. Prescribe diazepam
D. Admit to an acute psychiatric ward
E. Suggest 'weekly dispensing' of medication

4. A 29-year-old man has a diagnosis of antisocial personality disorder. He coldly tells his psychiatrist of his intention to kill his landlord following an argument about rent arrears, before describing a detailed plan on how he would stab him in the throat. What is the most appropriate next management step?

A. Ask him to return for review in 1 week
B. Prescribe diazepam
C. Warn the police and the intended victim
D. Admit to psychiatric hospital under detention
E. Refer for anger management

Chapter 29 The neurodevelopmental disorders

1. A 23-year-old man is diagnosed with an autism spectrum disorder. Which medication can be prescribed to reduce the core symptoms of his disorder?

A. Fluoxetine
B. Methylphenidate
C. None
D. Risperidone
E. Sodium valproate

2. A 7-year-old boy has recently been diagnosed with attention deficit hyperactivity disorder (ADHD). It is having a substantial impact on his behaviour at school, and he is at risk of expulsion. What is the first-line treatment?

A. Atomoxetine
B. Cognitive-behavioural therapy
C. Dexamfetamine
D. Methylphenidate
E. Parent-training/education programme

3. A 12-year-old boy has multiple motor tics and repeatedly shouts 'Batman!' when he is stressed or excited. He had to leave the cinema once because of this but is otherwise not troubled by his symptoms. What is the first-line treatment for this disorder?

A. Clonidine
B. No treatment
C. Pimozide
D. Psychoeducation
E. Risperidone

Chapter 30 Child and adolescent psychiatry

1. For the past 6 months, a 12-year-old boy has repeatedly been in trouble with the police. Recently, he has been violent towards his sister and has killed her pet hamster. His mother sought help after he deliberately set the garden shed on fire. What is the most likely diagnosis?
   A. Antisocial personality disorder
   B. Conduct disorder
   C. Oppositional defiant disorder
   D. Reactive attachment disorder
   E. Substance misuse

2. An 8-year-old girl presents with encopresis. During examination by the junior doctor, genital warts and vaginal trauma are noted. What is the next most appropriate step in management?
   A. The child should be sent home and seen in outpatients
   B. The parents should be confronted by the nurses
   C. The child should be directly asked what happened
   D. Police should be contacted to question the girl
   E. The duty social worker and on-call paediatrician should be alerted

3. A 16-year-old girl presents with a 2-month history of low mood and fatigue. She no longer enjoys playing netball and feels her friends do not like her any more. She is still attending school but is no longer doing well academically. What treatment should she be offered first line?
   A. Citalopram
   B. Cognitive-behavioural therapy
   C. Fluoxetine
   D. Sertraline
   E. Watchful waiting

4. A 16-year-old girl presents with low mood. She has had episodes of low mood for most of her life, often varying from good to bad and back again within a day. She has never had any close friends because she feels her peers have always rejected her. She has self-harmed by cutting since the age of 13 years, and often makes herself sick after meals. She says she feels angry and empty at the same time. After her father took an overdose she started hearing his voice inside her head telling her to do it too. Her body mass index is 22 kg/m². What is the most likely diagnosis?
   A. Bipolar affective disorder
   B. Bulimia nervosa
   C. Depressive episode
   D. Emotionally unstable personality disorder
   E. Schizophrenia

Chapter 31 Older adult psychiatry

1. A 74-year-old woman gives a 6-month history of low mood, anhedonia and fatigue associated with difficulty concentrating and remembering. Neighbours have noticed she is forgetting to put her bins out and no longer cooks meals for herself. Her score on the Addenbrooke's Cognitive Examination (ACE-III) is 72/100. What is the best management option?
   A. Antidepressant
   B. Cholinesterase inhibitor
   C. Memantine
   D. Refer for aromatherapy and massage
   E. Refer for counselling

2. A 72-year-old widow has presented to her general practitioner 20 times in the last month with minor physical concerns. Previously she attended infrequently. During consultations she is restless, wrings her hands and seems to struggle to remember advice given to her. Her friends are struggling to cope as she telephones them throughout the night to check they are alright. Her score on the Abbreviated Mental Test (AMT) is 10/10. What is the most likely diagnosis?
   A. Mild cognitive impairment
   B. Generalized anxiety disorder
   C. Depressive episode
   D. Late onset schizophrenia
   E. Hypochondriacal disorder

3. A 71-year-old widower has a 3-month history of low mood, fatigue and anhedonia associated with anorexia. He was transferred from a general hospital to a psychiatric hospital 4 weeks ago after an episode of acute kidney injury precipitated by poor oral intake. He has been commenced on an antidepressant but is poorly concordant and his presentation has changed little. His kidney function has not returned to baseline as he continues to drink little fluid. What is the best management option?
   A. Electroconvulsive therapy (ECT)
   B. Continue current oral antidepressant
   C. Commence depot medication with antidepressant properties
   D. Change to an alternative oral antidepressant
   E. Change to lithium

4. An out-of-hours general practitioner calls for advice about a patient who has been 'behaving oddly'. The computer system is down, so their past psychiatric history is unknown. Which of the patients below is most likely to have late-onset schizophrenia?
   A. A diabetic man who reports that the police are stealing his thoughts
   B. A deaf woman who lives alone and reports that the police are trying to rob her

C. An obese woman who lives alone and is thought disordered

D. A blind woman who lives alone and reports seeing policemen in her living room every night

E. A man with ischaemic heart disease who can hear talking on the police radio in all the rooms in his house

5. A 76-year-old woman who started mirtazapine for a depressive episode 4 weeks ago attends her general practitioner. Her son also has depression and noticed improvement after 2 weeks of an antidepressant. She has not noticed any benefit or side-effects from mirtazapine and is wondering if she should change treatment. What would be the best management option?

A. Change to the antidepressant that worked for her son

B. Augment mirtazapine with the antidepressant that worked for her son

C. Change to a tricyclic antidepressant

D. Continue mirtazapine for at least 8 weeks

E. Discontinue mirtazapine and observe without antidepressant

6. A 77-year-old lady with a history of bipolar affective disorder no longer requiring medication is brought to the accident and emergency department by her family. In the past 24 hours she has started behaving very oddly – getting dressed in the middle of the night, dropping to the ground and shaking her leg about and shouting irritably at people when she is asked questions about her orientation. Her Abbreviated Mental Test score is 2/10. What is the most likely diagnosis?

A. Lithium toxicity

B. Manic episode

C. Hypomanic episode

D. Somatization disorder

E. Delirium

7. A general practitioner (GP) pays a home visit to a 74-year-old man with a long history of schizophrenia. The man mentions that he is more bothered by auditory hallucinations than normal. The GP notices little piles of olanzapine tablets on saucers in the kitchen and living room. The man admits that he is struggling to keep track of whether he has taken his medication or not. What would be the best way to improve concordance?

A. Start a depot antipsychotic

B. Dispense medication weekly in a labelled dosette box

C. Refer for a support worker to prompt medication

D. Arrange daily dispensing at the local pharmacy

E. Change the time of olanzapine so he can take it in the morning with his other medication

8. An 82-year-old widow with no past psychiatric history presents to her general practitioner (GP) requesting a repeat prescription of trazodone. Her supply should not have run out yet, and she admits she took six extra tablets at the weekend in the hope of 'going to sleep and not waking up'. In the event she just overslept, and no harm was done. She feels foolish now and would just like to go home and stop wasting the GP's time. What is the best management option?

A. Ask her to attend accident and emergency (A&E)

B. Review by GP in a week

C. Refer to the local lunch club

D. Refer to psychiatric outpatients

E. Refer for urgent, same day, psychiatric review

Chapter 32 Forensic psychiatry

1. A 32-year-old man with substance misuse problems reports he is thinking of taking up mugging to fund his habit. Which of the following factors in his history places him at highest risk of future violence?

A. Having a mental disorder

B. Using substances

C. Previous violence

D. Experiencing command hallucinations

E. Childhood abuse

2. A 19-year-old gentleman has been charged with a serious assault. He appears incredibly distracted and distressed and is openly responding to auditory hallucinations. The forensic psychiatrist has been asked to assess his fitness to plead. What finding on mental state exam would suggest he was fit to plead?

A. He is unable to say why he is in custody

B. He asks for most questions to be repeated as he is distracted by hallucinations

C. He is thought disordered, with loosening of associations such that his answers are very hard to follow

D. He believes he has been abducted by aliens and his answers will determine the fate of the universe

E. He is able to give a coherent account of events leading up to the offence but denies memory of the offence itself

3. A 36-year-old man with schizophrenia has committed a crime. He asks his lawyer if he can be considered to have had diminished responsibility. What is the only charge diminished responsibility applies to?

A. Arson

B. Rape

C. Theft

D. Grievous bodily harm

E. Murder

4. A 21-year-old man has been charged with assaulting a police officer. He has a lengthy history of police contacts from adolescence onwards, mainly for impulsive acts of aggression. He dropped out of school at 14 years of age because he struggled to concentrate. He is angry with himself for getting into trouble with the police again and is asking for help in controlling his bursts of anger. What diagnosis should he be further assessed for?

A. Antisocial personality disorder
B. Attention deficit hyperactivity disorder (ADHD)
C. Autism spectrum disorder
D. Bipolar affective disorder
E. Emotionally unstable personality disorder

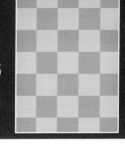

Extended-matching questions (EMQs)

Each answer can be used once, more than once or not at all.

Chapter 2 Pharmacological therapy and electroconvulsive therapy

Management of antipsychotic-induced extrapyramidal side-effects

A. Intramuscular procyclidine
B. Oral procyclidine
C. Propranolol
D. Stop anticholinergics
E. Oral olanzapine
F. Intramuscular haloperidol
G. Resuscitation
H. Baclofen
I. Dantrolene
J. Quinine

For each of the following patients, select the ONE best management option from the list above.

1. A 22-year-old woman recently commenced on an antipsychotic who is pacing her bedroom and says she feels very restless.
2. A 22-year-old woman recently commenced on an antipsychotic who is staring at the ceiling and clenching her jaw tightly.
3. A 22-year-old woman recently commenced on an antipsychotic who is collapsed in her bedroom with a fast pulse, low blood pressure, reduced consciousness level and stiff limbs.
4. A 26-year-old man who commenced antipsychotics a month ago. His face shows little expression, and he does not swing his arms when he walks. He does not have a tremor, and his gait is not shuffling.
5. A 34-year-old man who has been on antipsychotics and regular procyclidine for over a decade. He makes frequent darting movements with his tongue but seems unaware of this.

Mechanism of action of antidepressants

A. Agomelatine
B. Amitriptyline
C. Bupropion
D. Citalopram
E. Duloxetine
F. Moclobemide
G. Phenelzine
H. Pramipexole
I. Reboxetine

Select the antidepressant whose mechanism is best described by the descriptions below:

1. 5-HT 2C receptor antagonist and melatonin receptor agonist.
2. Inhibits serotonin and noradrenaline reuptake pumps; does not affect acetylcholine receptors.
3. Inhibits serotonin and noradrenaline reuptake pumps; also blocks acetylcholine receptors.
4. Reversible inhibition of monoamine oxidase A.
5. Inhibits dopamine and noradrenaline reuptake pumps.

Chapter 3 Psychological therapy

Modalities of individual psychotherapy

A. Psychoanalysis
B. Cognitive-behavioural therapy
C. Mentalization-based therapy
D. Psychodynamic psychotherapy
E. Dialectical behaviour therapy
F. Exposure and response prevention
G. Eye movement desensitization and reprocessing
H. Cognitive analytic therapy
I. Systematic desensitization
J. Mindfulness-based cognitive therapy
K. Interpersonal therapy

For the examples below, select the ONE most appropriate modality of psychological therapy from the list above.

1. A 28-year-old man has a diagnosis of emotionally unstable personality disorder. He reports that he often finds it difficult to know what others are thinking about him and tends to expect the worst and act accordingly. He sometimes has difficulty knowing what he is thinking and feeling.
2. A 57-year-old lady has a depressive disorder of moderate severity. She attributes her symptoms to the fact that her father has been taken into a nursing home, her daughter has left home to attend university and she was recently made redundant from her job in the bank.
3. A 35-year-old woman has a diagnosis of agoraphobia. She wants to start a practical sort of therapy in which she does not need to talk about her difficult past.
4. A 24-year-old ex-soldier has a diagnosis of posttraumatic stress disorder. He requests a talking therapy. In the past, he tried treatment with a therapist

who 'made me look at moving lights while I talked about what happened,' and found this unhelpful.

5. A 42-year-old gentleman has a diagnosis of obsessive-compulsive disorder and is mainly troubled by having to check switches and locks in his home. He feels that a therapy that is 'more practical than talking' would be helpful.

Psychodynamic psychotherapy

A. Acting out
B. Projective identification
C. Hypnosis
D. Catharsis
E. Parapraxis
F. Transference
G. Rationalization
H. Counter-transference
I. Dream interpretation
J. Working through

For each of the following, select the ONE most appropriate descriptor from the list above.

1. A 32-year-old woman, who has previously been very punctual, has arrived late and slightly inebriated for the past six sessions since the therapist was on leave.
2. The therapist of a 59-year-old woman realizes that he has been talking to her as if she were a mother figure.
3. A 43-year-old man feels better after his first psychotherapy session, because he has 'got it off his chest.'
4. A 21-year-old says 'I'm glad we're almost finished.' She intended to say 'I'm sad we're almost finished.'
5. A 29-year-old man has been avoiding his psychotherapist for the past few weeks, following what he considered to be a 'clash of personalities.' He decided to return and is keen to uncover his unconscious reasons behind this.

Chapter 4 Mental health and the law

Legislation

A. Mental health legislation
B. Mental capacity legislation
C. Forensic mental health legislation
D. Criminal legislation
E. No legislation required
F. Common law

Which type of legislation could help in the management of the following cases?

1. A 26-year-old man with schizophrenia and comorbid depression. He is currently severely depressed with an active plan to commit suicide by hanging. He lives

with his mother who does not feel he is safe to go home. He is refusing admission because he thinks the doctors want to torture him.
2. A 26-year-old man with schizophrenia. He has been charged with attempted murder after he attacked his mother, who he believed to be trying to torture him by whispering derogatory comments to him all night, even while he was staying at a friend's house.
3. A 26-year-old man with schizophrenia. He has been charged with a breach of the peace after he repeatedly shouted in the street at 2 a.m. He told the police he was telling the voices to go away. Because it did not work, he is now considering suicide.
4. A 26-year-old man with schizophrenia. He has been brought into the accident and emergency department by ambulance after an attempted hanging. He is unable to speak and has stridor and low oxygen saturations.
5. A 26-year-old man with schizophrenia. He suffered a hypoxic brain injury after attempting to hang himself and now has very poor short-term memory. He needs treatment with antibiotics for a urinary tract infection, but he does not realize he has one. The need for antibiotics has been explained to him on three different occasions, but he does not recall the information by the time he is due to receive treatment.

Chapter 5 Mental health service provision

Choice of service provision for mental disorder

A. Acute general adult inpatient unit
B. Assertive outreach team
C. Community mental health team
D. Day hospital
E. Early intervention in psychosis team
F. Home treatment team
G. Liaison psychiatry review
H. Outpatient clinic
I. Primary care
J. Rehabilitation unit

For each case below, select which service they should be referred to:

1. A 24-year-old man with a first episode of moderate depression.
2. A 24-year-old man who is an inpatient on a gastroenterology ward with inflammatory bowel disease. He is low in mood and fatigued.
3. A 34-year-old man with schizophrenia. Today he attempted to hang himself because he is terrified the secret services are planning to torture him.
4. A 34-year-old man with schizophrenia who is currently an inpatient on a general adult ward. He has been taking a therapeutic dose of clozapine for 12 weeks

but has ongoing auditory hallucinations. He has not been in employment since the onset of his illness.

5. A 34-year-old man with schizophrenia who is homeless and injects heroin. He frequently attends A&E reporting auditory hallucinations but has not attended numerous appointments with his CPN and psychiatrist.

Chapter 6 The patient with thoughts of suicide or self-harm

Mental disorder and self-harm

A. Obsessive-compulsive disorder
B. Anorexia nervosa
C. Alcohol-dependence syndrome
D. Lesch–Nyhan syndrome
E. Mania with psychotic symptoms
F. Emotionally unstable personality disorder
G. Depressive episode, moderate severity
H. Schizophrenia
I. Generalized anxiety disorder
J. Depressive episode, severe with psychotic features
K. Dissocial personality disorder

For each of the following patients, select the ONE most likely mental disorder from the list above.

1. A 19-year-old woman states that she is going to kill herself because 'the voices in my head are telling me to'. These started troubling her this morning after an argument with her mother. Yesterday, she felt fine with no voices. She has no symptoms of depression. She insists that 'it will be all your fault when I commit suicide' and demands admission to a psychiatric ward. She has a history of self-harm by cutting and is well known to mental health services from previous emergency presentations.

2. A 50-year-old male bank manager who tried to gas himself in his car is found in a remote forest clearing at 4:30 a.m. by a dog walker. Typed letters to his wife and children (currently on holiday) were found on the passenger seat. He has no psychiatric history. He appeared intoxicated; however, he states he is not a big drinker. He described recent weight loss and wakening early in the morning. He is convinced that a recent financial crisis is all his fault.

3. A 22-year-old man presents with his mother. She is concerned that he has burned his chest with cigarettes multiple times and appears to have created the image of a crucifix. He insists that he is the second coming of Jesus Christ and has special powers of healing that command respect. You note that he is dishevelled, topless, talking very fast about loosely related ideas, and is very distractible. There is no history of substance misuse. He has never been to church.

4. A 62-year-old woman reports that she took a 'handful' of her antidepressant tablets then told her husband what she had done. She is unsure whether she wanted to die. She has been in intermittent contact with the community mental health team several times during her adult life with periods of poor motivation and alterations in her sleep pattern; however, she has also had long periods of being well and managing to work in the local supermarket. She reports strong feelings of guilt and recent social withdrawal. At interview, you feel that her affect is flat and she is tearful. She does not drink alcohol or use drugs.

5. A 15-year-old girl was found having tried to hang herself in the family bathroom. She left a suicide note and was discovered by chance by the family cleaner. You notice that she looks thin. Her parents report that she has been 'picky' with food over the past few months, but they have not noticed anything else because of their busy jobs as lawyers. On examination, you note that she is wearing very baggy clothes and has fine hairs over visible skin areas. She has actively resisted physical examination. She tells you that nothing is wrong at all, and that she just wants to get home to study for her forthcoming exams.

Immediate psychiatric management of the patient who has inflicted harm upon themselves

A. Admission to psychiatric intensive care unit (PICU/IPCU)
B. Admission to inpatient psychiatric ward
C. Admission to medical assessment/short stay ward
D. Discharge with immediate outreach team involvement
E. Discharge with community mental health team later in the week
F. Discharge with outpatient psychiatry clinic appointment next month
G. Discharge with appointment with alcohol addictions services
H. Discharge to police custody
I. Discharge with information on non-NHS support services
J. Discharge with prescription for antidepressant medication
K. Discharge to the care of general practitioner

For each of the following cases, select the ONE most appropriate management option from the list above.

1. A 57-year-old, unemployed, divorced man who lives alone took an overdose of a benzodiazepine. A scribbled suicide note was left, and he called emergency services before falling unconscious. He saw his keyworker from the alcohol addictions team earlier that day who provided him with benzodiazepines for a community detoxification.

She felt that he was in 'good humour' when she saw him. He has presented numerous times in the past with minor overdoses. At interview, he appears very drowsy and smells strongly of alcohol. He is inconsolably tearful, stating that he is 'ruined' and wants to die.

2. A 20-year-old, unemployed, single woman took an overdose of dihydrocodeine. She was found collapsed in the street and required naloxone. Her urine drug test is positive for cannabis and cocaine. Upon wakening, she threatens to kill the nurse who has taken her cigarettes. She continues to be physically, verbally and racially aggressive to A&E staff. She has had one short admission to a psychiatric ward 2 years ago, and was discharged after assaulting a member of staff. On discharge, the consultant concluded 'no signs of mental illness'. At interview, she screams at you to supply her with more dihydrocodeine, and threatens to kill herself if you do not comply.

3. A 33-year-old, married taxi driver (male) was found by his wife in the loft, holding a nail gun to his head. He was slightly intoxicated and broke down in tears while agreeing to attend hospital. He has no history with psychiatric services, and—despite having taken a drink tonight—does not usually drink alcohol. He described feeling like he 'can't be bothered' since he had his pay severely cut about 2 months ago, and has since been burdened by creditors calling him. At interview, he described poor sleep, weight loss, lack of energy, and guilt about his loss of libido. While he described ongoing suicidal feelings, he described his daughter and wife as strong protective factors, is regretful that 'things have come to this', and glad that his wife found him before he did 'something stupid'. He seems a bit more optimistic after assessment.

4. A 67-year-old, retired widow with no psychiatric history, took an overdose of four of her blood pressure tablets. She waited until after her daughter went on holiday, and was only discovered when her neighbour visited unexpectedly and saw a suicide note addressed to her daughter on the coffee table, stating that she could not go on without her recently deceased husband. She later told the psychiatrist that she was 'just a silly old lady' and denied any suicidal intent. She just wanted to go home to look at her wedding photographs.

5. A 26-year-old, single, mature student, who lives with flat-mates, presents at the accident and emergency department requesting sutures for a self-inflicted laceration on her inner thigh. She has previously been involved with mental health services due to self-harming, but disengaged with them 2 years previously because she did not agree with their diagnosis of emotionally unstable personality disorder. She is on no medication. She is reluctant to talk to a psychiatrist; however, you manage to engage her

and she tells you that she is not suicidal. She reports that her self-harm was previously improving, but has recently become more frequent due to academic pressures. She is keen to go home, and refuses to have any involvement in the future with mental health services.

Chapter 7 The patient with impairment of consciousness, memory or cognition

Differential diagnosis of cognitive impairment

A. Delirium
B. Dementia
C. Mild cognitive impairment
D. Subjective cognitive impairment
E. Depression ('pseudodementia')
F. Psychotic disorders
G. Mood disorders
H. Intellectual disability
I. Dissociative disorders
J. Factitious disorder and malingering
K. Amnesic syndrome

For each of the following patients, select the most likely diagnosis from the list above.

1. A 62-year-old teacher presents to her general practitioner (GP) because she feels she is not remembering the names of the children in her class as well as she used to. She is worried she has dementia like her mother. She has no difficulties in activities of daily living and her mood is normal. She scores 100/100 on ACE-III.

2. A 62-year-old teacher presents to her GP because she feels she is not remembering the names of the children in her class as well as she used to. She is worried she has dementia like her mother. She has no difficulties in activities of daily living and her mood is normal. She scores 80/100 on ACE-III.

3. A 62-year-old teacher presents to her GP because she feels she is not remembering the names of the children in her class as well as she used to. She is worried she has dementia like her mother. She has noticed herself getting lost in the school corridors sometimes and her husband now does all the shopping because she kept getting disorientated in the supermarket. Her mood is normal. She scores 80/100 on ACE-III.

4. A 62-year-old teacher presents to her GP because she feels she is not remembering the names of the children in her class as well as she used to. She is worried she has dementia like her mother. She has no difficulties in activities of daily living and scores 90/100 on ACE-III, losing marks only in the domain of memory. She admits she has been low in mood recently, is not enjoying work any more, is fatigued, has lost weight and is not sleeping well.

5. A 62-year-old teacher presents to her GP because she feels she is not remembering the names of the children in her class as well as she used to. She is worried she has dementia like her mother. She has no difficulties in activities of daily living and scores 90/100 on ACE-III, losing marks only in the domain of memory. She admits she has drunk alcohol to excess for several years, as did her mother. During a recent admission with pancreatitis she was noted to show signs of alcohol withdrawal.

Potentially reversible causes of dementia

A. Subdural haematoma
B. Brain tumour
C. Normal pressure hydrocephalus
D. Hyperthyroidism
E. Hypothyroidism
F. Hyperparathyroidism
G. Hypoparathyroidism
H. Cushing syndrome
I. Addison disease
J. Vitamin B_{12} deficiency
K. Folate deficiency

For each of the following patients, select the most likely diagnosis from the list above.

1. A 74-year-old woman presents to her general practitioner (GP) with her husband who is concerned that over the last 8 weeks she has become increasingly forgetful and disorientated. She has burnt a couple of pans after leaving them unattended. Some days she takes afternoon naps, which is new for her. When pressed he recalls she was hit on the head by a football around 3 months ago while watching her grandson's team but seemed fine afterwards. Past medical history includes atrial fibrillation and asthma. ACE-III is 70/100 and neurological exam shows normal conscious level and a subtle right hemiparesis.

2. A 76-year-old widower attends his GP because of urinary incontinence. As he walks into the room he has a broad based, stiff-legged gait. He is very slow to answer questions and seems not to be paying close attention to what is asked. He says he cannot remember when his incontinence started or how often it occurs. Past medical history is of a duodenal ulcer only. ACE-III is 74/100 and neurological exam is normal apart from his gait.

3. A 52-year-old woman presents to her GP with memory and concentration problems. She reports feeling tired and sluggish for the last 6 months. She feels low in motivation and mood and has quit her running club because she can't be bothered to keep up any more. Past medical history is unremarkable. ACE-III is 98/100. Physical examination is normal apart from dizziness when she gets off the examination couch.

4. A 43-year-old traffic warden presents to her GP with weight gain and amenorrhoea. She is surprised to be going through the menopause so soon as her mother's occurred in her late 50s. She is finding herself forgetful at work, checking cars on the same streets repeatedly. She has got into trouble for this and feels very low in mood. ACE-III is 80/100. Physical examination shows hypertension, a plethoric complexion and central obesity.

5. A 76-year-old woman attends her GP with a 12-month history of gradually worsening memory problems and low mood. Past medical history includes renal calculi and abdominal pain for which no cause has been identified. ACE-III is 76/100. Physical examination is normal.

Subtypes of dementia

A. Alzheimer dementia
B. Vascular dementia
C. Mixed dementia
D. Frontotemporal dementia
E. Lewy body dementia
F. Parkinson disease with dementia
G. Progressive supranuclear palsy
H. Huntington disease
I. Creutzfeldt–Jakob disease
J. Neurosyphilis
K. HIV-related dementia

For each of the following patients, select the most likely cause from the options above.

1. A 77-year-old woman has a 9-month history of gradual onset, gradually worsening cognitive impairment. She forgets recent events and people's names. She can no longer manage her finances. Past medical history is of psoriasis and asthma. Head computed tomography (CT) showed generalized atrophy, particularly marked in the medial temporal lobes.

2. A 74-year-old man has a 10-month history of progressive cognitive impairment. His family notice he seems to worsen suddenly and then plateau before abruptly worsening again. He has marked word-finding difficulties and an abnormal gait. Past medical history is of ischaemic heart disease, hypertension and diabetes. He is a current smoker. CT of the head shows generalized atrophy, small vessel disease and an old lacunar infarct.

3. A 67-year-old retired chef has a 12-month history of gradual personality change. He was previously polite and considerate but has become very rude and tactless. He is having an affair with a waitress from his old restaurant. His wife of 40 years is thinking of leaving him but he says he does not care. Head CT shows generalized atrophy, particularly marked in the frontal lobes.

4. An 81-year-old man has an 18-month history of fluctuating cognitive impairment on a background of a gradual cognitive deterioration. He has been investigated for delirium but no cause found. Sometimes he is very drowsy during the day. He is increasingly stiff and finds it hard to roll over in bed. He also finds it hard to keep his balance and has had a lot of falls recently. Sometimes he experiences visual hallucinations of cats and mice. Head CT shows generalized cerebral atrophy.

5. A 71-year-old man was diagnosed with Parkinson disease 5 years ago. He has a 1-year history of cognitive impairment causing him to forget people's names and where he has left his clothes. Sometimes he has hallucinations of former work colleagues walking around the room. CT of the head shows generalized cerebral atrophy.

Clinical features in cognitive impairment

A. Apraxia
B. Agnosia
C. Aphasia
D. Amnesia
E. Perseveration
F. Disinhibition
G. Dyscalculia
H. Dyslexia
I. Apathy

For each of the following patients, select the clinical feature described from the options above.

1. When shown a pair of scissors a woman states they are scissors but cannot work out how to cut with them. She can mimic the correct action when shown.
2. When shown a pair of scissors a woman states they are 'those things used for cutting paper' but cannot name them.
3. A woman uses scissors to cut a piece of paper into squares as asked. When asked to then cut triangles, she keeps cutting squares.
4. When shown a pair of scissors a woman is unable to name them or describe their function. When she is allowed to touch them she quickly identifies what they are. She has normal visual acuity.
5. When given a pair of scissors inside a covered box, a woman turns them around in her hands but is unable to name them. When she is allowed to look at them she quickly identifies them. She has normal sensation in her hands.

Chapter 8 The patient with alcohol or substance use problems

A. MDMA
B. Cannabis
C. Heroin

D. Amphetamine
E. Diazepam
F. Cocaine
G. Ketamine
H. Mephedrone
I. Buprenorphine
J. Lysergic acid diethylamide

For each of the following statements, select the most appropriate answer from the options above.

1. Deviated nasal septum
2. Depersonalisation
3. Bacterial endocarditis
4. Memory impairment, particularly if taken long-term
5. Precipitated opioid withdrawal

Chapter 9 The patient with psychotic symptoms

Differential diagnosis of psychosis

A. Delusional disorder
B. Dementia/delirium
C. Depressive episode, severe, with psychotic features
D. Manic episode with psychotic features
E. Neurodevelopmental disorder
F. Personality disorder
G. Psychosis secondary to a general medical condition
H. Psychosis secondary to psychoactive substance use
I. Schizoaffective disorder
J. Schizophrenia
K. Schizophrenia-like psychotic disorders

For each of the following patients, select the ONE most likely diagnosis from the list of options above.

1. The mother of a 22-year-old man asks for a home visit from their general practitioner (GP). For the last 6 weeks her son has barely left his room and seems to be collecting tinfoil. She is adamant that he has never used drugs. He is in second year at university, having passed first year with a distinction, but 6 months ago he lost interest and stopped going to lectures. He tells the GP that a terrorist organization is trying to brainwash him into becoming a terrorist and he needs the tinfoil to make it more difficult for them to beam thoughts into him.

2. A 45-year-old man has recurrent episodes of low mood associated with third person auditory hallucinations in the form of an abusive running commentary. These symptoms do not occur separately.

3. A 52-year-old man has recurrent episodes of low mood associated with second person auditory hallucinations in the form of abusive comments. He has noticed his mood starts to dip first, and the hallucinations emerge as his mood worsens.

4. A 47-year-old teacher presents to his GP for the 25th time in 6 months convinced he has bowel cancer, despite having had a normal colonoscopy and abdomen/pelvis computed tomography. He tells his GP he knows logically he cannot have bowel cancer but at the same time he is certain he does. His mood is normal and he is still working.

5. A 37-year-old man who is brought to accident and emergency by the police for assessment after he called them to say his neighbour is persecuting him by refusing to move her wheelie-bin. The police note multiple previous calls over the last decade about previous neighbours. The man agrees it is possible the neighbour has some other reason for not wanting to move the wheelie-bin, but thinks it is most likely because she wants to spite him. He is angry with the police for bringing him to see a doctor, stating he plans to contact his lawyer about their behaviour.

6. A woman requests a GP home visit for her 78-year-old father who has no previous psychiatric history. She is concerned that he has told her he can hear his mother and sister, who are both dead, talking. She is also concerned that he seems very forgetful and does not seem to be looking after himself properly. He is quite cheerful and enjoys speaking with his relatives.

Psychosis secondary to a general medical condition or psychoactive substance use

A. Amphetamine
B. Cerebral tumour
C. Cocaine
D. Corticosteroids
E. Cushing syndrome
F. L-dopa
G. Neurosyphilis
H. Huntington disease
I. Hyperthyroidism
J. Hypothyroidism
K. Thiamine deficiency
L. Vitamin B_{12} deficiency

For each of the following patients, select the ONE most likely cause from the options above.

1. A 62-year-old retired navy officer is brought to his general practitioner (GP) by his wife. She is concerned that his personality has changed over the last few months. He has been unusually cheerful and keeps mentioning that he expects to be knighted for his naval service. He has become very extravagant, wanting to sell their home and give half the proceeds to charity. He forgot their wedding anniversary. On examination he has unusually brisk reflexes.

2. A 57-year-old accountant is brought to accident and emergency by the police after going to the supermarket in swimming trunks and flippers. He does not see what the problem is. He states he wore the flippers because he has a constant headache which worsens when he bends down to tie his shoelaces. He has no psychiatric history or previous encounters with the police.

3. A 46-year-old vegan goes to her GP because for the last 6 months she has found herself unusually clumsy, tripping over rugs and stairs in a way she never did before. She feels like everyone is watching her when she stumbles in the street and is sure she heard a group of strangers commenting on how they planned to rob her.

4. A 42-year-old man is admitted for emergency surgery following a road traffic accident. Two days after admission he becomes agitated and asks the charge nurse why there are so many insects in the ward (there are none). He keeps rubbing his skin and saying, 'get away, get away'. He has a stumbling gait and his eyes make rapid small movements to the side and back again.

Mental state examination in psychosis (perceptual disturbance)

A. Audible thoughts
B. Extracampine hallucination
C. Gustatory hallucination
D. Hypnagogic hallucination
E. Hypnopompic hallucination
F. Kinaesthetic hallucination
G. Olfactory hallucination
H. Pseudohallucination
I. Second person auditory hallucination
J. Tactile hallucination
K. Third person auditory hallucination
L. Visceral hallucination

For each of the following patients, select ONE clinical feature described from the list of options above.

1. I hear a man saying 'you idiot' in the corner of the room but no one's there.
2. I hear a man saying 'you idiot' inside my head.
3. I hear a man in Newcastle talking to me even though I live in Edinburgh.
4. My spleen is moving around inside me.
5. As I'm drifting off to sleep I catch a glimpse of a ginger cat beside the bed, but I have no cat.
6. I taste rotting meat all the time.

Mental state examination in psychosis (thought disturbance)

A. Delusion of control
B. Delusion of infidelity
C. Delusion of misidentification
D. Delusion of reference
E. Erotomania
F. Grandiose delusion
G. Loosening of association
H. Nihilistic delusion
I. Persecutory delusion
J. Somatic delusion

For each of the following patients, select ONE clinical feature described from the list above.

1. 'I'm sure I'm being spied on by the government, I can tell because of the amount of junk mail I get'.
2. 'My boss definitely loves me, even though he denies it every time I remind him.'
3. 'I can't understand why that woman has dressed up as my wife and keeps referring to me as her husband'.
4. 'The newsreader on the radio keeps reading out my name for some reason'.
5. 'I don't need to eat because I'm already dead'.
6. 'Someone else's thoughts are inside my head.'
7. 'Why should the cat indeed bend that carrot tomatoes are red.'

Chapter 10 The patient with elated or irritable mood

Differential diagnosis of elevated or irritable mood

A. Hypomanic episode
B. Manic episode without psychotic features
C. Manic episode with psychotic features
D. Mixed affective episode
E. Bipolar affective disorder
F. Cyclothymia
G. Schizophrenia
H. Schizoaffective disorder
I. Elevated or irritable mood secondary to a general medical condition
J. Elevated or irritable mood secondary to psychoactive substance use
K. Delirium/dementia

For each of the following patients, select the ONE most likely diagnosis from the list above.

1. A 40-year-old lawyer attends his general practitioner (GP) asking for a medication to reduce his sex drive because his wife is complaining. He is smartly dressed in a new suit and says he feels 'on top of the world'. He has been finding it hard to stay focused at work but so far no one has commented. Fortunately, he is able to stay up late catching up on work without feeling tired the next day. He denies any drug or alcohol use.

2. A 22-year-old trainee electrician is brought to Accident and emergency by the police after he was found breaking into an electronics shop. He states he needed the parts for a new jetpack he is designing—he plans to start a new business with it which will 'revolutionize transatlantic flight'. He has resigned from his apprenticeship in order to spend more time on this venture. He is irritable with the male police officer but flirtatious towards the female police officer. He denies drug or alcohol use.

3. A 37-year-old man with a history of bipolar disorder was admitted to a psychiatric ward one day ago. The nurses tell you he has been very elated and disinhibited so far today. When you interview him he seems low and tearful, but as the interview progresses he gets very irritable and starts to speak too quickly for you to ask him any more questions.

4. A 36-year-old secretary attends her GP because she is feeling unusually irritable at work. Sometimes she loves her job and sometimes she hates it, but forces herself to attend. Right now she is also feeling irritable with her family and neighbour. She has noticed her mood has seemed to cycle since her late teens, but it has never stopped her doing anything.

5. A 28-year-old doctor suffers from recurrent depressive disorder. He has recently started a stressful new job and his flatmates are worried because he doesn't seem to be eating or sleeping well, despite seeming quite cheerful. He paces the flat at night talking about new operative techniques he is designing. His consultant sent him home from work because he refused to scrub for theatre, stating 'I'm pristine already'.

Elevated or irritable mood secondary to a general medical condition or psychoactive substance use

A. Huntington disease
B. Multiple sclerosis
C. Parkinson disease
D. Cerebral tumour
E. Cushing disease
F. Hypothyroidism
G. Hyperthyroidism
H. Anabolic steroids
I. Corticosteroids
J. L-dopa
K. Cocaine
L. Amphetamine

For each of the following patients, select the ONE most likely cause from the options above.

1. A 66-year-old man with a shuffling gait and reduced facial expression has recently had a medication increase. Now he is elated, spends all his time playing online poker and asked his wife where all the monkeys in the kitchen had come from.
2. A 22-year-old student is brought to accident and emergency (A&E) by his friends from a party because he tried to fly off the roof. He is adamant he is Superman. He admits to having swallowed a pill earlier. On examination he is restless with dilated pupils.
3. A 28-year-old bodybuilder has recently become convinced he will win the next world championship. He is irritable with his girlfriend whenever she queries this. He is also hypersexual and forgetful and has been reprimanded at work.
4. A 62-year-old woman is an inpatient on an acute medical ward following a severe asthma exacerbation. The nurses notice she seems irritable and suspicious and keeps asking for a single room 'as befits someone of my status'. Her daughter says this is a complete change from normal.
5. A 45-year-old woman presents to A&E with palpitations. When not seen immediately she becomes extremely irritated and starts pacing in the waiting room. On examination she has a tremor, pupils are normal and electrocardiogram (ECG) shows sinus tachycardia. She shouts at the ECG technician for not being gentle enough when she removes the electrodes.

Mental state examination in elevated or irritable mood

A. Pressured speech
B. Flight of ideas
C. Tangential thinking
D. Poor concentration
E. Psychomotor retardation
F. Psychomotor agitation
G. Hyperacusis
H. Visual hyperaesthesia
I. Auditory hallucination
J. Visual hallucination

Lead in: For each of the following patients, select ONE clinical feature described from the list of options above.

1. There are no natural breaks in the conversation and it is impossible to interrupt the patient without speaking over them.
2. The patient comments she has never seen a blue as blue as the nurse's uniform before.
3. The patient speaks normally and initially starts to answer a question but quickly diverts onto related but unimportant topics.
4. The patient speaks rapidly and initially starts to answer a question but very rapidly diverts onto lots of other topics. It is very confusing to listen to but in retrospect there are links between the topics. Some of the links were rhyming words.
5. The patient is trying to complete serial 7s but keeps being distracted by the noise of hoovering.
6. The patient comments there is a beautiful blue bird in the corner of the room, but no one else can see anything there.

Chapter 11 The patient with low mood

Differential diagnosis of low mood

A. Mild depressive episode
B. Moderate depressive episode
C. Severe depressive episode without psychotic features
D. Severe depressive episode with psychotic features
E. Recurrent depressive episode
F. Dysthymia
G. Bipolar affective disorder
H. Schizoaffective disorder
I. Low mood secondary to a general medical condition
J. Low mood secondary to psychoactive substance use

For each of the following patients, select the ONE most likely diagnosis from the list above.

1. A 40-year-old man feels he has been depressed for 20 years. He cannot recall a lengthy period of normal mood since his early adulthood. Despite this, he is able to work as a supermarket manager, has a loving relationship with his wife and reports that he quite enjoyed his last holiday in Tenerife.
2. A 24-year-old waitress has had low mood and lethargy for 3 weeks. She finds it harder than normal to remember her customer's orders. She thinks this is because she has never been an intelligent person. She is eating normally, sleeping well and enjoyed going out to the movies last night.
3. A 71-year-old widowed woman who lives alone is brought to the surgery by her neighbour. The neighbour is shocked because the patient put a rude note through his door telling him to get his drains unblocked in order to get rid of the stench in the street. No one else has noticed a bad smell. Before her husband died the patient used to be very social and visited her neighbours frequently. On examination, she is unkempt and walks very slowly. When you ask her questions, she makes poor eye contact and does not answer for a long time.
4. A 35-year-old cashier presents to his general practitioner asking for a sick line. He feels he cannot continue at work because for the last month he has been low in mood and finds himself becoming easily

tired during his shifts. He is not enjoying talking with his colleagues as much as he used to. He finds himself wakening at 5 a.m. (he normally rises at 8 a.m.) and lies in bed worrying about the day ahead. His mood is a bit better in the evenings. He has been eating poorly and lost a stone in weight over the last month.

5. A 42-year-old construction worker reports intermittent low mood. Sometimes he is so low he is unable to go to work. On closer questioning it seems it is mainly Mondays he misses, and the weekends he feels low. The problem has come on over the last year, when he has been binge-drinking at the weekends after his wife left him. On weekends when he looks after his daughter he does not drink and feels fine.

Low mood secondary to a general medical condition

A. Huntington disease
B. Parkinson disease
C. Multiple sclerosis
D. Cerebral tumour
E. Cushing syndrome
F. Addison disease
G. Conn syndrome
H. Thrombocytopenia
I. Hypothyroidism
J. Hyperthyroidism
K. Systemic lupus erythematosus

For each of the following patients, select the ONE key diagnosis to exclude from the list above.

1. A 52-year-old care assistant presents to her general practitioner (GP) with a 6-month history of low mood and fatigue. She complains she has put on a lot of weight recently despite no changes in her diet or exercise. On examination she is obese, hypertensive and the blood pressure cuff leaves a bruise.
2. A 35-year-old traffic warden presents to his GP after he tripped over the curb and banged his knee. He also mentions a 3-month history of low mood. He is not sure why he tripped but has been stumbling more often than he used to and has given up football. He does not drink. He thinks he may have a family history of depression because his father went into a psychiatric hospital in his early 40s and died there 10 years later.
3. A 46-year-old florist presents because for the last 2 months she has felt tired all the time and low in mood. She feels ugly, her hair never seems to be glossy anymore and she thinks her skin is dry and flaky. On examination, her pulse is 52 regular.
4. A 26-year-old veterinary student presents with tingling in her left arm. She becomes tearful during the consultation, admitting she is finding the fourth year of her studies much more difficult than the

previous years. You see she attended 3 months ago with a sore eye and blurred vision which resolved spontaneously.

Mental state examination in low mood

A. Poor self-care
B. Malingering
C. Reduced range of reactivity
D. Incongruous affect
E. Low mood
F. Psychomotor retardation
G. Psychomotor agitation
H. Marche à petits pas
I. Negative cognition
J. Hopelessness
K. Complete anhedonia
L. Partial anhedonia

For each of the following patients, select ONE clinical feature described from the list of options above.

1. A 76-year-old widowed retired headmistress is brought to accident and emergency by her family who are concerned she has not been eating. She paces the cubicle, keeps buttoning and unbuttoning her coat and does not sit down when offered a chair.
2. A 44-year-old architect being treated for depression is upset because he has lost a contract after the company went bust. He says this means he will lose all his other contracts and never be asked to design another building.
3. A 22-year-old woman tells her general practitioner (GP) she has passed a recent exam but does not smile or appear pleased. Later she mentions she has broken up with her partner but does not look sad or relieved. She describes both things in a similar tone of speech.
4. A 36-year-old sales assistant attends his GP straight from work for a prescription of citalopram. He has greasy hair and stains on his shirt and is slightly malodorous.
5. A 55-year-old lorry driver tells his GP he has lost interest in everything he used to enjoy. He no longer plays darts or watches football as he does not care who wins now. However, he did enjoy spending time with his grandson at the weekend.

Chapter 12 The patient with anxiety, fear or avoidance

Differential diagnosis of anxiety, fear or avoidance

A. Agoraphobia with panic disorder
B. Agoraphobia without panic disorder
C. Social phobia

D. Generalized anxiety disorder
E. Panic disorder
F. Depressive episode
G. Acute stress reaction
H. Posttraumatic stress disorder
I. Adjustment disorder
J. Personality disorder
K. Anxiety secondary to a general medical condition
L. Anxiety secondary to psychoactive substance use

For each of the following patients, select the ONE most likely diagnosis from the list above.

1. A 25-year-old librarian avoids being with others whenever possible. He does all his shopping online and always volunteers to reshelve books rather than deal with enquiries. When he is forced to interact with people he can feel himself blushing and sweating. He feels they are scrutinizing and judging him critically, even though he knows he is not really a bad person.
2. A 43-year-old woman feels she has been on edge for 2 years. She spends most of each day worrying about many trivial topics and sometimes she feels something bad is going to happen for no reason. She lies awake at night thinking about these things. She often has a dry mouth, epigastric discomfort and a bilateral frontal headache.
3. A 28-year-old secretary presents to her general practitioner with weight loss. Six months ago in a supermarket she suddenly felt like she was going to die. She had pain in her chest, was short of breath and her arms and lips tingled. She rushed outside and the feeling subsided, but now she does not like to go into any large shops and is eating less well. She is still going to work but now walks 5 miles each way as she does not want to be on a bus and have another attack. As long as she is in her house or with her friends she is relaxed.
4. Over the last 3 months, a 35-year-old builder has experienced several episodes of sudden onset shortness of breath, palpitations, sweatiness, nausea, feeling that the world is unreal and feeling he is about to die. These feelings resolve spontaneously over 20 minutes. He cannot identify any triggers. In particular, they are not brought on by exercise and he can continue to do his active job. His electrocardiogram (ECG) is normal.
5. A 37-year-old professional violinist finds himself unable to play concerts. He can play well when alone but starts to sweat and shake such that he cannot play properly when in the presence of others. He has had to cancel a tour. These symptoms came on after he received a series of negative reviews. In general, he is a relaxed person who enjoys socializing.
6. A 42-year-old policeman has experienced low mood, anhedonia, fatigue, early morning wakening and anorexia for the last month. He has free-floating anxiety

most of the time and has had two panic attacks. These symptoms had onset after he witnessed an armed robbery but he denies flashbacks and still buys milk in the shop where he witnessed the robbery.

Anxiety secondary to a general medical condition or psychoactive substance use

A. Cushing syndrome
B. Hypoglycaemia
C. Hyperthyroidism
D. Pheochromocytoma
E. Caffeine
F. Alcohol
G. Cannabis
H. Amphetamine
I. Fluoxetine
J. Mirtazapine
K. Trazodone

For each of the following patients, select the ONE most likely cause from the options above.

1. A 63-year-old shopkeeper with hypertension has periodic episodes of anxiety, tachycardia, sweating and pallor. She can identify no triggers but recalls her mother having a similar problem. Her random glucose is elevated.
2. A 48-year-old scientist with a past medical history of vitiligo presents with a 3-month history of anxiety, increased appetite and heat intolerance. Her hands are shaky, and she has knocked over a lot of test tubes recently.
3. A 25-year-old joiner has recently been diagnosed with depression and commenced an antidepressant 4 days ago. Since then he has been very restless and agitated and frequently called his friends for reassurance. His sleep has worsened further.
4. A 23-year-old man has started a new job as a welder. He has noticed that he gets very irritable and anxious by the end of the day and has had to go home early a couple of times. He sweats a lot while working so is drinking a lot of his favourite soft drink, 'Go-Man'.
5. A 19-year-old man is brought to accident and emergency by his friends. He is pacing the cubicle, is tachycardic, hyperventilating, sweating and has dilated pupils. He jumps when his name is called. His friends saw him swallow a white tablet earlier in the evening.

Chapter 13 The patient with obsessions and compulsions

Differential diagnosis of obsessions and compulsions

A. No mental illness
B. Obsessive-compulsive disorder

C. Depressive episode
D. Phobia
E. Agoraphobia with panic disorder
F. Agoraphobia without panic disorder
G. Social phobia
H. Panic disorder
I. Eating disorder
J. Personality disorder
K. Hypochondriacal disorder

For each of the following patients, select the ONE most likely diagnosis from the list above.

1. For the last year, a 27-year-old woman has experienced repetitive images of soiled hands that she acknowledges are from her own mind. Washing her hands reduces her fear that her hands are dirty, but now she spends around 2 hours a day washing and is developing contact dermatitis. She has tried to wash less but this makes her very anxious.

2. For the last year, a 27-year-old nurse has been influenced by a National Health Service advertising campaign featuring soiled hands spreading infection. Washing her hands reduces her fear that they are dirty. Now she washes her hands before and after every patient contact, up to 100 times a day, and is developing contact dermatitis.

3. For the last 4 months, a 27-year-old woman has experienced repetitive images of herself having sexual encounters with children. This makes her feel extremely guilty and unclean. Showering reduces her fear that she will engage in such behaviour, but she now has to spend several hours a day in the shower. She describes herself as worthless and hopeless and admits that 6 months ago she started to feel low in mood, anhedonic and fatigued.

4. After a bad experience as a child, a 27-year-old woman has been terrified of illness. Most of the time she has no problems, but if she meets anyone who is unwell she avoids them and washes her hands thoroughly to reduce her risk of contracting their illness. If she cannot get away from the person, she feels overwhelmingly anxious and may have a panic attack.

5. For the last 4 months, a 27-year-old woman has experienced recurrent thoughts of herself as being fat and ugly. She feels these thoughts are her own, and are appropriate, as she believes she is fat and ugly. She has been avoiding food and exercising lots. Her periods have stopped and her body mass index is 17. She still views herself as overweight.

Differentiating types of repetitive or intrusive thoughts

A. No mental illness
B. Obsession

C. Rumination
D. Pseudohallucination
E. Hallucination
F. Over-valued idea
G. Delusion
H. Thought insertion
I. Flashback

For each of the following descriptions, select the ONE most likely psychopathology from the options above.

1. 'I keep seeing images of germs crawling on my skin. I try to stop my mind showing them to me, but I can't'.

2. 'After I got viral gastroenteritis, I became much more careful about hygiene. I'm worried I'll get it again. Now I autoclave every utensil and piece of crockery I use. I had to give up my job at the hospital, it wasn't worth the risk'.

3. 'I lie awake at night thinking about all the ways I could have avoided getting sick. I think about it from all the different angles but never reach a conclusion'.

4. 'I keep hearing a voice inside my head saying, "you're dirty". I don't know who it is but I think they're probably right'.

5. 'I keep hearing a voice outside my head saying, "you're dirty". I don't know who it is, but I think they're probably right'.

6. 'Someone puts ideas in my head. like thoughts of germs, and of being ill. I don't know how they get in there, but they're not my thoughts'.

7. 'When I saw a picture on TV of germs crawling on someone's skin, I knew that I was fatally ill. The doctor told me I was fine, but I know my days are numbered'.

Chapter 14 The patient with a reaction to a stressful event

Dissociative disorders

A. Stupor
B. Dissociative anaesthesia
C. Depersonalization disorder
D. Functional seizures
E. Functional paralysis
F. Psychogenic amnesia
G. Fugue state
H. Hysterical blindness
I. Dissociation secondary to psychoactive substance use
J. Dissociative identity disorder

Assuming physical causes have been excluded, which of the above would be the most likely diagnosis for the following?

1. A 29-year-old mother of two, with a history of depression and a family history of epilepsy, has recently started having seizures, which last for less than a minute, and do not cause tongue-biting, incontinence or post-ictal confusion. She denies alcohol or drug use and seems indifferent to her predicament. Her husband tells you that this started when he told his wife of his new job on an oil rig. He now feels he cannot leave home for fear that she will be seriously harmed by the seizures.

2. A 46-year-old businessman from a distant city is brought to hospital by the police, after apparently trying to withdraw money from a building society and being unable to remember his name. At interview, he seems unable to recall any personal details about himself and has no idea where he is. He is carrying a bundle of business cards for a company that was recently reported to have gone bankrupt.

3. A 21-year-old male prisoner complains of lack of sensation in his right arm, anterior abdomen and left leg. Neurological examination is otherwise normal. The prison guard tells you that he has been moved to protective custody because a senior gang member has threatened to kill him.

4. An 18-year-old tells you that she feels like she is 'in a bubble' and feels that everything around her appears to be unreal and distant from her life. She has no psychiatric history and was fine until yesterday. Her parents tell you that she returned home from a 'rave' party only a couple of hours ago.

Diagnosis following stressful events

A. Acute stress reaction
B. Posttraumatic stress disorder (PTSD)
C. Moderate depression
D. Adjustment disorder
E. Bereavement response
F. Acute/transient psychotic disorder
G. Alcoholic hallucinosis
H. Panic disorder
I. Conversion disorder
J. Temporal lobe epilepsy
K. Musculoskeletal injury

From the options above, which of the diagnoses would be the most appropriate for the scenarios below?

1. The wife of a 35-year-old Royal Air Force pilot has been hearing the voice of her husband, who was recently killed on duty in Syria. She has been feeling very low in mood since his death.

2. An 18-year-old man complains of pains in his neck and right shoulder that seem to have developed shortly after he was driving a car that had a head-on collision with a lorry. He feels lucky to be alive, and you are unable to elicit any other psychopathology.

3. A 52-year-old deep sea diver has felt constantly 'on edge' for the last 3 months since he was involved in an incident involving loss of oxygen flow while deep under the sea. He was convinced that he was going to die. He reports vivid nightmares and has been unable to return to work.

4. A 27-year-old woman is referred from the neurosurgical unit 4 months after a fall from a first-floor balcony. She reports episodes of derealization, followed by visual hallucinations, loss of memory and extreme tiredness.

Chapter 15 The patient with medically unexplained physical symptoms

Diagnosis of medically unexplained physical symptoms

A. Munchausen syndrome by proxy
B. Body dysmorphic disorder
C. Factitious disorder
D. Somatic delusional disorder
E. Schizophrenia
F. Hypochondriacal disorder
G. Somatization disorder
H. Malingering
I. Severe depression with psychotic features
J. Dissociative disorder

For each of the following scenarios, select the most appropriate diagnosis from the list above.

1. A 23-year-old quit her job as a dancer 2 years ago because she is preoccupied with the idea her breasts are misshapen. Now she barely leaves the house, wears baggy clothes and is requesting surgical augmentation. The cosmetic surgeon noted no abnormalities.

2. An 8-year-old girl is drowsy. Her mother tells you that it is sudden onset. On examination, you find subcutaneous needle marks between her toes. One of the nurses finds an insulin syringe on the bedside while her mother is at the bathroom.

3. A 21-year-old man is preoccupied by a small scar behind his ear, which he believes is where the government have implanted a microchip to insert thoughts.

4. A 65-year-old man in a surgical ward with abdominal pain believes that he is dead and rotting from the inside.

5. A 45-year-old man complains of whiplash following a road traffic accident and asks you to complete a medical report. He tells you he has been disabled permanently and alway wears a neck brace. You saw him getting off the bus earlier that morning wearing no neck brace.

Chapter 16 The patient with eating or weight problems

Psychiatric causes of low weight

A. Schizophrenia
B. Specific phobia
C. Depression, severe without psychotic symptoms
D. Bulimia nervosa
E. Alcohol dependence
F. Alzheimer dementia
G. Acute psychotic episode
H. Anorexia nervosa
I. Obsessive-compulsive disorder

For the case vignettes below, pick the most likely psychiatric cause from the list above.

1. A 42-year-old man with schizophrenia has a body mass index (BMI) of 17, with evidence of rapid weight loss. He denies any problems with body image. He says he is a little lonely as his mother died recently, and they used to live together. However, his mood is not pervasively low and there are no acute psychotic symptoms.
2. A 19-year-old male student was admitted to a general medical ward after collapsing in the street. He denies any problems and tells you it was 'probably just a funny turn'. His BMI is 22, serum potassium is 2.1 mmol/L, there are U waves on his electrocardiogram (EKG) and you notice that his parotid glands appear swollen.
3. A 16-year-old girl has lost 15 kg in the last 3 months, giving her a BMI of 16. She denies any body image concerns but tells you that she is only able to eat food prepared in a specific, time-consuming manner. She knows this is irrational; however, if she doesn't do this the prospect of contamination with food-borne pathogens causes her to have unpleasant panic attacks.
4. A 62-year-old ex-model has recently begun to lose weight, and her BMI is 18. She has a past history of anorexia nervosa. She reported that she could not bring herself to eat because of intense worry that she would vomit. Any time that she has tried to eat, she has suffered a panic attack and has ended up vomiting. She suffered from a severe case of norovirus about 6 weeks ago.
5. A 21-year-old plumber with no past psychiatric history has recently lost 12 kilograms, causing his BMI to fall to 15. He appears incredibly frightened and tells you that the owners of all the food shops in his locality are poisoning his food on behalf of government agents, who want him dead because of his involvement in recent terrorist attacks.

Physical consequences of eating disorders

A. Lanugo
B. Caries
C. Xerosis
D. Russell's sign
E. Onychorrhexis
F. Alopecia areata
G. Cheilitis
H. Acrocyanosis
I. Striae distensae

For the statements below, select the most appropriate descriptive term from the list above.

1. The fine, downy hair often seen on the body of sufferers of anorexia nervosa.
2. Erosion of dental enamel caused by repeated vomiting.
3. Dry nails, often associated with anorexia nervosa.
4. Stretch marks on the abdomen, associated with rapid changes in body weight.
5. A callus on the knuckle that may develop as a result of self-induced vomiting.

Chapter 17 The patient with personality problems

Diagnosis of personality disorder

A. Paranoid personality disorder
B. Schizoid personality disorder
C. Schizotypal personality disorder
D. Borderline personality disorder
E. Antisocial personality disorder
F. Narcissistic personality disorder
G. Histrionic personality disorder
H. Dependent personality disorder
I. Avoidant (anxious) personality disorder
J. Anankastic personality disorder

For the following, select the most appropriate personality disorder from the list above. Assume absence of mental illness and that a diagnosis of a personality disorder is appropriate.

1. A 24-year-old accountant wears inappropriate clothes to work. Her colleagues feel that she is always flirtatious and always seeks to be the centre of attention. When this does not happen, she tends to become very upset and dramatically displays emotion.
2. A 47-year-old housewife refuses to leave her abusive partner, despite having recently been hospitalized after he assaulted her. She feels that she could never manage without him.
3. A 26-year-old unemployed man is constantly preoccupied by the mischief of local youths and is

concerned that he is a 'marked man'. He cannot hold down a job as he always becomes concerned that colleagues are talking about him behind his back. His last girlfriend left him 3 years ago after he accused her of cheating on him.

4. A 49-year-old successful entrepreneur feels that others have trouble getting on with him. His fourth marriage has recently ended because of his affairs. He has always been incredibly confident and able to succeed.

5. A 35-year-old website designer has difficulty making friends because of his fear of others criticizing, rejecting or disliking him. Instead, he socializes mainly using social networking sites and will not physically meet others until he is sure they will like and accept him.

Traits of personality disorder

A. Callous unconcern for the feelings of others
B. Excessive sensitivity to setbacks and rebuffs
C. Consistent preference for solitary activities
D. Perfectionism that interferes with task completion
E. Over-concern with physical attractiveness
F. Frantic efforts to avoid real or imagined abandonment
G. Allowing others to make most of one's important life decisions
H. Excessive preoccupation with being rejected in social situations

For the personality disorders listed below, pick a common trait from the above examples.

1. Histrionic personality disorder.
2. Schizoid personality disorder.
3. Obsessive-compulsive personality disorder.
4. Paranoid personality disorder.
5. Dependent personality disorder.

Chapter 18 The patient with neurodevelopmental problems

Functional estimation of IQ in intellectual disability

A. >100 (above average intelligence)
B. 86–100 (below average intelligence)
C. 71–85 (borderline intellectual disability)
D. 50–69 (mild intellectual disability)
E. 35–49 (moderate intellectual disability)
F. 20–34 (severe intellectual disability)
G. <20 (profound intellectual disability)

For each of the scenarios below, select the ONE most appropriate estimation of IQ and level of disability from the list above.

1. A 24-year-old woman lives alone and works in a bakery. She cannot serve customers as she finds it very difficult to use the cash register or give the correct change. She needed extra help at school with reading and writing and did not achieve any qualifications.

2. A 19-year-old man lives alone, does not see his family and is unemployed. He has no support at home and spends much of his time writing programmes on his computer and reading about the mathematics of quantum mechanics. He has always found social interactions to be difficult and strongly dislikes socializing with others. There were no problems with language development.

3. A 14-year-old boy is wheelchair-bound and incontinent. He lives with his mother, who is his main carer. He is unable to undertake any activities of daily living and his mother has to feed him.

4. A 35-year-old woman lives in sheltered accommodation and requires support to cook meals, to keep her flat tidy and to do laundry. She has a job at a local toy factory, where she works on a production line and is closely supervised by a trained support worker.

5. A 22-year-old man lives with his family, who are his main carers. He requires some assistance getting dressed and tending to his personal hygiene; however, he can do this by himself on good days. He can feed himself and spends his days watching children's television programmes and playing with Lego.

Differential diagnosis in adults presenting for attention deficit hyperactivity disorder (ADHD) assessment

A. ADHD
B. Bipolar affective disorder
C. Depressive episode
D. Dissocial personality disorder
E. Emotionally unstable personality disorder
F. Generalized anxiety disorder
G. Intellectual disability
H. No mental disorder
I. Traumatic brain injury
J. Substance abuse, harmful

Select the most likely diagnosis for the situations below.

1. A 24-year-old woman reports her thoughts are racing and she is unable to sit still for more than a few minutes. She has felt this way for the past week. She denies any substance abuse. She had a similar, milder, episode a few months ago.

2. A 31-year-old man has had five jobs in the last 2 years. He keeps getting fired for making careless mistakes. He says he has always been this way. He is fidgety in the interview. He uses cocaine most weekends.

3. A 42-year-old man cannot concentrate and feels extremely irritable. He is pacing his house and having thoughts of suicide. These feelings began after his wife left him a month ago.
4. A 26-year-old man has just been released from prison for assaulting a police officer while on a night out. He was expelled from school for bad behaviour (talking too much, disturbing other pupils, not doing homework). He regrets the assault and would like to go to college but keeps losing the application form.
5. A 39-year-old man struggles to concentrate on tasks such as paying his bills. He has started gambling. At interview his speech is hard to interrupt and his thought form tangential. He has had to give up his job as an accountant following involvement in a road traffic accident.

Chapter 19 Dementia and delirium

Management of dementia

A. Donepezil
B. Rivastigmine
C. Galantamine
D. Memantine
E. Citalopram
F. Methylphenidate
G. Quetiapine
H. Trazodone
I. No treatment recommended by current guidelines

For each of the following patients, select the best treatment for maintaining cognition from the options above.

1. A woman with a recent diagnosis of Alzheimer dementia who continues to live at home with support workers visiting daily.
2. A woman with a diagnosis of Alzheimer dementia who lives in a nursing home and is aphasic.
3. A woman with a diagnosis of Alzheimer dementia who continues to live at home with support workers visiting daily. Her past medical history includes sick sinus syndrome, chronic obstructive pulmonary disease (COPD) and an active peptic ulcer.
4. Parkinson disease with dementia.
5. Frontotemporal dementia.

Chapter 20 Alcohol and substance-related disorders

Pharmacological management of opioid dependence

A. Naloxone
B. Dihydrocodeine
C. Levacetylmethadol
D. Buprenorphine
E. Lofexidine

F. Naltrexone
G. Loperamide
H. Methadone
I. Paracetamol
J. Diazepam

For the following questions, select the most appropriate drug from the list above.

1. A 37-year-old man is admitted to A&E via emergency ambulance. He is Glasgow Coma Scale (GCS) 5/15, with pinpoint pupils and a respiratory rate of six per minute. He has syringes and hypodermic needles in his pocket.
2. A 22-year-old man wants to abstain entirely from opioids. He is not interested in substitution therapy. However, he asks if he can be prescribed something to 'take the edge off' the withdrawal state.
3. A 30-year-old woman is motivated to stop injecting heroin. However, she feels that she needs to be prescribed a substitute for the long-term. She was previously spending £100 per day on heroin.
4. A 27-year-old man is undergoing detoxification from dihydrocodeine, but he is troubled by profuse diarrhoea.
5. A 38-year-old lady who intermittently abuses opioids asks to be prescribed a drug to reduce the associated 'high', as she feels this will discourage her from using.

Prochaska and DiClemente Transtheoretical Model of Change

A. Precontemplative
B. Relapse
C. Preparation
D. Action
E. Contemplative
F. Maintenance
G. Termination
H. Recycling

For the following questions, select the most appropriate term from the list above.

1. A 31-year-old nurse has set a 'quit date' to stop smoking.
2. A 62-year-old salesman has been abstinent from alcohol for 30 years, and is no longer even tempted by the thought of drinking.
3. A 22-year-old female student does not consider her heavy cannabis use to be a problem.
4. A 29-year-old banker is considering stopping his cocaine use; however, he is worried about what his friends will say.
5. A 33-year-old unemployed man has been using heroin on a daily basis for the last 2 weeks since his partner left him. He had previously been clean for 3 years.

Treatment of alcohol dependence

A. Alcoholics anonymous
B. Lorazepam
C. Psychoeducational group
D. Disulfiram
E. Thiamine
F. Chlordiazepoxide
G. Naltrexone
H. Cognitive-behavioural therapy (CBT)
I. Acamprosate
J. Motivational interviewing
K. Diazepam

For the questions below, select the most appropriate treatment option from the list above.

1. A 55-year-old man, currently drinking 70 units of alcohol per day, requires a benzodiazepine during an inpatient detoxification. He suffers from severe chronic liver failure.
2. A 45-year-old woman with alcohol dependence is uncharacteristically confused, walking with an ataxic gait and has nystagmus. She does not smell of alcohol.
3. A 57-year-old woman with a history of alcohol dependence is currently abstinent. However, she wants help to 'avoid temptation'. She does not want drugs and is frightened by the prospect of group therapy.
4. A 36-year-old man is currently abstinent from alcohol but has experienced a couple of 'slips' that he attributed to powerful cravings. He is also prescribed tramadol for knee pain.
5. A 44-year-old man has recently stopped drinking and wants to remain abstinent for life. He considers alcohol to be a 'disease' and does not really want to be involved with health services. He is socially isolated and feels that he would benefit from meeting like-minded individuals.

Chapter 21 The psychotic disorders: schizophrenia

Antipsychotic choice in schizophrenia

A. Chlorpromazine
B. Haloperidol
C. Flupentixol depot
D. Clozapine
E. Quetiapine
F. Aripiprazole
G. Risperidone
H. No antipsychotic indicated

For each of the following patients, select the ONE best management option from the options above.

1. A 47-year-old woman with schizophrenia. She remembers a good response to haloperidol in her 20s and would like to try it again.

2. A 28-year-old model experiencing a first episode of psychosis. She is very keen to avoid weight gain.
3. A 33-year-old man experiencing his second episode of psychosis. He recalls very unpleasant tremor and rigidity with the antipsychotic he used previously and would like to avoid these symptoms.
4. A 36-year-old man with schizophrenia who has had multiple relapses after forgetting to take oral medication.
5. A 26-year-old woman who has tried 3 months of olanzapine and 3 months of risperidone at optimum doses but remains troubled by distressing psychotic experiences associated with functional impairment.

Presentation of antipsychotic side-effects

A. Photosensitivity
B. Postural hypotension
C. Hypersalivation
D. Dry mouth
E. Agranulocytosis
F. Parkinsonism
G. Akathisia
H. Dystonia
I. Somnolence
J. Hyperprolactinaemia

Select the ONE term used to describe the following side-effects from the list of options above.

1. A 27-year-old man wakes up each morning drooling onto a wet pillow.
2. A 57-year-old woman describes feeling dizzy. On examination, she has a supine blood pressure of 140 mmHg systolic and an erect blood pressure of 100 mmHg systolic.
3. A 22-year-old woman has noticed milk coming from her nipples bilaterally, but is not pregnant or breast-feeding.
4. A 43-year-old man collapses with a severe pneumonia. He has an undetectable neutrophil count.
5. A 30-year-old woman keeps crossing and uncrossing her legs during an interview. She also keeps smoothing her hair and handbag. She says she feels like she is 'crawling out of my own skin'.

Chapter 22 The mood (affective) disorders

Treatment setting for depression

A. Admit to psychiatric hospital
B. Admit to general medical hospital
C. Manage in primary care
D. Refer to psychiatric outpatients routinely
E. Refer to psychiatric outpatients urgently
F. Refer to crisis team

For each of the following patients, select the ONE best management option from the list above.

1. A 55-year-old man with a severe depressive episode who has sent goodbye emails to his family. A dog walker alerted the police after he found him in isolated woodland tying a noose to a tree.
2. A 55-year-old man with a moderate depressive episode which has not responded to adequate trials of two antidepressants. He denies suicidal ideas and maintains an oral intake.
3. A 55-year-old man with a severe depressive episode who reports derogatory second person auditory hallucinations. He denies suicidal ideas and maintains an oral intake.
4. A 55-year-old man with a severe depressive episode who has lost 3 stone in weight over 3 months and has refused food and fluids for the last 2 days.
5. A 55-year-old man with a mild depressive episode who has not benefited from self-help CBT.

First-line antidepressants

A. Selective serotonin reuptake inhibitor (SSRI)
B. Venlafaxine
C. Duloxetine
D. Mirtazapine
E. Amitriptyline
F. Lofepramine
G. Phenelzine
H. Moclobemide
I. Lithium

For each of the following patients with moderate to severe depression, select the ONE best first-line antidepressant from the options above.

1. A 49-year-old stunt man on long-term ibuprofen for back pain.
2. A 23-year-old shop assistant with no past medical history.
3. A 32-year-old teacher whose chief complaint is insomnia.
4. A 45-year-old butcher who says he will stop any antidepressant that affects his sexual function.
5. A 64-year-old librarian with stress incontinence.

Chapter 23 The anxiety and somatoform disorders

Management of posttraumatic stress disorder

A. Self-help
B. Watchful waiting
C. Cognitive-behavioural therapy (CBT) with exposure response prevention
D. Eye movement desensitization and reprocessing therapy

E. Applied relaxation
F. Selective serotonin reuptake inhibitor (SSRI)
G. Tricyclic antidepressant (TCA)
H. Benzodiazepine
I. Venlafaxine
J. Pregabalin

For each of the following patients, select the ONE best first-line management option from the list above.

1. A 23-year-old woman has symptoms of posttraumatic stress disorder (PTSD) following being raped 2 weeks ago. She is no longer attending classes at university as she avoids leaving her house.
2. A 23-year-old woman has symptoms of PTSD following being raped 2 weeks ago. She is still able to attend classes at university.
3. A 23-year-old woman has symptoms of PTSD following being raped 2 months ago. She is still able to attend classes at university.
4. A 47-year-old former soldier has tried trauma-focused CBT for PTSD but continues to have symptoms which markedly affect his functioning.
5. A 35-year-old survivor of an airplane crash has tried talking therapies and two first-line drug therapies for severe PTSD symptoms. She would like to try a further medication.

Management of generalized anxiety disorder and panic disorder

A. Self-help
B. Watchful waiting
C. Cognitive-behavioural therapy (CBT)
D. Eye movement desensitization and reprocessing therapy
E. Applied relaxation
F. Selective serotonin reuptake inhibitor (SSRI)
G. Monoamine oxidase inhibitor
H. Benzodiazepine
I. Pregabalin

For each of the following patients, select the ONE best first-line management option from the list above.

1. A 27-year-old female grocer has panic disorder. She has had to leave her shop on several occasions in the last month because of panic attacks.
2. A 27-year-old female grocer has panic disorder but does not feel it stops her from doing anything.
3. A 44-year-old zookeeper has generalized anxiety disorder and is unable to work. He has tried CBT in the past and would now like to try a different talking therapy.
4. A 44-year-old zookeeper has generalized anxiety disorder and is unable to work. He has tried CBT in the past and would now like to try a medication.

5. A 44-year-old zookeeper has generalized anxiety disorder and is unable to work. He has tried CBT and an SSRI in the past and would now like to try a different class of medication.

Chapter 24 Eating disorders

Treatment strategies for patients with eating disorders

A. Nutritional advice from general practitioner
B. High-dose fluoxetine
C. Voluntary sector referral
D. Motivational interviewing
E. Cognitive-behavioural therapy (eating disorder focused)
F. Interpersonal therapy
G. Family therapy
H. Community mental health team involvement
I. Intensive home treatment by specialist eating disorder service
J. Informal admission to general psychiatric ward
K. Forced, involuntary nasogastric feeding under mental health legislation

For the scenarios below, select the most appropriate management strategy from the list above.

1. A 23-year-old pole-dancer has a diagnosis of anorexia nervosa. Her weight has recently stabilized and is slowly increasing. She has previously appeared fairly bubbly and cheerful. However, she reports a 3-week history of tearfulness, loss of interest in all hobbies, early morning wakening and strong suicidal thoughts. When questioned directly, she tearfully discloses that she bought a rope and posted final letters earlier today and intends to hang herself this evening when her flatmate goes out to work. She says she is amenable to whatever management is suggested.
2. A 19-year-old male medical student has a diagnosis of bulimia nervosa.
3. A 16-year-old schoolgirl has a diagnosis of anorexia nervosa. She has been under the care of the specialist intensive team but has continued to lose weight. Her body mass index is currently 11.7 kg/m^2. On examination, it is noted that she has incredible difficulty concentrating. She is hypotensive and bradycardic. Blood tests show profound hypoglycaemia and hypokalaemia. There are U waves on electrocardiogram. She vehemently refuses to eat, refutes that she has a problem and categorically declines hospital admission. She just wants to be left alone to study for her A levels.
4. A 28-year-old lawyer has a diagnosis of anorexia nervosa. She is motivated to engage with treatment. She feels that a number of her past difficulties, including

the death of her mother, starting work in her current firm, and not being able to stand up to dominant male partners, have played a role in the development of her illness. She is keen to explore these.

5. A 14-year-old schoolboy was recently diagnosed with anorexia nervosa. It is noted that his parents consistently correct him when he is trying to tell his story. Mum is a consultant surgeon, and dad is a barrister, and both spend a lot of time at work. They have persistently told him that they want him to be a doctor when he grows up and have set high standards for him. However, when interviewed alone, he stated that he aspired to attend art college and hoped for a career in photojournalism.

Chapter 25 Sleep–wake disorders

Diagnosis of sleep–wake disorders

A. Circadian rhythm sleep disorders
B. Primary insomnia
C. Insomnia secondary to psychiatric disorder
D. Insomnia secondary to general medical condition
E. Insomnia secondary to substances
F. Narcolepsy
G. Non-rapid eye movement (non-REM) sleep arousal disorder
H. Primary hypersomnolence
I. REM sleep behaviour disorder
J. Sleep-related breathing disorder
K. Sleep-related movement disorder

What is the most likely diagnosis?

1. A 52-year-old man fractures his wrist after punching his wardrobe while asleep. His wife reports that he was repeatedly shouting 'Leave me alone!' When woken he recalls a vivid dream about being chased by terrorists. He has no past psychiatric history, uses no substances and is otherwise well.
2. A 14-year-old girl fractures her wrist after walking into her wardrobe while asleep. When woken she seems disorientated. In the morning she recalls nothing of the night's events. Her father experienced sleep terrors during childhood.
3. A 52-year-old man fractures his wrist after being in a road traffic accident caused by him falling asleep at the wheel. He reports excessive daytime sleepiness for the past 5 years. His wife reports that he snores. His body mass index is 37 kg/m^2 and his blood pressure is 180/100 mmHg.
4. A 27-year-old man fractures his wrist after leaping off a bus shelter to prove he can fly. He has not slept for the last 3 nights. He denies any use of substances and his urine drug screen is clear. He was depressed for 3 months the previous year.

5. A 23-year-old woman fractures her wrist after falling suddenly to the floor when her uncle makes a joke. She sleeps well at night, but also often falls asleep during the day without warning.

Chapter 26 The psychosexual disorders

Medication associated with psychosexual disorders

A. Clozapine
B. Fluoxetine
C. Mirtazapine
D. Paracetamol
E. Propranolol
F. Pregabalin
G. Ropinirole
H. Salbutamol
I. Trazodone

Select the medication most likely to cause the problem:

1. Difficulty in achieving orgasm.
2. Difficulty in achieving an erection.
3. Exhibitionism.
4. Prolonged, painful erection.

Chapter 27 Disorders relating to the menstrual cycle, pregnancy and the puerperium

Management of mental illness in the puerperium

A. Lithium
B. Sertraline
C. Maternal skills teaching
D. Doxepin
E. Reassurance and check-up in 1 week
F. Olanzapine
G. Sodium valproate
H. Electroconvulsive therapy
I. Mirtazapine

For the situations below, select the most appropriate management strategy from the list above.

1. A 17-year-old mother of a 3-month-old baby reports that she is finding motherhood to be a burden and is worried that she is not 'doing it properly'.
2. A 26-year-old lady appears weepy and reports feeling 'down' 3 days after the birth of her son.
3. A 24-year-old lady with a history of bipolar affective disorder is 1 week postpartum and presents with auditory hallucinations and ideas that the father of the child is Jesus Christ.
4. A 33-year-old lady with a history of depression is 4 weeks postpartum. She has marked

psychomotor retardation. Her husband reports that she has not been eating or drinking for the past week.
5. A 29-year-old mother of a 2-month-old girl is tearful and reports feeling low in mood. She is finding breastfeeding difficult. She has early morning wakening and has stopped running the mother-and-baby group she set up while pregnant.

Psychotropic medication in pregnancy

A. Haloperidol
B. Olanzapine
C. Diazepam
D. Aripiprazole
E. Imipramine
F. Lithium carbonate
G. Carbamazepine
H. Fluoxetine
I. Chlorpromazine

From the list above, select the medication described by each of the statements below.

1. Should not be prescribed to women of childbearing age, due to the high risk of neural tube defects.
2. Associated with increased risk of gestational diabetes.
3. May be continued in pregnancy if risks of discontinuation are high, but should be balanced against the increased risk of fetal heart defects.
4. May be continued in pregnancy if benefits outweigh risks, but associated with an increased risk of pulmonary hypertension in the neonate.
5. Likely to need dose adjustment during pregnancy.

Chapter 28 The personality disorders

Management of patients with personality disorders

A. Weekly dispensing of medication
B. Detention under mental health legislation
C. Informal, time-limited admission to psychiatric ward
D. Removal to police custody
E. Referral for mentalization-based therapy
F. Encouragement to engage with existing care plan
G. Referral to social work
H. Trial of antipsychotic medication
I. Advice regarding lifestyle choices
J. Day-hospital referral
K. Urgent multiagency meeting

Choose the most appropriate intervention for the cases below.

1. A 36-year-old lady with dependent personality disorder arrives at accident and emergency demanding admission to the hospital because she

feels that she is not coping at home. She has missed her last two appointments with the occupational therapist.

2. A 22-year-old lady with emotionally unstable personality disorder was brought to hospital by police after being restrained to prevent her from jumping from a railway viaduct. She is covered in bruises and reports that her partner assaulted her and threw her out of the house. She is inconsolably upset, extremely pessimistic and voicing ongoing suicidal intent and plans.

3. A 43-year-old man has paranoid personality disorder. He is socially isolated and has longstanding worries that he will be targeted by local youth gangs. He does not trust doctors; however, he has recently acknowledged that his concerns are perhaps unfounded.

4. A 19-year-old lady has a diagnosis of emotionally unstable personality disorder, and an extensive history of self-harm. She has recently developed a comorbid depressive illness that her general practitioner (GP) feels would benefit from treatment with an antidepressant. However, the GP is reluctant to prescribe because of previous overdoses.

5. A 39-year-old man with a diagnosis of anxious personality disorder reports recent initial insomnia. He attributed this to worries about his future. Since he was made homeless, he has been spending his days drinking complimentary coffee in the support centre. When he cannot sleep at night, he lies in bed and smokes cigarettes.

Chapter 29 The neurodevelopmental disorders

Psychosocial interventions in neurodevelopmental disorders

A. Anger management
B. Antivictimization intervention
C. Cognitive-behavioural therapy
D. Habit control
E. Nil recommended
F. Parent-training/education programme
G. Play-based social–communication intervention
H. Social learning program
I. Structured leisure activity
J. Supported employment programme

Select the psychosocial intervention which is recommended as first-line treatment for each of the cases below.

1. A 7-year-old boy with attention deficit hyperactivity disorder (ADHD)
2. A 27-year-old woman with ADHD
3. A 7-year-old girl with autism spectrum disorder (ASD)

4. A 27-year-old man with ASD
5. A 10-year-old girl with Tourette syndrome

Chapter 30 Child and adolescent psychiatry

Diagnosis of psychiatric disorders with onset in childhood or adolescence

A. Academic setting inappropriate to ability
B. Age-appropriate behaviour
C. Attention deficit hyperactivity disorder (ADHD)
D. Child abuse
E. Conduct disorder
F. Elective mutism
G. Oppositional defiant disorder
H. Reactive attachment disorder
I. Separation anxiety disorder
J. Social anxiety
K. Specific phobia

For each scenario below, choose the most likely corresponding option from the list given above.

1. A 6-year-old boy is referred by an educational psychologist, due to his behaviour at school. He seems to be unable to concentrate on his schoolwork and has been running around the classroom distracting fellow pupils from completing their work, often by jumping on tables and throwing chairs around. On one occasion, he flooded the play area when he broke a water pipe. His parents are very surprised, because he is entirely normal at home.

2. A 12-year-old boy has been incredibly disobedient, both at school and within the home. He has been dancing in front of the TV when his father has been watching the football. He has also been using swear words in the house, and—on two occasions in the last week—has run away from home after being confined to his room. His parents are surprised that he has not been bullying others, or in trouble with the police.

3. A 4-year-old girl watches other children playing at nursery but does not attempt to join in. When she falls over in the playground she cowers away when an adult offers first-aid. She has a sad demeanour but otherwise shows little emotion. She has been taken into care after experiencing physical abuse from both parents.

4. A 10-year-old girl has always been shy. Recently, her father worked away for a month. Now she is experiencing nausea and abdominal pain every morning, except at the weekends. She can be persuaded to go to school but only if her father walks with her to the school gates.

5. A 4-year-old boy has recently been adopted by his aunt and uncle after his parents died in a road traffic accident. He had normal language development and initially he seemed to settle in well to his new home.

However, he gradually stopped speaking at home. Nursery staff report he speaks normally there. During the consultation he initially does not speak but does so when his adoptive parents leave the room. His adoptive parents appear caring but anxious and unsure what to do. They have been arguing recently.

Chapter 31 Older adult psychiatry

Adverse drug reactions in older adults receiving psychotropic medication

A. Lithium
B. Sodium valproate
C. Diazepam
D. Lorazepam
E. Trazodone
F. Mirtazapine
G. Amitriptyline
H. Fluoxetine
I. Olanzapine
J. Haloperidol

For each of the following patients, select the medication most likely to be implicated in their presentation from the options above.

1. A 67-year-old woman complains of insomnia, anxiety and anorexia. She has tinnitus and keeps mistaking her oxygen tubing for a snake. She was admitted 10 days ago with a myocardial infarction and her sleeping tablet was stopped.
2. A 72-year-old man receiving treatment for depression presents with general malaise. His serum sodium is 126 mmol/L.
3. A 69-year-old man receiving treatment for bipolar affective disorder presents with vomiting and diarrhoea. His serum sodium is 151 mmol/L.
4. A 74-year-old man collapses. His electrocardiogram shows torsade de pointes. He was admitted 5 days ago with delirium requiring pharmacological management.
5. An 81-year-old woman has delirium. She has recently been started on analgesia for trigeminal neuralgia.

Chapter 32 Forensic psychiatry

Diagnosis of mental disorder in offenders

A. Othello syndrome
B. Paranoid schizophrenia
C. Antisocial personality disorder
D. Mania with psychotic symptoms
E. Severe depression with psychotic symptoms
F. Emotionally unstable personality disorder
G. De Clérambault syndrome
H. Delirium tremens
I. Obsessive-compulsive disorder
J. Mild intellectual disability
K. Drug-induced psychosis

For each of the following scenarios, select the most appropriate diagnosis from the list above.

1. A 35-year-old man was arrested after he assaulted a bus driver. He believed that the driver was trying to procure the services of his wife, who he is convinced is working as a prostitute. He has dismissed extensive reassurances from his wife and his own siblings. He reports that he has a sword in the back of his car and intended to 'get the truth out of her'. He has a history of alcohol abuse.
2. A 50-year-old man with no psychiatric history was arrested after committing a public order offence on a train home from a music festival. He assaulted three police officers and required restraint. At interview, he appears distressed and is clearly responding to auditory hallucinations. He is convinced that the police are Nazis who plan to use his brain for experimentation.
3. A 21-year-old woman has been charged with fraud. She has applied for several credit cards and bank loans in the last fortnight and has used a number of different names to do so. She says that she is a pop star and needs money to fund a world tour. She was recently discharged from hospital following a depressive episode.
4. A 44-year-old man is arrested and charged with murdering a sandwich shop clerk, who was on his way home from work. He has an extensive forensic history and is a well-known member of an organized criminal gang. He denies any psychiatric history and admits killing the man because he got his order wrong. He appears cold and emotionless.
5. A 30-year-old man is arrested and charged with setting his neighbour's caravan on fire. He appears to be from a distant town; however, he reports that he used to have contact with psychiatric services as a youngster. He thought his actions would please people in his neighbourhood because the flames were 'pretty'.

SBA answers

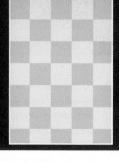

Chapter 2 Pharmacological therapy and electroconvulsive therapy

1. B. Looking at his prescription. Although the two syndromes have features in common, they can nearly always be easily distinguished by medication history (see Table 2.8). Clonus is another useful distinguishing factor, as it is present in serotonin syndrome but absent in neuroleptic malignant syndrome (where lead-pipe rigidity is common).

2. E. Assess ABC. This man is likely to be experiencing neuroleptic malignant syndrome. After ABC has been addressed, all antipsychotics should also be discontinued. The other answers are all possible treatment options, but none are first-line. Before they are considered, he needs initial resuscitation, and then is likely to need transfer to a general hospital for investigation and monitoring. See Table 2.8.

3. C. Weekly full blood counts (FBCs). Without monitoring, just under 3% of patients treated with clozapine develop neutropenia (low neutrophil count), and just under 1% develop agranulocytosis (negligible neutrophil count). This is most likely to occur early in treatment. Therefore, weekly FBCs are advised initially. As for all antipsychotics, she will also require regular checks of blood pressure, liver function, lipid profile and glucose. These parameters should be checked every 1–3 months initially, then annually.

4. E. Egg mayonnaise toastie is the only safe option, given the dietary restrictions required for irreversible monoamine oxidase inhibitors such as phenelzine. See Box 2.2. She should also avoid drinking Chianti wine with lunch.

5. E. 1.8 mmol/L. Her symptoms are consistent with lithium toxicity in the 1.5–2.0 mmol/L range. However, symptoms of toxicity can manifest at lower levels, particularly in older adults. Toxicity is likely to have been precipitated by the recent course of nonsteroidal antiinflammatory drugs. See Table 2.3.

Chapter 3 Psychological therapy

1. C. This man is suffering from a prolonged grief reaction. In the first instance, it would be helpful to refer him to bereavement counselling, which most commonly takes the form of person-centred counselling. In the United Kingdom, Cruse is a large voluntary sector service offering bereavement counselling. Psychodynamic therapy, cognitive-behavioural therapy and mindfulness-based cognitive therapy have little evidence to support their use in this instance. Exposure and response prevention is a behavioural therapy used in the treatment of obsessive-compulsive disorder.

2. C. Transference is the theoretical process by which the patient transfers feelings or attitudes experienced in an earlier significant relationship onto the therapist. Counter-transference refers to the feelings that are evoked in the *therapist* during the course of therapy. The therapist pays attention to these feelings, as they may be representative of what the patient is feeling, and so helps the therapist to empathize with the patient. Often, the therapist has undergone therapy themselves as part of their training: this helps the therapist to separate out what feelings belong to them, and what feelings belong to the patient.

3. E. This cognitive distortion is an example of magnification (also known as 'catastrophization'), where things get 'blown out of proportion.' An example of emotional reasoning in this context would be 'I feel so miserable, so I must have failed my exam.' An example of fortune telling would be 'I failed my exam, so in the future no one will employ me.' An example of personalization would be 'It is all my fault: I failed my exams.' An example of labelling would be 'I am stupid.' Note that more than one type of cognitive distortion can exist in the same patient in the same circumstances. See Table 3.3.

4. B There is a strong evidence base to support the use of interpersonal therapy in the treatment of mild to moderate depression. See Table 3.5 for modalities of benefit in the other conditions listed.

Chapter 4 Mental health and the law

1. D. She needs to notify the DVLA of her diagnosis. They will then ask for a doctor's report and potentially a driving assessment and are likely to arrange more frequent reviews of the licence than otherwise (e.g., annually). It is the DVLA's decision as to whether she is fit to drive or not. Many patients with mild dementia are found fit to continue to drive. Patient and partner reports of driving can be unreliable as patients can have poor insight and partners may not want to act in a way they perceive as harming the patient, or themselves. It is the patient's responsibility to notify the DVLA although doctors may need to do so if patients ignore this advice and present a significant risk to others through driving.

2. B. The patient lacks capacity as his low GCS means he will not be able to communicate his decision. He is also unlikely to be able to understand, to retain and to weigh up information, but this cannot be assessed in the absence of communication.

3. D. He is likely to lack capacity for any decisions requiring more consideration than is available in working memory as he will not be able to retain information for long enough to weigh it up. As a guide, someone should be able to retain information for as long as necessary to make a decision. A quick decision, e.g., meal choice, does not require a long time to make. A big decision, e.g., where to live, would normally be something that a person would consider and mull over for a few days at least.

4. C. She lacks capacity for the decision about surgery, as she does not believe the information because of a delusion. However, she is likely to have the capacity to make decisions about which she does not have delusions.

5. A. He should be assumed to have the capacity to make a decision about a statin, unless his psychotic symptoms relate to cholesterol (which is unusual) or he is very thought disordered.

Chapter 5 Mental health service provision

1. A. The other options demonstrate treatment resistance (B), bipolar disorder (C), significant risk to self (D) and diagnostic uncertainty (E), all of which means referral to secondary care should be considered.

2. B. Early intervention in psychosis team. This man may be experiencing prodromal psychosis. He does not currently appear to be at high enough risk to require home treatment or admission. As he does not have an established diagnosis of mental illness, an assertive outreach team is not appropriate. A community mental health team could manage him, but early intervention teams are expert at identifying early psychosis and are therefore best placed to monitor him.

Chapter 6 The patient with thoughts of suicide or self-harm

1. C. Measuring serum paracetamol levels (plus INR, liver function, other baseline bloods) to determine the requirement for potentially life-saving treatment is the priority in this case. This can be measured from 4 hours postingestion although levels become harder to interpret after 15 hours. The other options are all important aspects of psychiatric evaluation and risk assessment but are not urgent.

2. D. While researching methods is also worrying, acts of closure (such as making a will, organizing finances, writing suicide notes) are the most worrying signs and suggest strong suicidal intent. Contacting voluntary support agencies (such as the Samaritans) suggests emotional distress, but also a degree of ambivalence. Telling his wife of his plans may be a way of communicating his feelings to her but is not necessarily a final act. Disclosing plans to a health care professional does not reduce his risk.

3. C. Suspension hanging is the most common method of completed suicide in England, Wales and many other countries. Means are widely available and lethality is high. Self-inflicted firearm wounds are most common in the United States. Paracetamol is the most common drug of overdose in the UK; however, advances in medical treatment and public health measures have reduced mortality associated with this. Jumping from height is a fairly 'public' method of suicide, thus is often reported in the news (although media coverage of all suicides has reduced in recent years due to campaigns to reduce 'advertising' of suitable locations). Carbon monoxide poisoning used to be fairly common; however, catalytic converters on modern motor vehicles has reduced fatality of this method.

Chapter 7 The patient with impairment of consciousness, memory or cognition

1. D. Delirium. This is suggested by her acute onset objective cognitive impairment associated with sleep–wake cycle disturbance. Suspicion and visual hallucinations are common in delirium. Although Lewy body dementia is commonly associated with visual hallucinations it is excluded by the acute onset. Similarly, Alzheimer dementia is excluded by the acute onset. Late onset schizophrenia remains a possibility but is far less likely than delirium. Charles Bonnet syndrome would not account for all the features here, e.g., persecutory beliefs, sleep–wake cycle disturbance, cognitive impairment.

2. A. Amnesic syndrome. This man has an isolated long-term anterograde and retrograde memory impairment with intact working memory and other cognitive function. He is confabulating. A history of alcohol excess raises the possibility of Korsakoff syndrome as the cause. He does not have dementia because the impairment is not global or progressive.

3. A. This gentleman has a likely diagnosis of dementia. NICE (2006) recommends the blood tests this man has already received plus structural neuroimaging as a minimum assessment for reversible causes of dementia. However, there is some clinical judgement involved. Practice varies locally and some centres would not request a CT head unless there are neurological signs. There is no reason to think this man needs syphilis and HIV serology but

for other patients it may be appropriate. EEG and lumbar puncture are not recommended routinely in assessment of dementia but may be indicated in particular circumstances (e.g., if frontotemporal dementia or Creutzfeld-Jakob disease is suspected). See Table 7.7.

4. A. Delirium. This woman has recently been extremely unwell. Even though her UTI has been successfully treated, the brain can often lag behind the rest of the body when recovering from a serious illness. The fluctuation in her mental state may reflect a resolving or a new delirium. It would be wise to reassess for other causes that may have been missed initially or occurred since admission, e.g., a hospital acquired pneumonia. It may be that she will not regain her premorbid cognitive functioning and in due course will be diagnosed with dementia, but it is too early to make this diagnosis.

5. A. Amitriptyline. This man has a delirium. Anticholinergic medication is a common cause of delirium, as are opiates. Amitriptyline is sometimes used to reduce insomnia, although this is extremely inadvisable in an older adult, so this may be the precipitant. Starting or stopping any medication can potentially cause delirium but this does not occur commonly with the other medications listed.

Chapter 8   The patient with alcohol or substance use problems

1. B. Alcohol withdrawal would be suggested by symptoms of shakiness and sweatiness after a period of *not* drinking, not after having a drink. Onset of such symptoms after drinking is suggestive of a comorbid anxiety disorder or physical health problem (e.g., angina) which may be related to alcohol consumption (e.g., atrial fibrillation). The other options are all features of alcohol dependence (compulsion to drink, tolerance, persistence despite harm, neglect of other activities). The symptoms of dependence not listed are difficulties in controlling alcohol consumption and withdrawal symptoms. See Box 8.1.

2. D. This is classic alcoholic hallucinosis. Note the absence of memory or attentional problems, excluding delirium tremens or Wernicke–Korsakoff syndrome. Late-onset schizophrenia should be in the differential diagnosis, but is unlikely in this case. Social isolation is often a cause or consequence of alcohol misuse. Hepatic encephalopathy is excluded by her otherwise normal physical examination.

3. D. This man is delirious, and the history of heavy alcohol use suggests this is likely to be an alcohol withdrawal delirium. Note the visual 'Lilliputian hallucinations' of small figures (in his case, a horse), which are typical of alcohol withdrawal. Any surgical intervention should be delayed pending improvement in his delirium, unless it is felt that the fracture itself is a significant contributor to his presentation. The other options are all interventions which should be offered in delirium tremens. Benzodiazepines are used for alcohol withdrawal but not for other sorts of delirium. He should be empirically treated with parenteral thiamine as it is very difficult to exclude Wernicke–Korsakoff syndrome in delirious patients, and the consequences of missing it can be severe A full physical exam may highlight evidence of Wernicke–Korsakoff (ophthalmoplegia, ataxia) or highlight other contributors to the delirium (e.g., chest infection). Consistent nursing care will help to calm and orientate him.

4. E. Providing harm reduction advice is always important and can be effective immediately (e.g., directing him to a needle exchange service, offering screening for blood-borne viruses, offering a home naloxone injection kit). Prior to any substitute prescribing, it is vital to establish that the drug being substituted is actually being used, making urine drug testing the next essential step. Prescribing methadone to someone who is not opioid-tolerant can be fatal. Similarly, prescribing his previous dose of methadone could be fatal as he may be less opioid-tolerant now than he was previously. It is necessary for methadone doses to be initiated at a low level and gradually increased if required (titrated against withdrawal symptoms). Referring him to a drug counselling service may well be appropriate if he wishes to engage. See Chapter 20.

5. B. To calculate alcohol units, take the % ABV and multiply by volume (in litres): e.g., 40 × 0.350 = 14 units; 350 mL of a 40% ABV spirit contains 14 units. Six pints (3.408 L) of continental lager (5.3% ABV) contains 18 units; two bottles (1.5 L) of red wine (12.5% ABV) contains 18.75 units; 3 L of strong white cider (8.4% ABV) contains 25.2 units; and six bottles (1.980 L) of alcopops (4.9% ABV) contains 9.7 units. She should also be told that there is no 'safe' level at which to drink alcohol, merely lower to higher risk levels. If she plans to drink the full 14 units, it should be recommended that she spreads her alcohol consumption over around 3 days per week.

6. E. Drowsiness. Hyperalertness, tachycardia, hyperthermia, hypertension and psychotic symptoms arise commonly during cocaine use. Chest pain is a very concerning symptom suggesting arrhythmia or cardiac ischaemia due to coronary artery spasm. He should be advised to seek emergency medical care if this occurs after consumption.

Chapter 9   The patient with psychotic symptoms

1. B. Charles Bonnet syndrome. Based on the information given here, Charles Bonnet syndrome is the most likely diagnosis. However, it is crucial to

exclude delirium with a physical examination and cognitive assessment.

2. B. Ischaemic heart disease. This man has risk factors for ischaemic heart disease (age, male, smoker) and gives a description of exercise-induced chest pain with a classic 'weight on chest' description typical of cardiac ischaemia. People with schizophrenia are at increased risk of cardiovascular disease. Although this symptom could also be a tactile hallucination, it is important to exclude a physical origin before making this attribution.

3. E. Over-valued idea. Delusional jealousy is the key differential here, but the belief his wife is having an affair appears to be based on logical grounds, so he cannot be said to be delusional. The belief is not described as recurrent or intrusive so is not an obsession. However, the impact of the belief on this man's life is substantial as he has become preoccupied with it to an unreasonable extent. This is an over-valued idea.

4. B. Psychosis secondary to psychoactive substance use (a drug-induced psychosis). This is the most likely diagnosis; however, a definite diagnosis requires a longitudinal assessment. The diagnosis would be confirmed if he stops using substances and his symptoms resolve. However, chronic cannabis use is a risk factor for schizophrenia and if his symptoms persist despite abstaining from substances this may emerge as the diagnosis. At present he has not had the symptoms long enough to meet criteria for schizophrenia in any case.

5. B. Hebephrenic. This boy shows prominent thought disorder, incongruous affect and negative symptoms. Hebephrenic schizophrenia has an early onset and a poor prognosis.

Chapter 10 The patient with elated or irritable mood

1. A. Manic episode, with accelerated speech and probable thought disorder. Hypomania and cyclothymia are excluded by the significant functional impairment his symptoms have caused him. An agitated depression could be associated with an increased rate of speech, but the content should be understandable. Schizophrenia can be associated with thought disorder, but very rarely with accelerated rate of speech.

2. B. Bipolar affective disorder. An episode of depression is not necessary to meet criteria for bipolar affective disorder. Recurrent mania and hypomania are not diagnoses. No first-rank symptoms are mentioned, making schizoaffective disorder unlikely. Cyclothymia is excluded by the presence of psychotic symptoms.

3. D. Urine drug screen. This will demonstrate recent use of common recreational drugs (although it will not screen for novel psychoactive substances). The main differentials in a healthy young man are a manic episode or mania secondary to psychoactive substance use. Full blood count should be performed to check for evidence of infection, but is likely to be normal. Thyroid function test should be checked to exclude hyperthyroidism but is also likely to be normal. EEG and CT head should only be requested if there are neurological abnormalities.

4. D. Personality disorder. This woman describes a persistent pattern of maladaptive behaviour present since childhood associated with social and occupational dysfunction. This is most likely to be a personality disorder, with prominent impulsivity. It would be important to get a collateral history before making a definite diagnosis. The mood swings are faster than would occur within bipolar affective disorder and she has never had a period of euthymia, required for a diagnosis of a mood disorder. The symptoms cause marked functional impairment, excluding cyclothymia. Dysthymia is prolonged low mood, not mood swings. Although substance use can cause and worsen emotional lability it should not have onset in childhood.

Chapter 11 The patient with low mood

1. E. Prednisolone is the only medication listed commonly associated with depression. The others are not.

2. B. The midline neck swelling may represent a goitre. Given the patient's symptoms are mild, there is time to check her thyroid function before commencing treatment. If she is hypothyroid this should be treated first, which may normalize her mood without need for an antidepressant. Mild depression does not need referral to psychiatry. A neck ultrasound is likely to be needed also, but thyroid function should be checked first. She should not be sent away without investigation as the cause of the midline neck swelling needs determined.

3. D. The patient reports symptoms of depression alongside a mood-congruent nihilistic delusion. Therefore, the most likely diagnosis is a severe depressive episode with psychotic features. His lack of past psychiatric history makes schizoaffective disorder, schizophrenia and bipolar disorder unlikely, as onset at his age is rare. Early-onset dementia with behavioural and psychological symptoms is an unlikely possibility, but to check for this, his cognition, family history and ability to care for himself should be carefully assessed.

4. D. Suicidal ideation should be checked in everyone with a potential depressive episode. The other areas are all important but can be explored at a later review.

5. D. This patient is in a situational crisis. It is likely that her symptoms will resolve spontaneously. She

needs reassurance and to be offered a follow-up appointment to check on her progress. She cannot be diagnosed with depression as her symptoms are present for less than 2 weeks, and she is unlikely to benefit from an antidepressant. However, she may still be at risk of self-harm and should be screened for this. She does not need investigations or a mood diary unless her symptoms persist. Her symptoms are not severe enough to need referral to psychiatry at present.

Chapter 12 The patient with anxiety, fear or avoidance

1. D. Panic attack. This is the most likely diagnosis based on the history. However, it is important to take a full medical history (e.g., asthma, congenital heart disease) and family history (e.g., sudden death in young relatives) and to exclude other causes such as hyperthyroidism and hypoglycaemia, particularly given her repeat attendances. It would also be useful to know whether the attacks appear to have triggers (e.g., substance use/withdrawal, going to the library).

2. C. Blood-injection-injury phobia. This is suggested by his situational paroxysmal anxiety and avoidance. A myocardial infarction is unlikely to occur every time he is due to see the practice nurse. Hypoglycaemia, not hyperglycaemia, could cause these symptoms but is unlikely without a history of diabetes. Panic disorder does not have a specific trigger. Hypochondriasis is fear of having an illness, not fear of being investigated for one.

3. B. Airway, Breathing, Circulation. The first step in management is ABC. She is speaking to you, so her airway is maintained independently. The next step is to ascertain her breathing and circulation status. Although the differential includes a panic attack, she could also be experiencing a wide range of acute medical problems requiring urgent management. An ECG, ABG, blood tests and psychiatry referral may all be appropriate in due course.

4. E. Check blood sugar. Someone with type 1 diabetes will be receiving insulin. The description sounds very much like hypoglycaemia. If hypoglycaemia is confirmed it is important to treat the episode by consuming carbohydrate, and then examine his insulin/food/activity regime to reduce further episodes. If his blood sugars are normal, he may be experiencing panic attacks as part of panic disorder. Keeping a diary and deep breathing exercises may help with these (See Chapter 23 for management). Seeing a counsellor may help if he is experiencing a stressful life event, illness or bereavements. Diazepam is only recommended in social or specific phobia, for infrequent as required use.

5. D. Alcohol withdrawal. This man is drinking at least 60 units/week. He is experiencing physiological withdrawal symptoms after a few hours without alcohol, and the symptoms are relieved by further alcohol. Although anxiety in the morning may be part of diurnal variation in a depressive disorder, this man's mood is generally good, excluding depression. A phobia of something related to work is unlikely as the symptoms have only had onset recently (although enquiring regarding recent changes at work could be helpful). Hypoglycaemia secondary to diabetes is unlikely to present only in the mornings. Panic disorder is excluded by the clear relationship with alcohol.

Chapter 13 The patient with obsessions and compulsions

1. A. No mental illness. Lay people often use 'obsession' loosely. Her thoughts of the show are not obsessional as they are ego-syntonic, pleasurable and not resisted. She describes no compulsions. She is not delusional in that there is no evidence of irrational thinking. She is not socially phobic in that she has not reported anxiety in social situations. There is no evidence of a persistent pattern of perfectionism and rigid thinking, as would be expected in anankastic personality disorder. Calling in sick represents unethical behaviour rather than a mental illness.

2. C. Depressive episode. This man reports obsessions, but they are concurrent with the change in his mood, meeting the criteria for a depressive episode of moderate severity (five depressive symptoms). The obsessions are mood-congruent. Depression rather than obsessive-compulsive disorder is the primary diagnosis. Generalised anxiety disorder is unlikely as he does not report free-floating anxiety about many topics. Hypochondriacal disorder is unlikely as he is not worried about a particular condition, but being dead. A nihilistic delusion is not suggested as he tries to distract himself, suggesting he is resisting the image rather than accepting it as reality.

3. D. OCD with comorbid depressive episode. This man describes obsessions and compulsions associated with functional impairment of greater than 2 weeks duration, giving him a diagnosis of OCD. Superimposed on this he has developed a depressive episode of mild severity. Generalised anxiety disorder is unlikely as he does not report free-floating anxiety about many topics. There is no evidence of a persistent pattern of perfectionism and rigid thinking, as would be expected in anankastic personality disorder.

4. B. Obsessive-compulsive (anankastic) personality disorder. This is suggested by her lifelong history of unusual conscientiousness and perfectionism which

has caused some functional impairment (reduction of leisure time and being made redundant). Her thoughts of perfection are ego-syntonic and not resisted, meaning they are not true obsessions. Staying late to check is not a compulsion as it is not an unreasonable way to achieve her goal (assuming she does not check an excessive number of times). There is no evidence of low mood, excluding subsyndromal depressive symptoms. There is no evidence of social difficulties, making an autism spectrum disorder unlikely.

5. B. Pseudohallucination. She reports a perception in the absence of a stimulus from within internal space. A hallucination would occur in external space. An obsession would be attributed to herself. Thought insertion would be attributed to an external agency. A rumination is not experienced as a voice, but as a thought (see Table 13.1).

Chapter 14 The patient with a reaction to a stressful event

1. D. It is vital to robustly exclude physical aetiology prior to attributing symptoms to psychological causes. In this case, excluding intracranial haemorrhage secondary to head injury should take priority. This should include a history of the mechanism of assault (with corroboration from a witness if possible), full neurological examination and appropriate investigations (which may include a computed tomography brain scan).

2. C. This describes symptoms of fairly marked psychomotor retardation, which would be suggestive that a depressive illness has developed from the bereavement reaction. The other symptoms (wanting to be dead, poor concentration, intense guilt, hallucinations involving the deceased) are typical of normal bereavement.

3. B. This woman is suffering from an adjustment disorder, characterized by difficulty coping with a significant change in circumstances. Feelings of inability to cope are fairly typical of difficult adjustment. Note the duration of onset of symptoms (longer than for an acute stress reaction), and the fact that she has been signed off work, suggesting disruption to occupational functioning (which suggests that a diagnosis is appropriate, as opposed to 'no mental illness'). She does not appear to be suffering from other symptoms that would suggest depression or a conversion disorder.

4. A. This case is fairly typical of dissociative amnesia. She has no memory of a circumscribed period of her life, with intact memory for her past and the more recent present. While head trauma and Wernicke-Korsakoff syndrome (due to inadequate nutrition) is naturally a concern, she appears to have been able to

make her way to the UK and apply for asylum, which would suggest that cognitive impairment has not been global (excluding transient global amnesia), and she has been able to function at a reasonable level. She has no symptoms suggestive of posttraumatic stress disorder at this time, and the memory loss is more prolonged than would be expected in this disorder. In terms of stressful events, while she is unable to recall anything, she is seeking asylum from an area in which human rights violations are widely reported. The fact that she was pregnant with no recollection of conception or termination may suggest that she has been the victim of rape (which would be a traumatic stressor).

Chapter 15 The patient with medically unexplained physical symptoms

1. A. These situations are commonly encountered by GPs. The patient may well be developing multiple sclerosis; however, his symptoms are minimal and insufficient to make any diagnosis. Overzealous attempts to take his problems seriously by a well-intentioned doctor (such as referral to neurology, advanced investigations or arranging urgent follow-up) may reinforce his belief that something is wrong. However, dismissal by telling him it is 'all in his head' (or—at this stage—even empathic suggestion of psychiatric illness) is likely to cause him to seek a second opinion, and in any case is irresponsible given the inconclusive evidence. In the first instance, empathic acknowledgement and explanation, and inviting the patient to reattend if further symptoms arise (watchful waiting) is the most balanced option of the above.

2. D. This woman describes classic symptoms of body dysmorphic disorder. She is concerned with her appearance as opposed to an underlying disease (hypochondriacal disorder). If she did hold the over-valued idea with delusional intensity, somatic delusional disorder should be considered. Note that some patients may exaggerate (or even feign) psychological sequelae of imagined or minor flaws in their appearance to receive medical care (factitious disorder) or cosmetic surgery paid for by the state, which would be malingering.

3. D. This history is highly suggestive of factitious disorder (female, healthcare professional, symptoms without signs, broad knowledge, specific demands, far from home). It is imperative to contact previous hospitals to get more information; however, asking the patient for such contact details may yield vague answers (in some cases, requesting such details will result in the patient discharging themselves). Details of such patients are often shared between local

accident and emergency departments. It is not safe to prescribe pethidine or arrange a laparoscopy. It is not ethical to tell her she is lying without any definite evidence of this. It is too early to refer to psychiatry, although this may help in due course if she is willing to engage.

4. B. Onset of such symptoms in older people with no significant medical or psychiatric history is more likely to be indicative of insidious organic disease. Prior to attribution of symptoms to a psychological origin, physical disease needs to be thoroughly excluded. In this case, physical investigations have been inappropriate to exclude likely physical illnesses. At minimum he requires an electrocardiogram.

5. C. This presentation is classic somatization disorder. Note the multiple and changing symptoms, refusal to accept the absence of physical cause and duration of more than 2 years. Multiple sclerosis is possible, but more weight than normal should be placed on objective evidence before this is investigated. There is no evidence she is lying about her experiences, making factitious disorder unlikely. She is concerned about her symptoms rather than an underlying disorder, excluding hypochondriacal disorder. Generalised anxiety disorder is possible if she also reports anxiety about things other than physical symptoms.

Chapter 16 The patient with eating or weight problems

1. A. A body weight of at least 15% below expected for height is suggestive of anorexia nervosa. Patients with bulimia nervosa are often of normal or increased weight. Preoccupation with being thin, as well as a dread of fatness and a distorted perception of being too fat are associated with both anorexia and bulimia nervosa. Again, use of medication and exercise as means of controlling weight can occur in both disorders.

2. C. While patients with eating disorders often deny their symptoms, it is very important to exclude insidious physical illness as a cause of weight loss before attributing it to a psychiatric disorder. Physical causes can include malignancy, inflammatory disorders, infection and endocrine abnormalities. It would also be important to take a collateral history from his main caregiver, including psychosocial stressors.

3. E. Alcohol dependence. Self-neglect due to alcohol or substance use is a common cause of weight loss. Dependence is suggested by her withdrawal symptoms when she does not have access to alcohol (which are not panic attacks). Low mood is commonly associated with alcohol excess as alcohol is a depressant: the treatment is to stop alcohol. Anorexia and bulimia nervosa are excluded by the fact that she

is worried she has lost weight. Her vomiting sounds more likely to relate to gastritis secondary to alcohol excess, not purging.

4. E. potassium 2.1 mmol/L. She requires an electrocardiogram and cautious intravenous replacement of potassium. Hypoglycaemia, anaemia, hypercholesterolaemia and hypophosphatemia are all common in anorexia nervosa but the values given here are not dangerously low.

5. D. This woman has anorexia nervosa. She is dangerously underweight. While all of the listed mental illnesses can cause weight loss, they are differentiated from specific eating disorders by the presence of dread of fatness, distortion of body image and subsequent restriction of her dietary intake. The diagnosis of bulimia is excluded given her low body mass index.

6. E. Unable to rise from squatting without assistance. His blood pressure and heart rate place him at moderate risk but his capillary refill time and temperature are within the normal range. See The Royal College of Psychiatrists 'Management of Really Sick Patients with Anorexia Nervosa' (child and adult versions) for more details on physical risk assessment in anorexia nervosa.

Chapter 17 The patient with personality problems

1. A. Chronic feelings of emptiness is the only criterion listed here for borderline (emotionally unstable) personality disorder. According to DSM-5, a diagnosis of borderline personality disorder requires a pervasive pattern of instability of interpersonal relationships, self-image and affect, as well as marked impulsivity, beginning by early adulthood and present in a variety of contexts.

2. D. This man is likely to have schizoid personality disorder, as suggested by his stable and pervasive traits of social isolation and indifference to the opinions of others, with no evidence of an alternative mental disorder. It is important to exclude an autism spectrum disorder. See Table 17.1 for descriptions of the other personality disorders listed here.

3. C. This man is likely to have antisocial personality disorder. Antisocial personality disorder is very prevalent within prisons. However, a fuller psychiatric history would be needed prior to making this diagnosis.

4. E. In this case, there is too little information to make or exclude any diagnosis. The man is in a state of emotional distress following a significant life event (breakdown of a relationship, potential homelessness), which is compounded with acute intoxication. Initial management should focus on physical care, alleviating distress, ensuring his (and her) safety and achieving sobriety. Further psychiatric assessment (including collateral history) at a later

time is needed to establish a diagnosis or absence of mental illness.

5. A. It is likely that this man has borderline personality disorder. Note the link between childhood sexual abuse and borderline personality disorder.

Chapter 18 The patient with neurodevelopmental problems

1. C. Ensure he has an eye test. This boy may not be able to see the blackboard. Children can be embarrassed to admit this. ADHD and thyroid dysfunction are unlikely given that the symptoms are only present in one setting. Genetic testing is not yet indicated in ADHD and certainly cannot be used to exclude it. A collateral history from the teacher would be helpful if his eye test comes back normal.

2. E. Rett syndrome. The fact that she initially developed normally, then regressed, excludes autism and intellectual disability. Heller syndrome (childhood disintegrative disorder) is possible but unlikely as it is more common in males and usually has onset after the age of 2 years. Muscular dystrophy is also possible, but the child would be more likely to present with generalized muscle weakness, rather than only a reduced use of those muscles important for social interaction. It also mainly affects boys.

3. B. Autism spectrum disorder. This is suggested by his poor understanding of social cues and the hint that he has an unusually intense interest. To make this diagnosis definitive, a much fuller history would be required. Social phobia is unlikely as the problem is his poor social understanding, not him feeling that others are critical of him. Social anxiety is nonetheless common as a consequence of autism. Anankastic personality disorder is unlikely as this does not impair the ability to interact socially. A depressive episode might follow his redundancy but it is not the primary problem. Generalized anxiety is unlikely as he has not mentioned worrying about anything except social situations.

Chapter 19 Dementia and delirium

1. A. Aromatherapy. This woman has a behavioural and psychological symptom of dementia. Nonpharmacological options are recommended as a first line by NICE (2006), unless there is immediate risk of harm or severe distress. In the event of these risks, antipsychotics would be first line (after consideration of risk of stroke) and cholinesterase inhibitors second line. Antidepressants are only indicated if there is evidence of depression. Referral to speech and language therapy is unlikely to be of benefit given her severe dementia.

2. A. Antipsychotics. Antipsychotics can cause irreversible severe parkinsonian reactions in patients with Lewy body dementia. They are not absolutely contraindicated but should be used with even more caution than in other types of dementia and ideally under specialist advice. The other options may all potentially be of benefit – if his delusion is due to concurrent infection (antibiotics), depression (antidepressants) or worsening dementia – cholinesterase inhibitors can improve behavioural and psychological symptoms of dementia. Nutritional supplements may be of benefit whatever the cause if he is losing weight.

3. C. Co-codamol. This contains both codeine and paracetamol. Opiates are very common causes of delirium in older adults, both in their own right and due to their side-effect of constipation. Opiates are often started during acute admissions for pain or surgery. Any medication can potentially precipitate delirium, but opiates, benzodiazepines and anticholinergics are the commonest.

4. D. Acute medical ward. This lady is delirious. This is a medical emergency. She needs to be fully physically investigated. Her acute-onset psychotic symptoms are almost certainly due to her delirium, not a primary psychotic disorder.

Chapter 20 Alcohol and substance-related disorders

1. B. This man is currently contemplating changing his behaviour. He recognizes the need for change (he wants to give up), but he is ambivalent about it (worrying he will lose all his friends). Motivational interviewing may be helpful to allow him to progress to the next stage of preparation for change.

2. E. Prior to prescribing methadone, it is essential to confirm the use of opioids. A urine drug test can be used to do this. Admission to psychiatric hospital is not necessary, although dose titration should be undertaken in a controlled clinical environment with facilities to measure physiological response to opioids, and with emergency treatment for opioid toxicity (i.e., naloxone) close to hand. Viral serology testing and physical examination is important screening for health complications from intravenous drug use, but it is not necessary for a methadone prescription. Forcing a patient to identify a confidant for the purposes of corroboration can lead to problems, either placing false security in a possibly inaccurate historian or causing disengagement with services.

3. C. Naltrexone is an opioid receptor antagonist. This may control cravings and reduces the pleasurable effects of drinking alcohol, reducing 'reward' and – by

operant conditioning – can 'extinguish' the desire to drink (the 'Sinclair method'). Disulfiram causes an unpleasant reaction when taken with alcohol. Acamprosate may be helpful in controlling cravings. Long-term antidepressants or benzodiazepines are not recommended for the sole purpose of maintaining abstinence. However, antidepressants may be helpful for treating comorbid depression.

4. C. Buprenorphine (Subutex) is a partial opioid agonist and can be used for substitution therapy. The other drugs can be used in treating various stages of opioid dependence; however, none are true 'substitutes'.

Chapter 21 The psychotic disorders:
schizophrenia

1. B. If one parent has schizophrenia, the probability of their offspring having schizophrenia is 13%. The population lifetime risk is 1%. See Fig. 21.1.
2. E. If both parents have schizophrenia, the probability of their offspring having schizophrenia is 50%. The population lifetime risk is 1%. See Fig. 21.1.
3. C. This is a difficult question as there is little solid evidence about the optimum period of treatment for a first episode of psychosis. Without prophylactic antipsychotics following a first episode of schizophrenia, over half of patients will relapse within a year. The current recommendation is to continue antipsychotics for 1–2 years after a first episode. However, many patients wish to stop sooner. In this case, a gradual reduction over a few weeks reduces the risk of relapse. Alternatively, this man may prefer to switch to an antipsychotic less associated with weight gain.
4. D. Cognitive-behavioural therapy. The other modalities are not recommended in schizophrenia. Interpersonal therapy and cognitive-behavioural therapy are indicated in depression. Dialectical behavioural therapy is indicated in emotionally unstable personality disorder. Cognitive analytic therapy is indicated in eating disorders. Family therapy is also recommended if the patient lives with or is in close contact with their family.
5. D. Temperature, pulse, blood pressure, respiratory rate, hydration status and consciousness level should be checked every 15 minutes following parenteral administration of rapid tranquillization (until there are no further concerns about the patient's physical health status) where any of the following apply (NICE 2015):
    Patient appears to be asleep or sedated
    Patient has recently taken recreational drugs or alcohol
    BNF maximum doses for medication have been exceeded
    Patient has a pre-existing physical health problem
    Patient experienced any harm as a result of the intervention.

If none of the above have occurred, observations should be hourly until the patient is able to walk and interact normally. If the patient refuses or remains too behaviourally disturbed to allow observations, they should be regularly observed for respiratory effort, airway and consciousness level. See Fig. 21.2.

6. C. Transient hyperglycaemia secondary to stress may arise but is unlikely to be clinically important. All the other options are potentially life-threatening: benzodiazepines can cause respiratory depression, oversedation by any means can cause loss of airway, antipsychotics and hyperarousal increase the risk of arrhythmia, and benzodiazepines and antipsychotics can both cause hypotension. Additional life-threatening complications of antipsychotic use include seizures and dystonias. All these complications can occur with oral formulations also, but are more likely when large doses are given via a fast-acting method.

Chapter 22 The mood (affective) disorders

1. A. Someone who is not eating or drinking. ECT is indicated in options A–D, but not E. Treatment-resistant depression is an indication for ECT but if the patient has capacity and does not wish it, it is not given. No information is given to suggest s/he lacks capacity, which is presumed to be present in adults unless proven otherwise. Life-threatening reduction in oral intake, psychotic depression and previous good response to ECT are all other indications for ECT. If a prioritization has to be made, a life-threatening reduction in oral intake presents the highest risk and so should be treated first.
2. C. Admission under mental health legislation. This man is experiencing a manic episode with psychotic features. His psychotic beliefs place him at high risk of injury or death and are impairing his ability to make decisions regarding management of his mental health. It is not safe to let him go home and police custody is not appropriate given his behaviour is driven by illness. He may be persuadable to be admitted informally but if not, he would meet criteria for detention under mental health legislation (see Chapter 4).
3. D. Citalopram and quetiapine. This man has a severe depressive episode with psychotic features. A combination of an antidepressant and an antipsychotic is indicated. Citalopram is normally tried before amitriptyline as it has fewer side-effects. In addition, amitriptyline is more toxic than citalopram in overdose. Given his suicidal ideation it is best to choose the less toxic medication. Quetiapine or any other second-generation antipsychotic would be reasonable to treat his psychosis.

4. B. Olanzapine. Olanzapine, risperidone, quetiapine or haloperidol are the first-line antimanic agents recommended by NICE (2014). Lithium should not be started in the acute situation in someone with a history of nonconcordance. Valproate should be avoided where possible in a woman of childbearing age. Lamotrigine is not recommended during acute mania as it is ineffective. Citalopram, or any other antidepressant, should be discontinued in a manic patient. This woman is likely also to need rapid tranquillization with a benzodiazepine (see Fig. 21.2).

5. C. Individual CBT. Self-help CBT and structured group physical activity are recommended by NICE for mild depression (2011). Dialectical behaviour therapy is a psychological therapy for borderline personality disorder. Graded exposure therapy is used to treat obsessive-compulsive disease and phobias.

Chapter 23 The anxiety and somatoform disorders

1. B. Seeing patients with anxiety about their physical health on a regular basis can help contain their anxieties and reduce the total number and number of urgent appointments they need. However, this does not mean they should not be allowed access to urgent appointment slots – they will experience physical health problems along with somatization. Similarly, investigations should be carefully considered and avoided if possible, but some are likely to still be required to safely exclude other disorders. Benzodiazepines are not indicated for somatization disorder but may be indicated for some other reason. The nature of somatization disorder should be explained to patients, but it should not be done in a confrontational manner. Phrases such as 'all in the mind' should be avoided as patients are genuinely experiencing symptoms (see Box 23.1).

2. B. CBT with desensitization is recommended for phobias with mild to severe functional impairment. Trauma-focused CBT is for posttraumatic stress disorder. PRN diazepam would not be advisable given she is likely to come into contact with bodily fluids on a daily basis. SSRIs are not recommended for specific phobias.

3. C. An SSRI is the first-line drug therapy for obsessive-compulsive disorder. Clomipramine is a second-line drug therapy. Mirtazapine and pregabalin are not recommended by current guidelines. Self-help is recommended for mild symptoms but this woman's symptoms are associated with marked functional impairment. Talking therapies are first line for moderate to severe OCD and she should be encouraged to reconsider a talking therapy if a SSRI is ineffective.

Chapter 24 Eating disorders

1. B. Family therapy is the first-line psychological therapy for adolescents recommended by NICE (2017). The other therapies are all used in adults with anorexia.

2. E. Specialist supportive clinical management. This is one of the three psychotherapeutic modalities recommended first line by NICE (2017) for anorexia in adults. It is simply high-quality weekly outpatient treatment including psychoeducation about nutrition and weight, a positive therapeutic relationship and physical monitoring. Family therapy is first line for treating anorexia and bulimia in young people. Focal psychodynamic psychotherapy is a second-line treatment in anorexia. Interpersonal therapy is used to treat depression and exposure-response prevention is used to treat obsessive-compulsive disorder.

3. C. The presence of binge–purge symptoms is associated with a poorer prognosis in sufferers of anorexia nervosa, as is late age of onset, very low weight (not rapid weight loss), long duration of illness, personality difficulties and difficult family relationships. The presence of a family history of anorexia is not necessarily indicative of poor prognosis, neither is the rate of engagement with psychotherapy.

4. C. NICE (2017) recommends that people with anorexia nervosa should be encouraged to take a multivitamin and multimineral supplement. Selective serotonin reuptake inhibitors are no longer recommended in the management of eating disorders unless there is comorbid depression or anxiety, and these disorders are most likely to resolve with weight gain alone.

5. C. Phosphate 0.3 mmol/L. All the other blood results are in the normal range. Hypophosphataemia is the hallmark of refeeding syndrome and a low level indicates that replacement is required, along with frequent monitoring of phosphate, magnesium, sodium and potassium levels. Calcium levels are not generally affected in refeeding syndrome.

Chapter 25 The sleep–wake disorders

1. E. Pramipexole. Dopamine agonists such as pramipexole and ropinirole are recommended as first-line treatment for restless legs syndrome. The other medications listed are all potential causes of the syndrome.

2. D. Neuropathy. A peripheral neuropathy is suggested by her history of diabetes. Restless legs syndrome is unlikely as the pain is not brought on by inactivity. Iron deficiency is an uncommon cause of restless legs syndrome. Intermittent claudication is unlikely as exercise would worsen symptoms. Akathisia would not be limited to her legs.

3. D. Sleep hygiene advice. Everyone who is struggling with sleep should be given sleep hygiene advice, particularly those with depression. Her insomnia is likely secondary to depression and should improve over time as her mood improves. It is too early to increase the dose of fluoxetine. Hypnotics should be avoided where possible as patients can suffer from daytime drowsiness and develop tolerance. A sleep diary or referral is not indicated.

Chapter 26 The psychosexual disorders

1. A. Caressing without genital contact can improve sex. This is the kind of advice which may be given during sex therapy or in self-help materials related to sexual dysfunction. All the other pieces of advice are the opposite of what should be given: sexual dysfunction is common at all ages, physical problems are a rare cause of anorgasmia, medication may cause sexual dysfunction but should not be stopped immediately (a substitution may be required) and good communication with a partner about sex is associated with fewer sexual difficulties.
2. B. Check blood glucose. Erectile dysfunction is a common presenting symptom in diabetes, as is weight loss. Excluding diabetes is the priority here. All of the other options can also be appropriate management options in erectile dysfunction depending on the context (see Box 26.2).
3. B. Olanzapine. All the other agents are dopaminomimetic agents: levodopa is metabolized to dopamine, pergolide and pramipexole are dopamine receptor agonists and selegiline is a monoamine oxidase B inhibitor, reducing the breakdown of dopamine. High doses of dopaminomimetic agents have rarely been associated with new paraphilias in Parkinson disease, typically younger men with a long duration of illness. Olanzapine is a dopamine receptor antagonist which has been used to treat paraphilias in Parkinson disease.
4. D. Transvestic fetishism. This is the experience of sexual arousal due to dressing in clothing normally worn by members of the opposite sex. It is not a problem unless it is causing harm to the individual or others.

Chapter 27 Disorders relating to the menstrual cycle, pregnancy and the puerperium

1. A. Encourage exercise. This woman has mild premenstrual syndrome (PMS). One argument with her boyfriend is not evidence of significant functional impairment. For mild PMS, the National Institute for Health and Care Excellence (NICE; 2014) recommends healthy eating, stress reduction, regular sleep and regular exercise, particularly during the luteal phase. The oral contraceptive pill, ibuprofen and CBT are all options in managing moderately severe PMS. SSRIs are reserved for severe PMS.
2. E. Psychological therapy. While the woman in the case description attributes her symptoms to the menopause, the duration of the symptoms accompanied by the presence of suicidal thoughts are more suggestive of a depressive illness. The functional impact and suicidal thoughts suggest an episode of at least moderate severity. The National Institute for Health and Care Excellence (NICE; 2009) recommends a combination of an antidepressant and psychological therapy (cognitive-behavioural therapy or interpersonal therapy) as first line for treating moderate-to-severe depression. Counselling may also be useful if she has issues relating to relationships or bereavements she would like to reflect on, but it is not usually a treatment for depression. Dietary and lifestyle advice (avoiding alcohol, tobacco, eating a balanced diet, exercising) should be offered to everyone with mood symptoms but are unlikely to be sufficient in this case. Around the menopausal years, there can be an increase in psychosocial stressors (children leaving home, 'facing up' to growing older, changes in personal relationships, etc.), which may increase the risk of developing depression independently of the hormonal changes that arise during the menopause. Hormone replacement therapy can be useful in certain circumstances; however, it does not suit everyone, and should not be used as a substitute for recognized treatments in the management of major depression. Omega-3 fish oils may reduce menopausal vasomotor symptoms (hot flushes) but are not recommended as a treatment for depression.
3. E. Refer to perinatal psychiatry. This is a complex risk–benefit scenario that needs to be carefully discussed with the patient and which draws on the latest available evidence. Her history of bipolar disorder places this woman at high risk of postpartum psychosis, even with prophylactic treatment. Discontinuing treatment increases her risk of relapse at any time. A mentally unwell mother is harmful for the child *in utero* and once born. However, all the mood stabilizers are associated with teratogenic effects to various degrees (valproate > carbamazepine > lithium; see Table 27.1). The absolute risk of congenital abnormalities remains low with lithium but is unacceptably high with valproate or carbamazepine, so switching to them would not be helpful. Discontinuing lithium and remaining without prophylaxis may be an option depending on the severity of her previous mood episodes. Switching to olanzapine is also a reasonable option as it is thought to be safe in pregnancy but would depend on her past experience with this drug.
4. E. Refer to perinatal mental health team. Reassurance that she will not become unwell cannot be given.

This lady has a history of severe postnatal depression and is at greatly increased risk of suffering a further episode. She should be referred to the perinatal mental health team. Given this history, and her good response to medications in the past, commencing antidepressant treatment later in pregnancy or early postpartum may be beneficial. The perinatal mental health team would explore the risks versus benefits of this option. When choosing an agent, consideration should be given to previously effective drugs, and the mother's choice to breastfeed.

5. A. Detention in hospital under mental health act. This woman is experiencing a postpartum psychosis and is at very high risk of infanticide given the severity of her illness, the content of her delusion and the active steps she has taken towards killing her son. This risk is too high to be managed at home, however supportive her family. She lacks capacity to make decisions about her treatment due to her absent insight, therefore requiring admission under detention rather than informally. This should be to a mother-and-baby unit if available. Transfer to police cells is not appropriate as she requires intensive psychiatric care which cannot be provided there. Outpatient follow-up is not sufficient to manage her acute risk. A referral to social workers is likely to be helpful in due course as they may be able to identify additional supports for the patient, but the priority at the moment is to maintain her and her child's safety in hospital.

Chapter 28 The personality disorders

1. E. Drug treatment is not the main intervention. NICE (2009) does not recommend drug treatment for the core symptoms of emotionally unstable personality disorder. However, some medications can be helpful in reducing agitation during crises and in treating comorbid mental illness. The main intervention is psychological therapy.
2. A. All of the options have evidence supporting their use in emotionally unstable personality disorder, but dialectical behaviour therapy is the 'gold standard' and recommended by NICE (2009).
3. E. Ensure weekly dispensing of medication. This woman is probably suffering from a comorbid depressive episode. Management of this should be discussed with the patient – she may opt for 'watchful waiting' or it may be appropriate to start an antidepressant. As her risk of suicide has increased, it is sensible to reduce her access to means of suicide by suggesting weekly dispensing. Her risk is not so high that she needs admission. A urine drug screen may be helpful in excluding a substance-induced acute change in mood, but substance use (with the exception of alcohol) is unlikely to

account for a month of low mood. Benzodiazepines should be avoided where possible given the risks of dependence, particularly high in someone with persistent symptoms. Dialectical behaviour therapy is recommended for treatment of emotionally unstable personality disorder in the long term but will not help depression in the short–medium term.

4. C. Given the significant risk to another person, confidentiality needs to be broken in this case. The psychiatrist has a duty to immediately warn the police. In addition, the specific and detailed content of the threat necessitates that the intended victim be warned (see the Tarasoff case for further details). The responsibility for this falls on the doctor; however, in practice the police will usually be happy to facilitate this. Detention under mental health legislation would not be appropriate, as the threat should be addressed by law enforcement agencies in the first instance. Meticulous notes would need to be kept. It is likely that he would be held criminally responsible for his actions. Review in 1 week is too late. Anger management may be appropriate in due course but does not deal with the acute risk. Diazepam should be avoided given risks of dependence and absence of an indication.

Chapter 29 The neurodevelopmental disorders

1. C. There is no pharmacological treatment for the core symptoms of autism spectrum disorder. The first-line treatment is social skills training. The medications listed may be indicated to manage common comorbidities of autism spectrum disorder, anxiety or depression (fluoxetine), attention deficit hyperactivity disorder (methylphenidate), psychosis (risperidone) or epilepsy (sodium valproate).
2. D. Methylphenidate. NICE (2008) recommends this as first-line drug treatment for severe ADHD in school-age children. Dexamfetamine and atomoxetine are second line. Parent-training/education programmes are recommended as first line for school-age children with mild to moderate impairment. However, severe impairment is suggested by the fact this boy is at risk of losing his school place. Cognitive-behavioural therapy is recommended for older adolescents with mild to moderate ADHD.
3. D. This boy has Tourette syndrome. Psychoeducation is first-line treatment for this: speaking to him, his family and his teachers to explain the diagnosis and that the majority of cases improve by adulthood. The other options are all drug treatments that can reduce tics. However, as the tics are causing little interference with day-to-day activities, he may find the side-effects outweigh the benefits.

Chapter 30 Child and adolescent psychiatry

1. B. Conduct disorder. This is suggested by his major violations of societal norms (arson and severe aggression). Oppositional defiant disorder is often considered to be a 'milder' variant of conduct disorder, where defiant behaviour is characteristic, but this tends not to involve criminality or violating the rights of others. Conduct disorder is associated with the development of antisocial personality disorder, criminality and substance misuse in later life. He is too young to diagnose a personality disorder. Substance misuse is a possibility which should be explored but is unlikely to present with oppositional behaviour in isolation. Reactive attachment disorder presents under the age of 5 years with disordered social interaction.

2. E. Vaginal trauma and genital warts are not normal in an 8-year-old girl, and the findings should immediately raise suspicions of sexual abuse. The safety of the child is paramount, and steps should be taken to maintain this. While protocols vary slightly between areas, child protection procedures usually advise contacting the duty social worker and/or the local paediatrician on-call for child protection. If in any doubt about a possible child protection concern, either of these parties will usually be more than happy to offer guidance. The child should not be directly asked about what happened at this stage: a formal interview needs to be arranged involving the police, social workers and paediatric staff. Police will not question the girl just now. Parents should never be 'confronted' by medical staff; however, it is obviously courteous (if possible) to let them know what is going on and what will happen next. The child should not be allowed home until all relevant agencies are involved and safety at home can be ensured. This may not be possible, and an alternative place of safety may have to be sought. Should the parent remove the child from safety, it would be appropriate to contact the police given the magnitude of the concerns.

3. B. Cognitive-behavioural therapy. This girl has a probable diagnosis of depression, of moderate severity (based on her functional impairment). NICE (2005) recommends individual psychological therapy first line. Fluoxetine is the first-line antidepressant, sertraline and citalopram are second line. Watchful waiting is recommended only in mild cases.

4. D. Emotionally unstable personality disorder (EUPD). This is suggested by her long-term rapidly fluctuating mood, difficulties in relationships, self-harm, pseudohallucinations (the voice inside her head) and disturbed self-image (feeling empty). Childhood adversity is a risk factor for EUPD and suggested by a parental overdose. Bipolar affective disorder or a depressive episode would be associated with episodes of altered mood which lasted for days, not

hours. However, EUPD is a risk factor for comorbid depression. Disordered eating is common in EUPD. Bulimia is unlikely given the rest of the history, but it would be useful to check what her weight-related cognitions are to definitely exclude this (see Chapter 16). Schizophrenia is unlikely as she is not reporting any psychotic symptoms (she reports pseudohallucinations, not hallucinations).

Chapter 31 Older adult psychiatry

1. A. Antidepressant. The key issue here is the diagnosis. She presents with a common triad in older adults: depressive symptoms, cognitive impairment and functional impairment. It is often difficult to tease out whether someone is experiencing depression manifesting with cognitive impairment or an early dementia leading to comorbid depression. Ideally, depression is treated first, then cognition reassessed once mood is euthymic. An antidepressant would be first line in view of her cognitive impairment, but counselling or psychological therapy could still be considered in someone with this level of cognitive impairment.

2. C. Depressive episode. It is common for depression to manifest with prominent features of anxiety, psychomotor agitation and hypochondriacal ideas in older adults. Mild cognitive impairment is the next most likely differential – although her AMT score of 10/10 is reassuring, a more sensitive test such as the Addenbrooke's Cognitive Examination (ACE-III) may still show an objective impairment. Generalized anxiety disorder or hypochondriacal disorder is unlikely to have onset so late in life, and diagnosis would require a longer duration of symptoms. There are no psychotic features to suggest schizophrenia.

3. A. ECT. All of the suggested management strategies are reasonable, but ECT is preferable because of this man's potentially life-threatening poor fluid intake and poor medication concordance. Depot medication would get around the concordance problem but there are no depot medications licensed as antidepressants. ECT is the quickest and most effective treatment for depression known and seems to work particularly well in older adults.

4. B. All of these patients could potentially have late-onset schizophrenia. However, symptoms of late-onset schizophrenia are predominantly delusional, rather than bizarre or negative symptoms (as in patients A and C). Patient D is more likely to have Charles Bonnet syndrome. Late-onset schizophrenia is far more common in women than in men, and social deprivation and hearing impairment are also risk factors.

5. D. Continue mirtazapine for at least 8 weeks. Older adults can take longer to show response to

antidepressants, so an adequate trial is at least 8 weeks. Augmentation is not necessary at this stage and increases the risk of drug interactions. Tricyclics are not recommended as first line in older adults due to their side-effect profile.

6. E. Delirium. This lady has acute-onset cognitive impairment: delirium until proven otherwise. The history is concerningly suggestive of a focal seizure. She needs to be admitted to a medical ward for investigation. A manic or hypomanic episode would be highly unlikely to have such a rapid onset. Were she on lithium, it would be crucial to check a random lithium level as her presentation could also be due to lithium toxicity.

7. B. This is the simplest and easiest of the options. If concordance remains poor despite this, prompting by a carer could be considered. A depot could be useful if the patient wishes it, or his insight reduces and he requires compulsory treatment. Daily dispensing is normally reserved for methadone or for those at high risk of overdose. In general, simplifying medication regimes to once daily is a good idea, but unfortunately olanzapine is likely to be too sedating to allow use in the mornings. Potentially, his other once daily medication could be changed to the evening.

8. A. Ask her to attend A&E. It is unclear what dose of trazodone she has taken, or whether she has taken any other tablets. She needs examination, blood samples tested and an electrocardiogram. The next step would be for her to receive an urgent psychiatric review. This lady has recently attempted suicide. Older adults are at high risk of completed suicide. She may perceive taking extra trazodone as far more harmful than it actually is, as she may have memories of barbiturates – highly toxic sleeping tablets, which

are fatal in minor overdose. Her ongoing intent is unclear from the vignette. She may require admission or urgent community support from mental health services.

Chapter 32 Forensic psychiatry

1. C. The best predictor of future violence is past violence. The other options also increase his risk of future violence, particularly substance use.

2. E. An individual being considered unfit to plead through mental illness is relatively uncommon. The mental state findings given in A–D are all fairly extreme abnormalities suggesting that he would struggle to understand the difference between a plea of guilty and not guilty (D), understand the nature of the charge (D), instruct counsel (A and C), follow the evidence brought before the court (C) or challenge a juror (B and C). Amnesia (real or reported) for the offence itself does not necessarily impact on fitness to plead.

3. E. Murder is the only charge for which diminished responsibility may apply. If the accused is found to have diminished responsibility, the conviction is reduced to manslaughter (or culpable homicide in Scotland). This was particularly important historically when murder carried the death penalty.

4. B. ADHD. This is a typical history for someone with ADHD symptoms of impulsivity and emotional instability leading to offending behaviour. It may be that treatment for ADHD helps this young man (see Chapter 29). However, it would be crucial to gain collateral history from someone who knew him well during his development before making this diagnosis. The other options are also consistent with the majority of the vignette and important to consider. The final diagnosis that is imperative to explore is his use of substances.

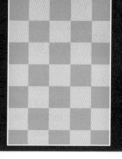

EMQ answers

Chapter 2 Pharmacological therapy and electroconvulsive therapy

Management of antipsychotic-induced extrapyramidal side-effects

1. C. Propranolol. This woman is probably experiencing akathisia. This is hard to treat, but propranolol or benzodiazepines can help. See Table 2.7. Ideally, the dose of antipsychotic is reduced. Quinine can be used for restless leg syndrome when in bed. The differential includes agitation secondary to psychosis.

2. F. Intramuscular procyclidine. This woman is experiencing a dystonia with an oculogyric crisis and trismus. Her clenched jaw means administering oral procyclidine is not possible. Baclofen and dantrolene should be used for chronic spasticity.

3. G. Resuscitation. This woman is acutely unwell. She needs ABC and probably a periarrest call/999 ambulance. She may have neuroleptic malignant syndrome or a range of other differentials (e.g., meningitis, substance intoxication). Dantrolene is not an emergency treatment and is not indicated until the diagnosis is clearer.

4. B. Oral procyclidine. This man has drug-induced parkinsonism. In the early stages, the features are different to idiopathic parkinsonism. Anticholinergics can help, but ideally the dose of antipsychotic would be reduced or an alternative antipsychotic trialled.

5. D. Stop anticholinergics. This man has tardive dyskinesia. This is hard to treat but stopping anticholinergics (in this case procyclidine) and reducing or withdrawing antipsychotics, if possible, can help.

Mechanism of action of antidepressants

1. A. Agomelatine.

2. E. Duloxetine. Venlafaxine also works this way. Tricyclic antidepressants are SNRIs, which also influence muscarinic, histaminergic and α-adrenergic receptors.

3. B. Amitriptyline. Tricyclic antidepressants are SNRIs, which also influence muscarinic, histaminergic and α-adrenergic receptors.

4. F. Moclobemide. Phenelzine is an irreversible inhibitor of monoamine oxidase A and B.

5. C. Bupropion. Pramipexole is a dopamine receptor agonist.

General feedback: See Table 2.1.

Chapter 3 Psychological therapy

Modalities of individual psychotherapy

1. C. Mentalization is the process by which we implicitly and explicitly interpret our and others' actions as meaningful on the basis of intentional mental states. Mentalization-based therapy is a treatment intended to improve the capacity to mentalize, which is often a specific difficulty in those with borderline personality disorder. This is thought to improve emotional regulation and interpersonal relationships. He may also find useful dialectical behaviour therapy, which incorporates mentalization training.

2. K. Interpersonal therapy is based on the assumptions that problems with interpersonal relationships and social functioning contribute significantly to mental illness. Main areas of focus include role disputes, role transitions, interpersonal deficits and grief. She may also find cognitive-behavioural therapy of benefit, for example, if interpersonal therapy is not available.

3. I. Systematic desensitization is a type of behavioural therapy that can be useful in the treatment of phobias. It involves compilation of a hierarchy of phobic stimuli (e.g., standing at the front door, going into the garden, going to the end of the street, going to the supermarket) and. with support from the therapist and the use of appropriate relaxation techniques. working through the hierarchy in order to face increasingly anxiety-provoking scenarios.

4. B. Trauma-focussed cognitive-behavioural therapy can be useful in the treatment of posttraumatic stress disorder, where the emphasis is on identifying and changing thoughts, feelings, sensations and behaviour related to the traumatic event. The 'dual attention stimulus' type of therapy that the gentleman in the scenario describes is eye movement desensitization and reprocessing, which can also be helpful for some.

5. F. Exposure and response prevention is a type of behavioural therapy in which the patient is

encouraged not to respond to the obsessional thought with a compulsive act. Relaxation techniques are used instead to overcome the anxiety associated with not carrying out the compulsion.

Psychodynamic psychotherapy

1. A. This is an example of acting out: behaving in a certain way in order to express thoughts or feelings that the person feels otherwise incapable of expressing.

2. H. Counter-transference is the process whereby the therapist unconsciously interacts with the patient as if they were a significant figure from the patient's past.

3. D. Catharsis is a Greek word meaning 'cleansing' or 'purging.' It is often used to describe a feeling of relief after an outpouring of emotive material.

4. E. Parapraxis is a term used to describe an error of memory, speech, writing, reading or action that may be due to the interference of repressed thoughts and unconscious features of the individual's personality. It is commonly referred to as a 'slip of the tongue' or a 'Freudian slip.'

5. J. Working through describes the concept of working over one's emotional difficulties from the past. In psychotherapy, it usually follows an 'impasse', which can be thought of as a therapeutic stalemate.

Chapter 4 Mental health and the law

Legislation

1. A. Mental health legislation. This man has evidence of mental disorder (depressive episode with psychotic symptoms) significantly affecting his ability to make decisions about his treatment (delusional belief that he will be tortured). He is at high risk (active plan of suicide by violent means, mental disorder, young male) and hospital is the least restrictive option (risk cannot be managed safely at home). He therefore meets the criteria for detention under the mental health act.

2. C. Forensic mental health legislation. This man has evidence of mental disorder (psychotic symptoms) and has been charged with a serious offence. The severity of his charge means he needs assessment and treatment under forensic, not civil, legislation.

3. A. Mental health legislation. This man meets criteria for detention under mental health

legislation as in case 1. Although he has been charged by the police, his offence is not severe enough to require management under forensic legislation.

4. F. Common law. It is in this man's best interests to receive aggressive airway management and oxygen. He currently lacks the capacity to consent as he is unable to communicate. Treatment under common law is indicated to sustain life and to prevent serious deterioration.

5. B. Mental capacity legislation. As this man needs treatment for a physical problem, mental health legislation is not appropriate. He lacks capacity as he is unable to retain information for long enough. It is not an emergency, so common law is not appropriate.

Chapter 5 Mental health service provision

Choice of service provision for mental disorder

1. I. Primary Care. Most episodes of depression are managed in primary care. Referral to secondary care should be considered in cases that are resistant to treatment or high risk or that present diagnostic uncertainty.

2. G. Liaison psychiatry review. Liaison psychiatrists provide psychiatric care to people admitted to general hospitals. This man may be experiencing a depressive episode, symptoms of physical illness, side effects from medication, or an adjustment reaction.

3. A. Acute general adult inpatient unit. This man is high risk and therefore requires hospital admission. He cannot safely be managed at home. As he has an established diagnosis of schizophrenia, the early intervention in psychosis team is unlikely to be needed.

4. J. Rehabilitation unit. This man has treatment-resistant schizophrenia with ongoing symptoms despite appropriate treatment. He also has functional impairment. A rehabilitation unit will be able to optimize his ability to live well despite ongoing symptoms.

5. B. Assertive outreach team. This man has schizophrenia with complex needs (homelessness, comorbid substance use), poor engagement, frequent use of crisis services and a need for intensive support (ongoing symptoms). A community mental health team is unlikely to be able to support him as well as an assertive outreach team.

Chapter 6 The patient with thoughts of suicide or self-harm

Mental disorder and self-harm

1. F. Emotionally unstable personality disorder. She is a young woman with a long history of self-harm, difficulties with interpersonal relationships and auditory pseudohallucinations at times of stress. Of note, she has no symptoms suggestive of a depressive illness.

2. J. Depressive episode, severe with psychotic features. This man has made a serious suicide attempt. Note that he went to some effort to prevent discovery (remote location, unsocial hour) and made acts of closure (typed letters imply that some thought had gone into these). He has biological and psychotic symptoms of depression. He may have intoxicated himself to reduce his inhibitions prior to the act and is not necessarily alcohol dependent.

3. E. Mania with psychosis. This young man's self-inflicted injuries are in keeping with his grandiose beliefs (of a religious nature), of which he is entirely convinced. He is disinhibited and feels that he has special powers. He also exhibits flight of ideas on mental state examination. Important differential diagnoses in this case would be a drug-induced state or an organic illness.

4. G. Depressive episode of moderate severity would be the most fitting of the listed diagnoses. Note the pattern of previous periods of illness, punctuated by periods of relatively good functioning. There is no mention of psychotic symptoms, and drugs or alcohol are not implicated.

5. B. Anorexia nervosa. Although a full history and physical examination would be required to definitively establish this diagnosis, the patient's history and presentation is suggestive of a serious eating disorder. Note the baggy clothes and the lanugo hair.

Immediate psychiatric management of the patient who has inflicted harm upon themselves

1. C. An admission to a medical assessment/short stay ward is necessary, with a psychiatric evaluation when he sobers up. He is currently too intoxicated (with drugs and alcohol) to undertake an adequate mental state examination and risk assessment, and admission to a psychiatric ward would not be appropriate due to potential medical complications of alcohol intoxication/ withdrawal. Discharging a patient in this state is unacceptable, as he is at risk of not only committing further acts of self-harm, but of medical complications. He is also possibly unable to look after himself and could be vulnerable from exploitation or accidents.

2. H. This person should be discharged to police custody. Her overdose does not appear to have been with strong suicidal intent (she was found in the street), and she is exhibiting drug-seeking and manipulative behaviour. While many patients like this do not require police involvement, she has committed physical, verbal and racial assaults on healthcare workers, and needs to face consequences for these actions. Admission to a psychiatric ward is unlikely to be beneficial, and may even prove detrimental by reinforcing the suggestion that behaviour of this nature is driven by mental illness.

3. E. This gentleman should be referred for urgent (later in the week) input from the community mental health team. He is likely to be suffering from a depressive illness, probably precipitated by financial and employment difficulties. While he is clearly remorseful about his suicidal behaviour, he appears to be struggling with his current situation, has some biological symptoms of depression, and could well benefit from input by the community mental health team. He has a concerned and supportive wife and a stable domestic situation, which is why immediate outreach team involvement is not necessary at present.

4. B. This lady most likely requires admission to a psychiatric ward for further assessment and management of her mental state and risk. Should she refuse, use of mental health legislation may need to be considered. Despite the overdose being relatively small, this is likely due to lack of knowledge and there appears to have been very clear suicidal intent. First presentations of self-harm in older adults should be considered to be with suicidal intent unless there is clear evidence to the contrary. Intensive outreach support in this case would be inappropriate given the very high risk of imminent further acts, despite her pleas that she will be fine.

5. I. Discharge with information on non-NHS support services. Despite her history and diagnosis, this woman appears to be functioning at a relatively high level (studying, not self-harming until recent stressors). She has made it clear that she is not wishing mental health service input; however,

it could be that she would benefit from non-NHS resources. Information on local student support agencies or voluntary support services for people who self-harm should be offered. Most of these agencies accept self-referrals and distribute leaflets to local mental health bases.

Chapter 7 The patient with impairment of consciousness, memory or cognition

Differential diagnosis of cognitive impairment

1. D. Subjective cognitive impairment. This woman presents with concerns about her memory but has a normal score on standardized cognitive assessment. This may reflect her high educational level. It would be important to clarify how old her mother was when she was diagnosed with dementia, to guide frequency of follow-up (above 65 years of age suggests the teacher has a 3-fold increased risk, under 65 years suggests the possibility of a stronger genetic risk).

2. C. Mild cognitive impairment. This woman has a below normal score on standardized cognitive assessment but no impairment in activities of daily living. This low score is quite concerning in view of her young age and high educational attainment and she should be referred to a young onset memory clinic for comprehensive investigation.

3. B. Dementia (early onset). This woman has a below normal score on standardized cognitive assessment and impairment in activities of daily living. She should be referred to a young onset memory clinic for comprehensive investigation. In view of her family history, genetic testing and counselling of any children may be considered.

4. E. Depression. This woman has symptoms of a depressive episode of moderate severity. This is likely to account for her cognitive symptoms and loss of marks on cognitive testing.

5. K. Amnesic syndrome. This woman has a specific memory impairment on standardized cognitive assessment. She recently experienced alcohol withdrawal which may have been complicated by unrecognized Wernicke encephalopathy, leaving her now with Korsakoff syndrome. She should be prescribed thiamine, undergo structural brain imaging and options for managing her alcohol use discussed with her. See Chapter 20.

Potentially reversible causes of dementia

1. A. Subdural haematoma. This woman has atrial fibrillation and so is likely to be on warfarin. There should therefore be a low threshold for suspecting an intracranial bleed after minor or no injury. A chronic subdural haematoma as opposed to neurodegenerative cause of dementia is suggested by her relatively quick cognitive deterioration, possible fluctuating conscious level (uncharacteristic afternoon naps), neurological signs and history of head injury. It is not uncommon for there to be a latent period of days to weeks between injury and symptoms. The next step should be brain imaging.

2. C. Normal pressure hydrocephalus. This is suggested by this man's incontinence, ataxia and cognitive impairment, the classic triad of 'wet, wobbly, wacky'. Often this disorder is idiopathic. The next step should be brain imaging.

3. I. Addison disease. This often presents insidiously with fatigue, loss of stamina, weight loss, apathy and memory problems. Postural hypotension is common and is suggested by her dizziness on rising. Hyperpigmentation of the palmar creases and buccal mucosa is often present but easy to miss. Addison disease is rare, so this woman is most likely to be suffering from depression, but it would be important to check urea and electrolytes (hyponatraemia, hyperkalaemia) and glucose (hypoglycaemia) and consider a short synacthen test (diagnostic test).

4. H. Cushing syndrome. This is suggested by the central obesity, amenorrhoea, hypertension, plethoric face and characteristic psychiatric symptoms of low mood and forgetfulness. Glucose is likely to be elevated. The next step would be to refer for a dexamethasone suppression test to confirm the diagnosis.

5. F. Hyperparathyroidism. Hyperparathyroidism causes hypercalcaemia. Mild hypercalcaemia (<3.0 mmol/L) is common in older women and often asymptomatic. Symptoms when present include low mood, abdominal pain, bone pain and renal calculi. Mild memory problems often occur, progressing to a delirium if calcium levels are very high (>3.8 mmol/L). The next step should be to check serum calcium and phosphate.

Subtypes of dementia

1. A. Alzheimer dementia. Medial temporal atrophy is an early change in Alzheimer.

2. B. Vascular dementia. Note this man's multiple vascular risk factors and evidence of cerebrovascular disease on imaging.

3. D. Frontotemporal dementia. This is particularly common in younger adults.

4. E. Lewy body dementia.
5. F. Parkinson disease with dementia. Parkinson disease is associated with an increased risk of dementia.

General feedback: see Table 7.4.

Clinical features in cognitive impairment

1. A. Apraxia (intact motor ability shown by her ability to mimic).
2. C. Aphasia (expressive nominal aphasia).
3. E. Perseveration (receptive aphasia is less likely as she understood the initial instructions).
4. B. Agnosia (visual).
5. B. Agnosia (tactile, also called astereognosia).

General feedback: See Table 7.1.

Chapter 8 The patient with alcohol or substance use problems

1. F. Chronic insufflation ('snorting') of cocaine can cause damage to the nasal septum.
2. G. Ketamine is a potent glutamatergic (NMDA receptor) channel blocker, and is a potent short-acting dissociative anaesthetic. It is legitimately used in veterinary surgery as an anaesthetic agent. It can also be used as an anaesthetic analgesic agent in human medicine.
3. C. Heroin. Intravenous drug use is a major risk factor for bacterial endocarditis, blood-borne virus infection, deep vein thrombosis and injection site cellulitis or abscesses. Other substances on the list can be injected, but heroin is the commonest injected recreational drug.
4. E. Diazepam. Like alcohol, benzodiazepine intoxication and long-term use is associated with memory impairment.
5. I. Buprenorphine is a partial opioid agonist. When taken by an opioid naïve person, it can cause euphoria, sedation, and other symptoms of opioid intoxication. However, when taken by someone who is opioid-dependent and already has a lot of circulating opioid receptor agonists present (e.g., heroin), it can displace these agonists from opioid receptors and cause withdrawal symptoms.

Chapter 9 The patient with psychotic symptoms

Differential diagnosis of psychosis

1. J. Schizophrenia. This man describes the symptom of thought insertion for greater than 1 month. The diagnosis is supported by his age and functional decline prior to the onset of symptoms. Although his mother does not think he misuses substances, it would be important to exclude this by asking the man himself and performing a urine drug screen.
2. I. Schizoaffective disorder. This man has concurrent mood symptoms and first rank symptoms of schizophrenia. His mood and psychotic symptoms are equally prominent, making a recurrent psychotic depression unlikely.
3. C. Depressive episode, severe, with psychotic features. This man has mood symptoms and psychotic symptoms which are not typical of schizophrenia (because they are second rather than third person). The mood symptoms appear to be more prominent than the psychotic symptoms, making schizoaffective disorder unlikely.
4. A. Delusional disorder. This man has a longstanding unshakeable belief arrived at through faulty reasoning: a delusion. He has insight into this. Schizophrenia is unlikely because the delusion is nonbizarre and functioning is intact.
5. F. Personality disorder. This man is not delusional as his belief is not fixed. He is suspicious and litigious. The history from the police of multiple previous calls suggests his difficulties are longstanding. This would be consistent with a paranoid personality disorder. However, a fuller background history would be required to make a definite diagnosis.
6. B. Dementia/delirium. This man has cognitive impairment, functional decline and auditory hallucinations. It is crucial to exclude delirium by clarifying the onset of these symptoms (acute or chronic), by assessing his consciousness level and by completing a full physical examination and basic investigations. Dementia can also be associated with hallucinations. A mood disorder is made less likely by the description of him as 'cheerful'; however, a severe depressive episode could also account for his symptoms. Schizophrenia is unlikely to have such late onset.

Psychosis secondary to a general medical condition or psychoactive substance use

1. G. Neurosyphilis. This is now a rare diagnosis in the UK but should always be considered in those with work or travel histories that may have placed them at risk of contracting syphilis.

Neurosyphilis is a type of tertiary syphilis that emerges several years after initial infection. Clinical features are diverse but can include personality change, grandiose behaviour and dementia, along with upper motor neurone abnormalities such as brisk reflexes and extensor plantars.

2. B. Cerebral tumour. This man is socially disinhibited with a headache suggestive of raised intracranial pressure. The presence of focal neurological signs would further support the diagnosis.

3. L. Vitamin B_{12} deficiency. As a vegan, this woman is at risk of vitamin B_{12} deficiency (which is present only in meat and dairy products). She describes ataxia and paranoia, both of which can be features of vitamin B_{12} deficiency.

4. K. Thiamine deficiency. This man is likely experiencing Wernicke encephalopathy. He is experiencing visual hallucinations and possibly tactile hallucinations of insects beneath the skin (formication). He is ataxic and has nystagmus. Thus, he has the classic triad for Wernicke: confusion, ataxia and ophthalmoplegia. Although this man's alcohol history is unknown, the time course of these symptoms is consistent with the onset of alcohol withdrawal and alcohol use may have predisposed him to being in a road traffic accident.

Mental state examination in psychosis (perceptual disturbance)

1. I. Second-person auditory hallucination.
2. H. Pseudohallucination.
3. B. Extracampine hallucination.
4. L. Visceral hallucination.
5. D. Hypnagogic hallucination.
6. C. Gustatory hallucination.

Mental state examination in psychosis (thought disturbance)

1. I. Persecutory delusion.
2. E. Erotomania.
3. C. Delusion of misidentification (Capgras syndrome).
4. D. Delusion of reference.
5. H. Nihilistic delusion.
6. A. Delusion of control.
7. G. Loosening of associations.

See Table 9.1 for explanation.

Chapter 10 The patient with elated or irritable mood

Differential diagnosis of elevated or irritable mood

1. A. Hypomanic episode. This man describes elated mood with a decreased need for sleep, poor concentration, increased energy, increased recent expenditure and increased libido. It is interfering with his social and occupational functioning, but these activities are not completely disrupted. We are not given information on past mood abnormalities, so the diagnosis of bipolar affective disorder is not appropriate.

2. C. Manic episode with psychotic features. This man has irritable mood, sexual disinhibition and grandiose delusions which have led him to commit an offence and quit his career. Schizophrenia is made less likely by the presence of mood symptoms and disinhibition. It would be important to check a urine drug screen to exclude mania secondary to psychoactive substance use. We are not given information on past mood abnormalities, so the diagnosis of bipolar affective disorder is not appropriate.

3. D. Mixed affective episode. This man shows rapid changes between an elated, low and irritable mood within 24 hours.

4. F. Cyclothymia. This woman describes alternating periods of mild elation and mild depression since early adulthood which do not impact on her functioning.

5. E. Bipolar affective disorder. Current episode mania with psychotic features. This man has a history of depression and now presents with reduced sleep, reduced appetite, psychomotor agitation and a grandiose delusion which has resulted in marked disruption to his occupational function.

Elevated or irritable mood secondary to a general medical condition or psychoactive substance use

1. J. L-dopa. This man probably has Parkinson disease and is likely to be treated with dopaminergic agents such as L-dopa, a precursor to dopamine. Excess dopamine is associated with euphoria, psychosis and a reduction in impulse control. Note it is the treatment rather than Parkinson's disease itself which is associated with these symptoms.

2. L. Amphetamine. Amphetamine intoxication can be associated with an acute psychosis. It is a sympathomimetic and so associated with dilated pupils. Cocaine can have similar effects but is normally smoked or snorted.

3. H. Anabolic steroids. These are commonly used by bodybuilders to increase muscle bulk but can be associated with changes in mood, arousal and cognition.

4. I. Corticosteroids. High dose corticosteroids are often prescribed for severe acute asthma. Mood changes and psychosis are common psychiatric complications of steroid use.

5. G. Hyperthyroidism. This is suggested by tremor, tachycardia and irritability. Substance use is an important differential although her normal pupils make use of a stimulant less likely.

Mental state examination in elevated or irritable mood

1. A. Pressured speech.
2. H. Visual hyperaesthesia. This is an increased intensity of perception.
3. C. Tangential thinking.
4. B. Flight of ideas.
5. D. Poor concentration (or distractibility).
6. J. Visual hallucination. A perception in the absence of a stimulus.

Chapter 11 The patient with low mood
Differential diagnosis of low mood

1. F. Dysthymia. This man describes subsyndromal symptoms of depression which emerged in adulthood and do not significantly interfere with his functioning. The lack of discrete episodes excludes recurrent depressive disorder.

2. A. Mild depressive episode. This woman has two out of three of the core symptoms of depression, poor concentration and poor self-esteem. There are no biological symptoms mentioned. She is able to continue her normal activities, meeting criteria for mild depression.

3. D. Severe depression with psychotic features. This woman has a clear change in functioning from her baseline, psychomotor retardation and what may be olfactory hallucinations of foul smells leading to the secondary delusional belief that her neighbour's drains are clogged. Although her mood is not reported, she is at risk of depression following a bereavement and these hallucinations are typical of severe depression.

4. B. Moderate depression. This man has the three core symptoms of depression and two further symptoms (disturbed sleep and appetite). He is having great difficulty continuing his normal activities, meeting criteria for moderate depression.

5. J. Low mood secondary to psychoactive substance use. This would normally be diagnosed as harmful use of alcohol (see Chapter 20). This man gives a clear history of low mood following alcohol excess. This is impacting upon his mental health and occupational functioning. He is easily able to abstain from drink, indicating he is not dependent.

Low mood secondary to a general medical condition

1. E. Cushing syndrome is an excess of cortisol. It can present with depression or psychosis. Clinical features include obesity, hypertension and easy bruising.

2. A. Huntington disease is an autosomal dominant neurodegenerative disorder beginning in the basal ganglia. Depression is often an early symptom. Increased clumsiness and poor coordination can be subtle early features of the movement disorder which progresses to marked ataxia with choreiform movements. Huntington disease is not always talked about in families and the description of the patient's father is more typical of the course of Huntington than of depression.

3. I. Hypothyroidism is suggested by this woman's fatigue, low mood, dry, thin hair, dry skin and bradycardia.

4. C. Multiple sclerosis would be an important differential. This is suggested by her two neurological symptoms separated in time and place. Depression is common in multiple sclerosis.

Mental state examination in low mood

1. G. Psychomotor agitation. This is a common feature of depression in older adults.

2. I. Negative cognition. When considering the loss of the contract this man has demonstrated Beck's cognitive triad: negative views of himself, the world and the future.

3. C. Reduced range of reactivity (blunted affect). This woman's affect does not vary as would be expected when discussing content of different types.

4. A. Poor self-care. This is particularly concerning as personal appearance is important to this man's job.

5. L. Partial anhedonia. This man reports a markedly reduced interest in all activities with loss of the ability to derive pleasure from most, but not all, activities he previously enjoyed.

Chapter 12 The patient with anxiety, fear or avoidance

Differential diagnosis of anxiety, fear or avoidance

1. C. Social phobia. This man has a generalized social phobia shown by his avoidance of social situations and marked anxiety and distress when in them.

2. D. Generalized anxiety disorder. This lady has experienced continuous anxiety and apprehension about minor matters associated with autonomic overactivity and muscle tension for over 6 months.

3. A. Agoraphobia with panic disorder. This lady had a panic attack in a supermarket and has now become increasingly avoidant of crowding and confinement. Her symptoms are restricted to these situations. The weight loss may well be explained by her reduced dietary intake and increased exercise, but other disorders should be screened for, i.e., hyperthyroidism.

4. E. Panic disorder. This man reports repeated nonsituational panic attacks including a sensation of derealization. His symptoms could be due to cardiac problems but his young age, lack of exercise-induced symptoms and normal ECG are reassuring.

5. C. Social phobia (specific to playing a musical instrument in concert). This man has a social phobia as shown by his situation-specific anxiety and avoidance. This is not a generalized social phobia but is limited to one specific situation. The Diagnostic and Statistical Manual of Mental Disorders, 5th Edition codes for generalized or performance only social phobias whereas ICD-10 does not differentiate.

6. F. Depressive episode. This man has the three core symptoms of depression and two further biological symptoms. His anxiety symptoms are concurrent with his depression so the primary diagnosis is of a depressive disorder rather than an anxiety disorder. Although his symptoms had onset following a traumatic event, they are too prolonged to be an acute stress reaction, too severe to be an adjustment disorder, and he denies two of the three key symptoms of posttraumatic stress disorder (flashbacks, avoidance and hyperarousal).

Anxiety secondary to a general medical condition or psychoactive substance use

1. D. Pheochromocytoma. Although, because of its rarity, this remains an unlikely diagnosis for the scenario, it is the most likely from the options given. The features suggestive of pheochromocytoma are the family history (not always present), hypertension, hyperglycaemia and intermittent episodes of increased catecholamine release. The history alone is not diagnostic: urinary or serum catecholamine assays and imaging of the adrenals would be required.

2. C. Hyperthyroidism. This lady already suffers from one autoimmune disorder (vitiligo) which increases her risk of another (Graves disease). Tremor, heat intolerance, anxiety and increased appetite are classic symptoms of hyperthyroidism.

3. I. Fluoxetine. Selective serotonin reuptake inhibitors can initially be alerting and agitating, particularly in young people. This can increase the risk of suicide in the severely depressed. Use of an alternative antidepressant should be considered.

4. E. Caffeine. Caffeine has anxiogenic effects. Many soft drinks contain large amounts of caffeine.

5. H. Amphetamine. This drug increases concentrations of dopamine and noradrenaline (norepinephrine), leading to increased sympathetic nervous system activation. Cocaine intoxication would give a similar presentation.

Chapter 13 The patient with obsessions and compulsions

Differential diagnosis of obsessions and compulsions

1. B. Obsessive-compulsive disorder. This woman has a greater than 2-week history of both obsessions and compulsions associated with functional impairment.

2. A. No mental illness. This woman is not experiencing obsessions or compulsions. She is responding to external influences and her handwashing may realistically reduce the feared outcome of infection transmission.

3. C. Depressive episode. This woman has the three core symptoms of depression and two further symptoms. Her obsessions and compulsions are concurrent with her depression so the primary diagnosis is of a depressive disorder rather than obsessive-compulsive disorder.

4. D. Phobia. This woman has situation-specific anxiety with avoidance and panic attacks. She does not have obsessional thoughts, rather her anxiety is brought on by external stimuli. Although she washes her hands to reduce her anxiety, it is not a purposeless or excessive action, meaning it is not a compulsion. She is not hypochondriacal as she does not believe she is ill.

5. I. Eating disorder. This woman's low body weight, self-induced weight loss, body image disturbance and amenorrhoea mean she meets criteria for anorexia nervosa. She is not experiencing obsessions as she describes ego-syntonic thoughts which she does not resist. Rather they are over-valued ideas as they are plausible beliefs which have come to dominate her life.

Differentiating types of repetitive or intrusive thoughts

1. B. Obsession. The patient knows the images originate from their mind and is trying to resist (see Table 13.1).

2. F. Over-valued idea. The fear of infection is logical but held with undue importance. It is not an obsession as it is not viewed as abnormal or resisted (see Table 13.1).

3. C. Rumination (see Table 13.1).

4. D. Pseudohallucination (see Table 13.1).

5. E. Hallucination (see Table 13.1).

6. H. Thought insertion (see Table 13.1).

7. G. Delusion (strictly, a delusional perception). This belief is fixed, was arrived at illogically, and is not amenable to reason. The patient experienced a normal perception but interpreted it with delusional meaning, termed a 'delusional perception'. This is a first rank symptom of schizophrenia.

Chapter 14 The patient with a reaction to a stressful event

Dissociative disorders

1. D. This woman appears to be suffering from functional seizures. This is suggested by the chronological association with a significant stressor (being told that she will be left alone when her husband starts work). These are often more common in those with a family or personal history of epilepsy.

2. G. This is a classic presentation of a dissociative fugue, or 'fugue state'. The man is unable to recount any personal details and appears to have travelled from a distant city. Note the possible severe stressor of being involved with a company that has recently been bankrupted.

3. B. Dissociative anaesthesia. This is suggested by the chronological association with a significant stressor, the nondermatomal distribution of signs and the otherwise normal neurological exam.

4. I. Dissociation secondary to psychoactive substance use. Given the history of onset, and the fact that she was at a party the previous evening, initial consideration should be given to substance-induced dissociation. Common substances associated with this include ketamine and tranquillizers; however, it can also occur following ingestion of less common substances such as mescaline or peyote.

Diagnosis following stressful events

1. E. Bereavement response. Note the chronological proximity to his death, and that the psychotic content features her husband.

2. K. Musculoskeletal injury. Note the distribution of injuries and given the fact he was a driver (in the UK, the driver's seatbelt crosses the right shoulder) this is likely to be a whiplash/seatbelt-related injury. There is no suggestion of psychogenic origin in this case.

3. B. PTSD is the likely diagnosis in this case. Note the hyperarousal, avoidance and nightmares. Also note the persistent duration of the symptoms.

4. J. These symptoms are fairly typical of temporal lobe epilepsy. Note the history of likely head injury (implied by the fact she was referred from the neurosurgical unit). She should be referred for electroencephalogram.

Chapter 15 The patient with medically unexplained physical symptoms

Diagnosis of medically unexplained physical symptoms

1. B. Body dysmorphic disorder.

2. A. This is highly suggestive of Munchausen syndrome by proxy. The safety of the child should be the immediate concern.

3. E. This is a first rank symptom of schizophrenia.

4. I. Psychotic depression (Cotard syndrome).

5. H. Malingering. While more information would ideally be required, this scenario is suggestive of malingering.

Chapter 16 The patient with eating or weight problems

Psychiatric causes of low weight

1. A. This man with schizophrenia may not be able to look after himself due to negative symptoms of schizophrenia impairing his motivation and executive function. His mother may have been providing substantial support with meal

preparation. He needs a functional assessment by an occupational therapist. It is also important to exclude depression, alcohol or substance misuse, or psychotic symptoms as an alternative cause for his weight loss.

2. D. Even though he has told you that he is fine, it is likely that he is suffering from bulimia nervosa. Both hypokalaemia and swollen parotid glands can be caused by excessive vomiting. The hypokalaemia is probably responsible for the U waves on the ECG.

3. I. This girl describes classic obsessive-compulsive symptoms: obsession (fear of infection); compulsion (having to prepare food in a specific manner), with awareness that it is irrational, but severe anxiety if the compulsion is not used to 'cancel out' the obsession.

4. B. Despite this woman's history of anorexia nervosa, her current presentation is not suggestive of relapse. She appears to have developed a specific phobia (with panic attacks) of vomiting, which has probably resulted from her recent physical illness (norovirus, the 'winter vomiting bug'). The link between the two could be understood as an example of psychological 'conditioning'.

5. G. The cause of weight loss in this case does not suggest any concern with body shape. Instead, this man appears not to be eating food because of a delusional belief that the food would be poisoned. He is suffering from an acute psychotic episode. More information is needed to make a diagnosis of schizophrenia or psychotic depression. Assessing for substance use is crucial.

Physical consequences of eating disorders

1. A. Lanugo
2. B. Caries
3. E. Onychorrhexis
4. J. Striae distensae
5. D. Russell's sign

General feedback: xerosis is dry skin, alopecia areata is spot baldness and acrocyanosis is blueness of the extremities. All of these signs can occur in anorexia nervosa. Cheilitis is inflammation of the lips, which can occur in bulimia or anorexia when associated with vomiting

Chapter 17 The patient with personality problems

Diagnosis of personality disorder

1. G. Histrionic personality disorder.
2. H. Dependent personality disorder.
3. A. Paranoid personality disorder.
4. F. Narcissistic personality disorder.
5. I. Avoidant (anxious) personality disorder.

General feedback: see Table 17.1

Traits of personality disorder

1. E. Over-concern with physical attractiveness.
2. C. Consistent preference for solitary activities. This differs from avoidant (anxious) personality disorder in that the latter tend to avoid social activities for fear of rejection or criticism, while the former appear to lack any real desire for social activities.
3. D. Perfectionism that interferes with task completion.
4. B. Excessive sensitivity to setbacks and rebuffs.
5. G. Allowing others to make the most of one's important life decisions. Note that 'Frantic efforts to avoid real or imagined abandonment' is a trait of borderline personality disorder. A trait of dependent personality disorder is the preoccupation with being abandoned rather than the frantic attempts to avoid it. Be aware that the disorders commonly overlap or exist together.

General feedback: see Table 17.1

Chapter 18 The patient with neurodevelopmental problems

Functional estimation of IQ in intellectual disability

1. D. This lady has a mild intellectual disability and will have an estimated IQ of 50–69. Individuals in this group represent the majority (85%) of all people with intellectual disabilities.
2. A. From the information given, this gentleman manages to live alone without support. His symptoms suggest that he may suffer from an autism spectrum disorder. His interests would suggest that he has above-average intelligence (IQ > 100).
3. G. This boy has a profound intellectual disability (IQ < 20). He is unable to care for himself and fully dependent on the support of others.
4. E. This woman has a moderate intellectual disability (IQ 35–49). She is able to live on her own, albeit in a supported housing complex with a great deal of support.
5. F. This gentleman has a severe intellectual disability (IQ 20–34). He lives with his family, who are his main carers and is able to perform simple tasks under supervision. His self-care skills are limited, but sometimes he seems able to contribute to these.

Differential diagnosis in adults presenting for attention deficit hyperactivity disorder (ADHD) assessment

1 B. Bipolar affective disorder. Her symptoms may represent hypomanic episodes. ADHD is excluded by the episodic nature of the symptoms. A urine drug screen would be helpful to support her report of no substance abuse.

2 J. Substance abuse, harmful. His behaviour while not under the influence of substances for a period of at least six months needs to be assessed before a diagnosis of ADHD can be considered. Cocaine use may well lead to making careless mistakes at work. His history of possibly having ADHD symptoms from childhood is not relevant unless he has on-going symptoms now.

3 C. Depressive episode. The acute onset of these symptoms excludes ADHD. Irritability and psychomotor agitation are common in depression.

4 A. ADHD. A fuller history would be needed to make this diagnosis definitive. However, ADHD is suggested by his problems with impulsivity and inattention present during childhood and adulthood. Dissocial personality disorder is unlikely as the assault sounds impulsive and he is now regretful of this.

5 I. Traumatic brain injury. This would need to be confirmed by checking the details of his injuries in the road traffic accident. ADHD is excluded by the lack of significant difficulties prior to the accident. He may be suffering neuropsychological sequelae post damage to his frontal lobes.

Chapter 19 Dementia and delirium

Management of dementia

1. A. Donepezil. This woman has mild to moderate dementia for which cholinesterase inhibitors are recommended. Donepezil is first line.

2. D. Memantine. This woman has severe dementia for which memantine is recommended.

3. D. Memantine. This woman has mild to moderate dementia for which cholinesterase inhibitors are recommended. However, she has a number of relative contraindications to cholinesterase inhibitor use. Their cholinergic effects can induce bradycardia, which may be particularly problematic in those with conduction defects. Similarly, cholinergic drugs can cause bronchoconstriction, which may be problematic in COPD and asthma. Cholinergic drugs can also increase gastric acid secretions, which could worsen peptic ulceration. Overall, it would probably be better to try memantine first for this woman.

4. B. Rivastigmine. This is the cholinesterase inhibitor with the best evidence for maintaining cognition in Parkinson disease with dementia and Lewy body dementia, although other cholinesterase inhibitors are also of benefit.

5. I. No treatment recommended by current guidelines. Unfortunately, no medications have yet been found to slow the progression of frontotemporal dementia.

Chapter 20 Alcohol and substance-related disorders

Pharmacological management of opioid dependence

1. A. It is likely that this man has overdosed on intravenous opioids, leading to respiratory depression and a reduced consciousness level. Naloxone is an opioid antagonist and needs to be given to reverse toxicity. Naltrexone is also an opioid antagonist, but it needs to be given orally so is not suitable for someone with a low GCS (risk of aspiration).

2. E. Lofexidine can be helpful in reducing the unpleasant symptoms of opioid withdrawal. It would not be advisable to prescribe benzodiazepines to someone who already has substance dependence.

3. H. While methadone, buprenorphine and dihydrocodeine are used as substitution therapy, this lady's heavy use of heroin means that she is likely to have severe withdrawal symptoms. As a partial opioid agonist, buprenorphine is likely to precipitate a withdrawal state given the magnitude of her usage. There is some evidence to suggest that dihydrocodeine can be as effective as methadone. However, because it is in tablet form, it is easier to divert and its use is therefore not widespread. Levacetylmethadol is a synthetic opioid similar to methadone, which is no longer prescribed due to dangerous arrhythmias.

4. G. This man could benefit from loperamide, which is a mu-opioid receptor agonist that acts only in the large intestine to reduce gut motility (and hence diarrhoea).

5. F. Naltrexone is an opioid receptor antagonist that can be used to reduce the euphoric effects of opioids. Naloxone would also have this effect, but it needs to be given parenteral and is short-acting, and therefore naltrexone is preferred.

Prochaska and DiClemente Transtheoretical Model of Change

1. C. Preparation.

2. G. Termination.

3. A. Precontemplative.

4. E. Contemplative.

5. B. Relapse.

General feedback: see Fig. 20.3

Treatment of alcohol dependence

1. B. Lorazepam. Given that benzodiazepines are metabolized in the liver and that impaired liver function can delay metabolism and excretion, drugs with a long half-life can accumulate and increase the risk of toxicity. From the three benzodiazepines listed, lorazepam has the shortest half-life and is therefore safest to use for detoxification in this case. Oxazepam is often used for the same reason.

2. E. Thiamine. From the history given, this lady is not intoxicated. She appears to be suffering from the triad of symptoms associated with Wernicke encephalopathy and needs urgent treatment with parenteral thiamine.

3. H. CBT, focusing on identifying cues and preventing relapse, could be very helpful for this lady. Motivational interviewing, with a focus on 'promoting change', may not be so useful as she is already abstinent. Psychoeducation tends to happen in groups and because she is not keen on this, there is a risk of early disengagement.

4. I. Acamprosate may be helpful in reducing cravings. Naltrexone is also thought to reduce cravings, but it is likely to reduce the efficacy of the tramadol.

5. A. Alcoholics Anonymous is a 12-step mutual programme that could be useful for this man. It is not run by health services, and consists of self-funded groups. Their ethos is one of complete abstinence and their system of peer support (or 'sponsorship') can be very beneficial for some.

Chapter 21 The psychotic disorders: schizophrenia

Antipsychotic choice in schizophrenia

1. B. Haloperidol. Although haloperidol is not first line for schizophrenia, patient preference is important in the choice of antipsychotic. She should have an electrocardiogram before recommencing as haloperidol can prolong the QTc.

2. F. Aripiprazole. This is the antipsychotic least likely to be associated with weight gain and the metabolic syndrome. First-generation antipsychotics would be the next best choice.

3. E. Quetiapine. From the options given, haloperidol, risperidone and chlorpromazine are most likely to be associated with extrapyramidal side-effects. Aripiprazole is less associated with extrapyramidal side-effects, but quetiapine has an even lower likelihood. Flupentixol is a depot medication and the majority of patients prefer oral. Clozapine is not indicated as the patient is not treatment resistant.

4. C. Flupentixol depot formulation. Long-acting intramuscular injections (depot formulations) administered 1–12 weekly are a good option for patients with poor concordance.

5. D. Clozapine. This woman has treatment-resistant schizophrenia as she has had two trials of antipsychotic at adequate doses for adequate durations, including at least one second-generation drug.

Presentation of antipsychotic side-effects

1. C. Hypersalivation. This is most commonly seen with clozapine. Most antipsychotics cause a dry mouth.

2. B. Postural hypotension. This is a side-effect of most antipsychotics, secondary to adrenergic receptor blockade.

3. J. Hyperprolactinaemia, causing galactorrhoea. This is a side-effect of most but not all antipsychotics, secondary to D_2 receptor blockade in the tuberoinfundibular pathway.

4. E. Agranulocytosis. Without monitoring, this is seen in just under 1% of patients taking clozapine.

5. G. Akathisia. This is frequent purposeless movement associated with a subjective inner restlessness. It is very unpleasant for patients, and a risk factor for suicide. It is a side-effect of most antipsychotics and some other psychotropics also. High doses are a risk factor.

Chapter 22 The mood (affective) disorders

Treatment setting for depression

1. A. Admission to psychiatric hospital. This man is at high risk of suicide because of his age, sex, violent method of planned suicide, final acts and mental disorder. The extremely high suicidal intent indicated by the circumstances of his presentation means hospital admission is the only safe management option.

2. D. Refer to psychiatric outpatients routinely. A psychiatric referral is advisable given his treatment-resistant depression. There is no suggestion of acute risk to necessitate an urgent referral.

3. F. Refer to crisis team. Even without evidence of risk to self or others, psychotic features are suggestive of a very severe depression that could worsen rapidly.

4. A. Admit to psychiatric hospital. This man has depression with poor oral intake. This is not manageable in the community. He needs an urgent physical examination and blood samples evaluation. If his renal function is acutely impaired, he may need transfer to a general hospital for intravenous fluids. If this man is in a general hospital at the time of mental health assessment, he should be physically assessed prior to transfer.

5. C. Manage in primary care. The next step for this man is to consider a higher intensity psychological intervention or an antidepressant.

First-line antidepressants

1. D. Mirtazapine. SSRIs increase risk of bleeding when coprescribed with nonsteroidals and anticoagulants. Mirtazapine is suggested as an alternative first-line antidepressant by NICE (2009).

2. A. SSRI. NICE (2009) recommends SSRIs as first-line antidepressants if there are no cautions.

3. A. SSRI. NICE (2009) recommends SSRIs as first-line antidepressants. Sleep disturbance often resolves as depression improves. A more sedating antidepressant such as mirtazapine would be a good second-line option.

4. D. Mirtazapine. Although first line, SSRIs often cause sexual dysfunction. If avoidance of this side-effect is very important to patients, an alternative such as mirtazapine can be considered.

5. C. Duloxetine. Duloxetine is licensed for both stress incontinence and depression. It is a joint serotonin and noradrenaline (norepinephrine) reuptake inhibitor. This action in the spinal cord leads to increased tone in the urethral sphincter. It would be reasonable to try to avoid polypharmacy by using one drug to treat both problems.

Chapter 23 The anxiety and somatoform disorders

Management of posttraumatic stress disorder

1. D. Eye movement desensitization and reprocessing therapy. This or trauma-focused CBT is recommended for moderate to severe PTSD even if the trauma occurred less than 4 weeks ago.

2. B. Watchful waiting. This is recommended for symptoms of mild PTSD within 4 weeks of the trauma.

3. D. Eye movement desensitization and reprocessing therapy. This or trauma-focused CBT is recommended for all severities of PTSD where the trauma occurred more than 4 weeks ago.

4. F. SSRI. Mirtazapine or paroxetine are recommended as first-line medications for PTSD.

5. G. TCA. Amitriptyline (a tricyclic antidepressant) and phenelzine (monoamine oxidase inhibitor) are second-line drug therapies for PTSD.

Management of generalized anxiety disorder and panic disorder

1. C. CBT. First-line therapy for moderate to severe panic disorder is CBT.

2. A. Self-help. First-line therapy for mild panic disorder is self-help materials.

3. E. Applied relaxation. This and CBT are the two psychological therapies recommended for moderate to severe generalized anxiety disorder.

4. F. SSRI. First-line drug therapy for moderate to severe generalized anxiety disorder is an SSRI.

5. I. Pregabalin. This is a second-line drug therapy for moderate to severe generalized anxiety disorder.

Chapter 24 Eating disorders

Treatment strategies for patients with eating disorders

1. J. Informal admission to general psychiatric ward. It would appear that this lady has developed a comorbid depressive illness. Her eating appears to have been improving. Therapeutic priority should be given to managing her depressive symptoms and her high risk of completing suicide. From the options listed, the most appropriate would be an informal admission to a general psychiatric ward. Outpatient or home treatment may be considered; however, given the levels of risk involved, admission to hospital would probably be more appropriate.

2. E. NICE recommends cognitive-behavioural therapy as the first-line intervention for bulimia nervosa. Initially, this should be delivered via guided self-help but if this is ineffective or inappropriate, then therapist-guided individual cognitive-behavioural therapy is recommended.

3. K. This girl is incredibly unwell, and her current physical condition poses a threat to her life. By virtue of her mental illness, and probably also her state of malnutrition, she clearly lacks capacity to make decisions regarding her healthcare. Immediate hospital treatment is required, and she should be transferred urgently under mental health legislation. In addition,

given her persistent refusal to eat, and her lack of capacity and insight, it is likely that involuntary nasogastric feeding will be required to save her life. This is both a clinically and medicolegally difficult situation and should be managed by a specialist.

4. E.   Cognitive-behavioural therapy (eating disorder focused). This is one of the first-line psychological therapies recommended by NICE (2017) for managing anorexia. Although this women's difficulties with relationships may suggest interpersonal therapy, this is not currently recommended for management of eating disorders.

5. G.   Family therapy; This boy lives in a family in which both parents are high-achievers, and subsequently feels pressured to live up to their expectations. Family therapy is likely to be useful in this case and is the first-line treatment recommended by NICE (2017) for anorexia in adolescents.

Chapter 25 The sleep–wake disorders
Diagnosis of sleep–wake disorders

1. I.   REM sleep behaviour disorder. This commonly presents in middle-aged men. Details of the dream are recalled. It is closely linked with synucleinopathies.

2. G.   Non-REM sleep arousal disorder. Sleepwalking and sleep terrors are both subtypes of non-REM sleep arousal disorders. Sufferers are disorientated on waking. The two subtypes are closely linked and run in families.

3. J.   Sleep-related breathing disorder. This increases the risk of road traffic accidents several fold. Obesity increases risk for it, and hypertension can arise as a consequence. His wife's account of snoring is suggestive of upper airway obstruction, but he would need further investigation to confirm the diagnosis.

4. C.   Insomnia secondary to psychiatric disorder. This history is suggestive of mania, likely secondary to bipolar disorder.

5. F.   Narcolepsy. This history is suggestive of cataplexy. Intrusive daytime sleepiness is the other core symptom of narcolepsy.

Chapter 26 The psychosexual disorders
Medication associated with psychosexual disorders

1. B.   Fluoxetine. Selective serotonin reuptake inhibitors are commonly associated with anorgasmia. Mirtazapine is the antidepressant

least likely to be associated with sexual side-effects.

2. E.   Propranolol. Antihypertensives including β-blockers can result in erectile dysfunction.

3. G.   Ropinirole is a dopamine agonist. Paraphilia is a rare side-effect of dopamine agonists.

4. I.   Trazodone. Priapism is a very rare side-effect of any drug which blocks α-adrenergic receptors.

Chapter 27 Disorders relating to the menstrual cycle, pregnancy and the puerperium
Management of mental illness in the puerperium

1. C.   This woman may benefit from maternal skills teaching. The health visitor can be an invaluable resource for providing this.

2. E.   This woman appears to be suffering from the 'baby blues'. Simple reassurance should be given. This will likely pass after 10 days or so, but follow-up is important to ensure that she is not developing postnatal depression.

3. F.   This woman appears to be developing a puerperal psychosis. Given her symptoms, the use of an antipsychotic medication is indicated. Olanzapine is widely used for puerperal psychosis. Electroconvulsive therapy may be required if she does not respond to pharmacological treatment. These interventions would need to be delivered on an inpatient basis, preferably in a mother-and-baby psychiatric unit.

4. H.   This woman is likely to have a severe postnatal depressive illness. Given her presentation and her poor oral intake, her illness should be considered to be potentially life-threatening. Electroconvulsive therapy should be considered.

5. B.   This woman is likely to be suffering a depressive episode with some functional impairment suggesting it is of moderate severity. The National Institute for Health and Care Excellence (NICE; 2014) recommends she should be offered antidepressant medication or a high-intensity psychological intervention (e.g., cognitive-behavioural therapy). Should she wish to start an antidepressant, sertraline is a good choice as very little is excreted in breast milk. Doxepin should be avoided in breastfeeding mothers but in general tricyclics are probably safe in breastfeeding. She may also benefit from referral to the health visitor for support with breastfeeding.

Psychotropic medication in pregnancy

1. I.   Both carbamazepine and sodium valproate are associated with the development of neural tube defects. It is not recommended to prescribe carbamazepine or sodium valproate to women of childbearing age, and less teratogenic alternatives should be considered. If it is considered absolutely necessary (e.g., treatment-resistant mania), reliable contraception is essential.

2. B.   Olanzapine is associated with an increased risk of gestational diabetes. It should be prescribed with caution in all pregnant women, and alternatives should be used in women who are already at increased risk of gestational diabetes (e.g., obesity, gestational diabetes during previous pregnancy, strong family history of diabetes). In any case, blood and/or urinary glucose should be regularly monitored.

3. F.   The use of lithium during pregnancy has been associated with an increased risk of fetal heart defects, including but not limited to Ebstein anomaly (displacement of the opening of the tricuspid valve). Cardiac abnormalities occur in around 1 in 100 live births, increasing twofold to 2 in 100 live births in children exposed to lithium. There is a dose–response effect, with higher doses associated with greater risk. This risk needs to be balanced against the risk of relapse of illness associated with discontinuation of lithium, as untreated affective/psychotic illness can place the fetus at greatly increased risk.

4. H.   A class effect of selective serotonin reuptake inhibitors taken in the third trimester is an increased risk of persistent neonatal pulmonary hypertension (absolute risk increased from 1 in 1000 to 3 in 1000 live births). This needs to be balanced against the risk of untreated anxiety or depression on the developing fetus.

5. F.   Lithium. Lithium levels should be checked every 4 weeks during pregnancy. Physiological changes during pregnancy mean doses have to be increased on average by 50% during the third trimester to remain within the therapeutic range.

Chapter 28 The personality disorders
Management of patients with personality disorders

1. F.   Encourage to engage with existing care plan. Patients with dependent personality disorder can quickly become institutionalized, and alternatives to admission should be preferred. In this case, the lady should be empathically reassured, and encouraged to engage with her occupational therapist.

2. C.   Informal, time-limited admission to psychiatric ward. She is clearly distressed and—in the short term—at incredibly high risk of completing suicide or otherwise harming herself. It would also appear that there is no safe place to which she could be discharged. A short 'crisis' admission to a psychiatric ward, of agreed duration and with clear goals and boundaries, would allow for her distress and short-term risk to be managed, and longer-term support organized. Discharging her to police custody is not appropriate.

3. H.   It may be worth offering this gentleman a trial of antipsychotic medication. While psychotherapeutic measures would be more likely to be effective in the long term, he appears to be untrusting of services, and it would be unlikely that he would engage with this. A small dose of an antipsychotic may be enough to reduce his paranoia to the extent that he may engage with a psychotherapist and may also provide a reason for ongoing contact with doctors such that trust and rapport can be established.

4. A.   Weekly dispensing. Depression arising in patients with personality disorders can be amenable to drug treatment; however, the benefits of this need to be balanced with the risk of overdosing on potentially harmful drugs. Antidepressants dispensed on a weekly/twice-weekly/three times weekly/daily basis can, to some degree, modify this risk.

5. I.   This gentleman could benefit from lifestyle advice. His situation has recently changed, which may explain his increased anxiety. However, it is likely that his caffeine consumption is contributing to his insomnia, and that smoking cigarettes all night is perpetuating the problem. Advice regarding caffeine, nicotine, diet and exercise should be given in the first instance.

Chapter 29 The neurodevelopmental disorders
Psychosocial interventions in neurodevelopmental disorders

1. F.   Parent-training/education programme is first line for children of school age.

2. E.   Nil recommended. Although cognitive-behavioural therapy may be helpful in adults with ADHD, particularly in those with residual symptoms after medication, there is insufficient evidence for NICE to currently recommend its standalone use as first line.

3. G.   Play-based social–communication intervention. First-line intervention for children of school age with ASD.

4. H.   Social learning program. First-line intervention for adults with ASD.

5. D.   Habit control. Psychoeducation, habit control or exposure and response prevention are recommended first line for Tourette syndrome.

Chapter 30 Child and adolescent psychiatry

Diagnosis of psychiatric disorders with onset in childhood or adolescence

1. A.   Academic setting inappropriate to ability. While many of the behaviours are suggestive of the core symptoms of ADHD, note that they appear to be limited to the academic setting (he appears fine at home). ADHD is pervasive rather than situational, and this case is suggestive that the boy may be having difficulties with schoolwork (either because it is too difficult or too easy).

2. G.   Oppositional defiant disorder is similar to conduct disorder in that behaviour is negativistic, rebellious, defiant and disruptive. However, unlike conduct disorder, the behaviour associated with oppositional defiant disorder does not violate the rights of others and troubles with the law are less common.

3. H.   Reactive attachment disorder. This is suggested by the child's history of abuse, marked fearfulness and social withdrawal. The diagnosis is not child abuse alone, as not all children who are abused respond in this way or go on to experience mental disorder.

4. I.   Separation anxiety disorder. This is suggested by the child's fear of removal from a major attachment figure, triggered by a time apart. She is more anxious about this than would be expected of a 10-year-old. She is experiencing somatic symptoms of anxiety.

5. F.   Elective mutism. This is suggested by the child's normal language development and ability to speak in some situations. Elective mutism often follows emotional trauma (such as separation from parents, war, severe illness) and situations where there is conflict at home.

Chapter 31 Older adult psychiatry

Adverse drug reactions in older adults receiving psychotropic medication

1. C.   Diazepam. Abruptly discontinuing benzodiazepines can result in withdrawal symptoms. These can have onset within a day of stopping a short-acting benzodiazepine (e.g., lorazepam) or up to 3 weeks for a longer acting drug (e.g., diazepam). Symptoms include insomnia, anxiety, anorexia, tremor, perspiration, tinnitus and perceptual disturbances. such as this woman's visual illusion.

2. H.   Fluoxetine. All antidepressants, but particularly selective serotonin reuptake inhibitors, can be associated with the syndrome of inappropriate secretion of antidiuretic hormone, leading to hyponatraemia. This is particularly likely in older adults.

3. A.   Lithium. Lithium can induce nephrogenic diabetes insipidus, leading to hypernatraemia if fluid intake cannot be maintained, e.g., due to diarrhoea and vomiting. Dehydration increases the risk of lithium toxicity (which is renally excreted) so a random lithium level should also be urgently checked for this man.

4. J.   Haloperidol. This man is likely to have received haloperidol to manage his delirium. Haloperidol can cause prolongation of the QT interval. In extreme cases this can lead to torsade de pointes. Olanzapine is less likely to have this side-effect.

5. G.   Amitriptyline. Anticholinergic medication is a big risk factor for delirium. Amitriptyline is often prescribed for neuropathic pain.

Chapter 32 Forensic psychiatry

Diagnosis of mental disorder in offenders

1. A.   This man has delusional jealousy. He is convinced that his partner is being unfaithful, despite extensive reassurances and evidence to the contrary. The name 'Othello syndrome' is derived from the play Othello by William Shakespeare, in which the protagonist murders his wife (Desdemona. which means 'the unfortunate' in Greek). Othello syndrome is associated with alcohol misuse and violence. Treatment includes antipsychotic medication and psychotherapy; however, given the very poor prognosis, it is often said that the most effective treatment is 'geographical' (i.e., relocation of the spouse to a distant area).

2. K.   The symptoms present in this man (delusions and hallucinations) are suggestive of a paranoid psychotic state. Given his age, the implied rapid onset of symptoms and the fact that he has no psychiatric history, this is unlikely to be a first presentation of paranoid schizophrenia. The fact that he has been at a music festival should be a pointer that substances may be implicated in his presentation. His symptoms are not typical

of an alcohol-withdrawal delirium; however, this is an important differential.

3. D. This lady is likely to be suffering from a manic illness. She has grandiose delusions (that she is a pop star). Note that she has recently been hospitalized with a depressive illness: her mania may be associated with drug treatment or may signify the presence of a bipolar illness. Crimes related to mania include financial offences and occasionally aggression.

4. C. The nature of this crime (killing a man in retribution for a mistake in making a sandwich) is alarming. The fact this man has an extensive forensic history, is actively involved with organized crime and appears cold and emotionless in the face of

a crime of such magnitude is strongly suggestive of dissocial/antisocial personality disorder. It could be that the man also scores highly on the Hare Psychopathy Checklist Revised (the 'gold standard' for assessing psychopathy). Further assessment would be required to confirm this diagnosis.

5. J. There is an association between fire-setting and mild intellectual disability. This should be differentiated from arson (deliberate fire-raising for secondary gain, e.g., insurance money), pyromania (compulsion to set fires, followed by a 'release of tension'), wilful destruction of property (e.g., in antisocial personality disorder) or fire-setting driven by other mental disorders.

Affect Affect refers to the transient ebb and flow of emotion in response to particular stimuli, for example, smiling at a joke or crying at a sad memory. It is assessed by observing the patient's posture, facial expression, emotional reactivity and speech. The two components that should be assessed are the appropriateness of the affect and its range. See Chapter 1.

Anxiety Anxiety is a mood state. It is a response to an unknown, internal or vague threat. This is distinct from fear, which is defined later. The experience of anxiety consists of both apprehensive or nervous thoughts and the awareness of a physical reaction to anxiety. See Chapter 12.

Attempted suicide An episode of deliberate self-harm, which did not end in death but was driven by suicidal intent. This is in contrast to episodes of nonfatal deliberate self-harm driven by other motivations. See Chapter 6.

Capacity Capacity is the ability of an individual to make their own decisions. See Chapter 4.

Circumstantiality Circumstantiality describes over-inclusive speech that is delayed in reaching its final goal. This is because of excessive detail and diversion. However, the final goal will be reached, which distinguishes it from flight of ideas. Circumstantiality can be found in the normal population but is increased in anxiety disorders and hypomania. See Chapter 9.

Compulsions Compulsions can be defined as repetitive mental operations (such as counting) or physical acts (such as checking) that a patient feels compelled to perform in response to their own obsessions. The motivation for compulsions is the reduction of anxiety generated by an obsession. The compulsion may be either unrelated to the preceding obsession (e.g., counting) or an unnecessarily excessive response to the obsession (e.g., handwashing). See Chapter 13.

Delusion A delusion is the most severe form of an abnormal idea. It is a fixed belief arrived at illogically and is not amenable to reason. It is not accepted in the patient's cultural background. The presence of a delusion signifies a psychotic disorder. See Chapter 9.

Delusional perception Experiencing a normal perception but interpreting it with delusional meaning. For example, 'I heard the clock chime and I knew that meant the aliens were planning to kill me'. This is a first-rank symptom of schizophrenia. See Chapter 9.

Depersonalization Depersonalization is feeling yourself to be strange or unreal.

Derealization Derealization is feeling that external reality is strange or unreal.

Depression A depressed mood is when a patient describes feeling depressed, sad, dejected, despondent or low. A depressive disorder is a specific psychiatric condition diagnosed if the mood change is sufficiently severe and chronic and occurs with other symptoms.

Dissociation Dissociation is an altered state of consciousness in which normally integrated experiences or processes are disrupted. For example, walking to work on 'autopilot' and not noticing a new shop front – the sensory information has not been integrated with the conscious experience. Depersonalization and derealization are dissociative symptoms (see definitions above). Extreme dissociative states can be associated with disorders including non-epileptic seizures and fugue. See Chapter 14.

Dysphasia Dysphasia is an impairment of language abilities despite intact sensory and motor function. See Chapter 7.

Dyspraxia Dyspraxia is an impairment of the ability to carry out skilled motor movements despite intact motor function. See Chapter 7.

Dysgnosia Dysgnosia is an impairment in the ability to interpret sensory information despite intact sensory organ function. See Chapter 7.

Echolalia Echolalia is when a patient senselessly repeats words or phrases that have been spoken near them. It can be viewed either as a form of disorganized thinking or as an abnormality of speech. It occurs in a range of psychiatric conditions such as schizophrenic catatonia, autism and dementia.

Fear Fear, similar to anxiety, is an alerting signal in response to a potential threat. It differs from anxiety in that it is a response to a known, external or definite object. Anxiety and fear are discussed on Chapter 12.

First-rank symptoms First-rank symptoms were described by Schneider who suggested that the presence of one or more first-rank symptoms, in the absence of organic disease, was sufficient to diagnose schizophrenia. These symptoms still feature strongly in modern diagnostic criteria for schizophrenia. See Chapter 9.

Flight of ideas Flight of ideas can be described as either a disorder of thought form or an abnormality of speech. It describes thinking that is markedly accelerated and results in a stream of loosely connected concepts. The link between concepts can be normal, tenuous or through puns and clanging. It differs from circumstantiality in that the links between concepts are more tenuous and the final goal is less likely to be reached. In its extreme form, speech can become unintelligible or approach the incoherent thought disorder of schizophrenia. See Chapter 9.

Functional symptoms Functional symptoms are physical symptoms without identifiable physiological or structural cause. They may arise due to dysfunction of high-level cortical processing of motor and sensory information. They are genuinely experienced, involuntary and not necessarily related to past or current trauma. See Chapter 14.

Hallucination Hallucinations are perceptions that occur in the absence of external stimuli and are indistinguishable from normal sensation. See Chapter 9.

Illusion Illusions are misperceptions of real external stimuli. For example, spots on the carpet are perceived as insects. Illusions can occur in healthy people particularly when tired, not concentrating, experiencing strong emotions or intoxicated with substances.

Insight Insight describes a patient's understanding of the nature and degree of his or her mental illness and the recognition of the need for treatment. An assessment of insight is an integral part of the mental state examination. See Chapter 1.

Mood Mood is sustained emotion over a period. This differs from a 'feeling', which is a short-lived experience, and 'affect', which is the external expression of transient emotion.

Neologism Neologism is an example of disorganized thinking. It is a new word created by the patient, often combining syllables. It is classically associated with schizophrenia and can also occur in organic brain disorder. They also arise in popular culture, for example, 'webinar' (a seminar on the Web) or 'staycation' (staying at home for a vacation).

Obsession An obsession is an involuntary thought, image or impulse, which is recurrent, intrusive, unpleasant and enters the mind against conscious resistance. Patients recognize that the thoughts are a product of their own mind even though they are involuntary and repugnant. See Chapter 13.

Over-valued idea An over-valued idea is an incorrect belief that is not impossible (in contrast to some schizophrenic delusions), is held with marked emotional investment but not with unshakable conviction. See Chapter 9.

Panic attack Panic attacks are discrete episodes of short-lived (usually less than 1 hour), intense anxiety. They have an abrupt onset and rapidly build up to a peak level of anxiety. They are accompanied by strong autonomic

symptoms, which may lead patients to believe that they are dying, having a heart attack or going mad. See Chapter 12.

Paranoia Paranoia has a range of meanings. Strictly it means that someone is falsely relating things to themselves [e.g., fears that someone wishes to harm them (persecutory delusions, feelings that the TV/radio/Internet is specifically designed to communicate with them (delusions of reference)]. It is used by lay people to mean that someone feels persecuted or at risk 'I've felt awfully paranoid recently, I don't feel safe outside'. Paranoid schizophrenia is a subtype of schizophrenia.

Perseveration Perseveration is when a patient inappropriately repeats an initially correct action. For example, unnecessarily repeating a word or phrase, or applying the rules of one task to a second task.

Pseudohallucinations Pseudohallucinations are perceptions that occur in the absence of external stimuli but are experienced in the internal world rather than the external world. For example, hearing a voice 'inside my head'. See Chapter 9.

Psychosis Psychosis is the presence of hallucinations, delusions or thought disorder.

Psychotherapy Psychotherapy is an umbrella term for psychological or talking therapy. There are a large number of psychological therapies; the most common ones include supportive therapy, cognitive-behavioural therapy, psychodynamic psychotherapy, family therapy and group therapy. It is sometimes used to refer to a subtype of psychological therapies only: psychodynamic psychotherapy and psychoanalysis.

Psychotropic medication Psychotropic medication influences cognition, mood or behaviour. All medications used to treat psychiatric disorders are psychotropic.

Rumination Repeatedly thinking about the causes and experience of previous distress and difficulties. Voluntary thinking which is not resisted.

Self-harm Self-harm is a blanket term used to mean any intentional act done in the knowledge that it was potentially harmful. It can take the form of self-poisoning (overdosing) or self-injury (cutting, slashing, burning, etc.). See Chapter 6.

Suicide Suicide is the act of intentionally ending one's own life.

Thought disorder Thought disorder is speech so disorganized that it becomes difficult to understand what is meant. The coherency of patients with disorganized thinking varies from being mostly understandable in patients exhibiting circumstantial thinking to being completely incomprehensible in patients with a word salad phenomenon. See Chapter 9.